AIDS Drugs for All

Markets provide a mechanism for allocating goods and services, but they don't always work in the way that political and economic agents deem to be consistent with their interests. Take pharmaceutical products, the main topic of this book. Should drugs be allocated by free markets and priced accordingly, or should public agencies and the private sector seek to make them widely available according to some definition of need? Because the answers to such questions are open to debate – as exemplified by the fact that societies around the world approach the issue of access to health care quite differently – markets may become contentious, as governments, firms, and consumers all seek a hand in shaping patterns of supply, demand, and price.

This is a book about market transformations and, more specifically, about how social advocacy movements have inserted themselves into market processes with the objective of changing their outcomes or distributive effects. The particular case that we examine focuses on how the AIDS treatment movement was able to catalyze a profound transformation in the market for antiretroviral (ARV) medications at the turn of the millennium, from one whose business model was "high price, low volume" to one characterized instead by "universal access," meaning that everyone, everywhere should be able to obtain ARVs regardless of their nationality or income level. In short, ARVs were transformed from private goods into what we call "merit goods."

How and why did that dramatic change occur in the marketplace for ARV drugs? And what are the lessons for other issue-areas? These are the central questions we raise in these pages. In so doing, we offer a theory of strategic moral action, which provides the conditions under which advocates are most likely to be successful in achieving sustained market transformations. Accordingly, in addition to examining the prospects for market transformation in other areas of global health, we also compare the AIDS story against a range of cases where advocates have tried to influence economic behavior and outcomes such as climate change.

ETHAN B. KAPSTEIN is Arizona Centennial Professor of International Affairs, and Senior Director for Research at the McCain Institute for International Leadership, Arizona State University. He is also a Visiting

Fellow at the Center for Global Development in Washington DC. A former naval officer and international banker, Kapstein is the author or editor of ten books and scores of professional articles, including *The Fate of Young Democracies* (Cambridge University Press, 2008).

JOSHUA W. BUSBY is an Associate Professor in the Lyndon B. Johnson School of Public Affairs at the University of Texas at Austin. He is also the Crook Distinguished Scholar at the Robert S. Strauss Center for International Security and Law, and a Fellow with the RGK Center for Philanthropy and Community Service. He has published widely on social movements, global health, climate change, and US foreign policy, including *Moral Movements and Foreign Policy* (Cambridge University Press, 2010).

AIDS Drugs for All:

Social Movements and Market Transformations

Ethan B. Kapstein and Joshua W. Busby

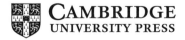

CAMBRIDGE
UNIVERSITY PRESS

CAMBRIDGE
UNIVERSITY PRESS

University Printing House, Cambridge CB2 8BS, United Kingdom

Published in the United States of America by Cambridge University Press, New York

Cambridge University Press is part of the University of Cambridge.

It furthers the University's mission by disseminating knowledge in the pursuit of education, learning and research at the highest international levels of excellence.

www.cambridge.org
Information on this title: www.cambridge.org/9781107632646

© Ethan B. Kapstein and Joshua W. Busby 2013

First published 2013

Printed in the United Kingdom by Clays, St Ives plc

A catalogue record for this publication is available from the British Library

Library of Congress Cataloguing in Publication data

Kapstein, Ethan B., author.
AIDS drugs for all social movements and market transformations / Ethan B. Kapstein and Joshua W. Busby.
    p. ; cm.
Includes bibliographical references and index.
ISBN 978-1-107-03614-7 (Hardback) – ISBN 978-1-107-63264-6 (Paperback)
I. Busby, Joshua W., author. II. Title.
[DNLM: 1. Acquired Immunodeficiency Syndrome–drug therapy. 2. HIV Infections–drug therapy. 3. Anti-Retroviral Agents–economics. 4. Social Change. 5. Social Marketing. WC 503.2]
RC606.5
362.19697'92–dc23   2013005994

ISBN 978-1-107-03614-7 Hardback
ISBN 978-1-107-63264-6 Paperback

Contents

Preface

> We must lay hold of the fact that economic laws are not made by nature.
> They are made by human beings.
> Franklin D. Roosevelt, Presidential Nomination Address, 2 July 1932

Markets provide a mechanism for allocating goods and services, but they don't always work in a way that participants deem to be consistent with their interests. Take pharmaceutical products, the main topic of this book. Should drugs be allocated to patients according to free market dictates, or instead be guided by some overarching set of social norms such as "need"? Should all drugs be made universally available or only the select few that are "essential" or "life-saving"? Because the answers to such questions are open to debate, the markets for drugs, among other products and services, may become fields of contention, as governments, firms, and consumers all seek to influence patterns of supply, demand, and price.

In fact, recent years have seen an explosion in the number of advocacy campaigns aimed at changing the behavior of multinational corporations. Among other objectives, these campaigns have sought to limit fossil fuel emissions, promote "fair trade," protect global fisheries, prevent exploitation of workers, and reduce habitat destruction. What these diverse movements have in common is an effort to change the way that markets currently function.

This is a book about market transformations, or efforts by social movements to change global market processes and their distributive effects. Our main case study is drawn from the pharmaceutical industry, and, more narrowly, we examine how social activists and policy entrepreneurs in the public and private sectors (whom we collectively refer to as "advocates") decisively shaped the market for the antiretroviral drugs (ARVs) that are used to combat HIV/AIDS. Specifically, we are interested in the profound changes that occurred in this market at the turn of the millennium, from one whose initial business model was "high price, low volume" to one that was characterized by "universal access to treatment," meaning that everyone, everywhere should have access to ARVs, no matter their location or income.

How and why did that dramatic shift in the market occur? How were ARVs transformed from private goods into what we call "merit goods," or products that nobody should be denied? What are the lessons from HIV/AIDS for other issue-areas where advocates seek market changes, as in climate change and carbon markets? These are some of the questions we seek to address in the chapters that follow.

Despite a recent resurgence of scholarly interest in market contention, this area of research has been surprisingly dormant for most of the postwar era. Perhaps that reflects the rending of the market from its social environment by modern economics in an effort to build more tractable mathematical models. The consequences of that separation, however, have not gone unnoticed, even by some leading economists themselves. As the Nobel Prize winner Gary Becker wrote many years ago, "the emphasis of earlier economists" on how social relations shaped economic behavior "deserved to be taken much more seriously" by the profession (Becker 1974).

To take an example from the AIDS case, economists have generally argued that what brought down the price of ARVs around the world was entry by low-cost generic producers, just as these producers have driven prices down on many medications that are now on offer (see, e.g., Hellerstein 2004). In this version of events, the market acts "naturally" or "spontaneously," with new entrants forcing competition upon the incumbent firms. What this perspective overlooks, however, is that the groundwork for generic entry was laid by advocates who sought to show in the first instance that ARV delivery in the developing world was effective and who then helped to pool demand in order to create a market sizeable enough to be of commercial interest. Finally, they helped spur industrialized world governments to increase foreign aid funds that were earmarked for AIDS treatment, so that developing world governments could acquire the drugs at these reduced prices. Generic drugs, in short, did not "drop by parachute" into the developing world; their entry was catalyzed by advocates, that at a minimum helped save many lives by speeding drug delivery.

In this book we examine in detail the campaign that was dedicated to ensuring "universal access" to ARV treatment for all People Living with AIDS (PWAs). Imagine the audacity of such a movement whose objective was nothing less than the creation of the world's first global entitlement regime, of providing drugs to all who needed ARVs for their entire lifetime (Over 2008, 2011; Piot 2012). As we will show, providing something approaching universal access required what must be called, without hyperbole, a heroic effort on the part of social activists, policy entrepreneurs, and sympathetic corporate executives, for it required profound changes in the supply and demand of ARVs and in the way these drugs would be priced. It also required a set of new and innovative domestic programs and international institutions to support the universal access to treatment regime. In short, the move toward universal access to treatment required a profound transformation in how the market for these essential, life-extending drugs operated.

We believe that this book is among the first to trace in detail how a product market was altered by a social advocacy movement; how supply, demand, price, and institutions were decisively shaped by political agitation (for a book with some parallels, see Rao 2008). In so doing, we hope to contribute to social science by digging deep into market processes and outcomes in an effort to find the "moving parts" that are amenable to external manipulation. One phrase we often heard during our research from those we interviewed was that "the stars were aligned" in the AIDS case on behalf of the universal access to treatment regime (Piot 2009). This astrological vision suggests that the possibilities for market transformation might be few and far between, demanding those rare moments when Jupiter aligns with Mars. The issue that we raise is: what are the forces or moving parts that advocates themselves can harness to help align those stars?

There is, of course, a growing literature that examines market-oriented social movements and the conditions under which (anti-) corporate campaigns have "succeeded" in influencing firm-level behavior (Spar and La Mure 2003; O'Rourke 2005). This literature has generated a number of hypotheses about the conditions under which firms are most likely to bend to non-market pressures. These include the degree of brand recognition (the better known the brand, the more susceptible it is to pressure); the costs of changing production processes (the higher the costs, the less likely that firms will submit); and the competitive position of the firm (the better situated the firm is to use "corporate social responsibility" as a source of competitive advantage, the more likely it will negotiate with the advocates). We believe these provide useful starting points for analyzing movement activity.

We build on that literature by developing our own view of the role of advocates in spurring market transformations, what we call a theory of *strategic moral action*. Our theory argues that market transformation in the case of ARVs required the following: *first*, a market structure or favorable set of underlying economic and industrial conditions that provided opportunities or openings for an advocacy movement; *second*, the elaboration by the AIDS movement of a compelling frame that pitted drug company profits against global access to life-saving ARV medications; *third*, a political and organizational consensus or coherent "ask" on the part of the social movement that treatment should receive the highest policy priority, trumping, for example, prevention; *fourth*, a feasible strategy (defined in this case as one that minimized the costs of market transformation to the major players) for how a universal access to treatment market could be made to operate; and *finally*, a set of institutional arrangements to help set the rules for the transformed market and to stabilize its operations.

The AIDS movement thus presented a strong argument for universal access to treatment by appealing both to the emotions and to the intellect of its intended audiences in business, government, international organizations, and civil society; in other words, the movement combined a powerful ethical story about what constituted justice and fairness with what seemed to be a compelling or feasible business case. In the introductory chapter, we frame this argument in more precise terms by generating a set of hypotheses about the conditions under which social movements are most likely to be successful in generating market changes.

When one looks at the ARV example from this analytical perspective, it illuminates why some other movements – like those which seek to tackle climate change – have had greater difficulty in advancing their cause. In addition to the fact that the costs for many firms (like oil companies) of adjusting to climate change could be quite high, leading them to balk at movement demands to reduce their carbon footprint, climate change activists among themselves have, after converging on a politically intractable set of legally binding targets and timetables, subsequently divided over the appropriate "solution" or "ask" to the problem. Throughout, they have struggled to articulate a strong business model that provides a pathway from the present to the future. Some climate change activists focus on the need for deep, short-term legally binding emissions reductions by advanced industrialized countries and compensation for affected poor countries, while others emphasize more phased-in, voluntary pledges of emissions reductions by all countries, including fast-growing countries like China and India. We would argue, at a minimum, that the climate change movement will need to achieve a clearer strategy regarding its policy "ask" if it is to have a profound impact on the energy market.

This book unfolds in eight chapters. First, Chapter 1 provides an overview of the literature on social movements and market contestation, before turning to our own theoretical argument and specific hypotheses about the conditions under which these movements are most likely to catalyze market transformations. In Chapter 2, we examine the structure of the pharmaceutical industry and market for ARVs that provided advocates with "openings" for their campaign. Chapters 3 and 4 examine how advocates made a compelling moral argument and cohered around a common set of demands. In Chapter 5, we explore how advocates sought to address the concerns by governments and firms about the costs of their policy "ask" for expanded treatment access. Chapter 6 then turns to the institutions that were developed to help stabilize the new access to treatment regime. We try to generalize from the AIDS case in Chapter 7 by examining the potential for market transformation in several other issue-areas that have been the focus of advocacy movements, while Chapter 8 presents our conclusions and "take-aways" for the public policy, business, and advocacy communities, as well as our ideas concerning next steps for a research program on market politics. For readers less familiar with the history of AIDS and the AIDS treatment movement, we provide a brief summary of key events and an accompanying timeline of key dates as appendices to Chapter 1.

During the writing of this book we have accumulated the usual pile of debts that overwhelms each and every author. This research was supported by a grant from Merck & Co., Inc. We thank the Merck Foundation for its generous sponsorship, and in particular, we wish to thank Leslie Hardy at the Foundation and Clinton Riley at Merck Corporation for all the help they provided. The book, however, does not in any way reflect the views of either the Merck Foundation or Merck Corporation, and we are solely responsible for its content.

Our work came to the attention of the Merck Foundation thanks to Dr. Jeffrey Sturchio, who was formerly at Merck and was deeply involved in many of the issues tackled in this book. Jeff has generously replied to every request we made of him for interviews, for material, and for his views on the accuracy and quality of our work. We cannot begin to express our gratitude for the efforts he made on our behalf and only hope that the finished product provides him with some small gratification.

One of the authors (Ethan B. Kapstein) worked on this book during a stint as a Fellow of the Niehaus Center on Governance and Globalization at Princeton University. He wishes to thank the Center's Director, Professor Helen Milner, and its Assistant Director, Patricia Trinity, for their warm hospitality. He also benefited from his association with the Department of Management at the Wharton School, University of Pennsylvania, and in particular he thanks Professor Mauro Guillen, who (with Charles Perrow) wrote an early and courageous book aptly entitled *The AIDS Crisis*. Joshua Busby benefited from feedback on the work from presentations at George Washington University, Knowledge Ecology International, Loyola Marymount University, the University of Texas, and Uppsala University, while Ethan Kapstein presented early drafts at the London School of Hygiene and Tropical Medicine, Yale University, and the University of California at Santa Barbara. Both authors also wish to thank their academic home they shared during the writing of this book, the Lyndon Baines Johnson School at the University of Texas at Austin.

A great joy in writing this book was that it led us to interview a truly remarkable group of individuals, who combined great passion with acute strategic and political acumen as they moved the international community to embrace the universal access to treatment regime. Dr. Peter Piot, formerly director of UNAIDS and now director of the London School of Hygiene and Tropical Medicine, was a tremendous supporter of this project from its inception, and was incredibly generous with his time. His own memoir of his time at UNAIDS, *No Time to Lose*, also provided a useful chronicle to draw upon. Others who assisted our efforts include Zackie Achmat, Christoph Benn, Daniel Berman, Nancy Birdsall, Paul Boneberg, Kate Condliffe, Mark Dybul, Dai Ellis, Richard Feachem, Loon Gangte, Laurie Garrett, Mauro Guarinieri, Gregg Gonsalves, Ian Grubb, Bill Haddad, Yusuf Hamied, John S. James, Sandeep Juneja, Karyn Kaplan, Michel Kazatchkine, Kate Krauss, Bob Lederer, William Looney, Ira Magaziner, Mark Milano, Stavros Nicolaou, Mead Over, Bernard Pécoul, Shailesh Pednekar, Carmen Perez-Casas, Joseph Perriëns, Ben Plumley, John Riley, David Ripin, Asia Russell, Badara Samb, Eric Sawyer, Ken Shadlen, Anil Soni, Ellen 't Hoen, Andre van Zyl, and Brenda Waning. Of course, they bear no responsibility for the final product. We also had the assistance of numerous public officials, many of whom prefer to remain anonymous. We would like to thank Dylan Mohan Gray and David France, the directors, respectively, of *Fire in the Blood* and *How to Survive a Plague*, for allowing us to screen their films before wider public release. We would also like to thank Anne-christine d'Adesky, Shanti Avirgan, and Ann Rossetti for making additional interview material from the documentary *Pills, Profits, and Protests* available to us. We would also like to thank Bob Lederer and John Riley for sharing additional foundational material from Health GAP's early meetings and emails. We hope all of them will feel we have made good use of the time and materials they generously shared with us.

We further thank Matthew Flynn for research assistance on the project and Linda Busby for her careful line editing of the entire manuscript. We are appreciative of John Haslam and the editorial team at Cambridge University Press as well as the anonymous reviewers who read earlier drafts of the manuscript. Finally, we would like to thank our spouses, Benedicte Callan and Bethany Albertson, who are more expert than us on several of the topics treated here and were constant sources of support. Benedicte provided key insights on health and IP protection and made a significant contribution to Chapter 2, while Bethany was a source of guidance on survey experiments.

Figures

Tables

Abbreviations

3TC – Lamuvidine
AAI – Accelerated Access Initiative
ABC – Abacavir
ACT UP – AIDS Coalition to Unleash Power
AIDS – Acquired immunodeficiency syndrome
APIs – active pharmaceutical ingredients
ARV – Antiretrovirals
AZT, or ZDV – Zidovudine
BMS – Bristol Myers Squibb
CAN – Climate Action Network
CDC – Centers for Disease Control
CHAI – Clinton HIV/AIDS Initiative (later the Clinton Health Access
       Initiative)
d4T – Stavudine
DAI – Drug Access Initiative
ddl – Didanosine
EFV – Efavirenz
FDA – Food and Drug Administration
FDC – Fixed-dose combinations
FTC – emtricitabine
GAO – Government Accountability Office
GAVI – Global Alliance for Vaccines and Immunisation
GSK – GlaxoSmithKline
HAART – Highly Active Anti Retroviral Therapy
HIV – Human immunodeficiency virus
IP – Intellectual property
IPR – Intellectual property rights
ITPC – International Treatment Preparedness Coalition
MPP – Medicines Patent Pool
MSF – Médecins sans Frontières (Doctors without Borders)
NIH – National Institutes of Health

NNRTIs – Non-Nucleoside Reverse Transcriptase Inhibitors
NRTIs – Nucleoside Reverse Transcriptase Inhibitors
NVP – Nevirapine
PEPFAR – the President's Emergency Plan for AIDS Relief
PI – Protease inhibitors
PWAs – People living with HIV/AIDS
TAC – Treatment Action Campaign
TDF – Tenofovir
TRIPS – Trade-Related Aspects of Intellectual Property Rights
UNAIDS – Joint United Nations Programme on HIV and AIDS
UNFPA – United Nations Population Fund
UNICEF – United Nations Children's Fund
WHO – World Health Organization
WTO – World Trade Organization

1 Introduction: global markets and transnational social movements

In the beginning there were markets.
Oliver Williamson, *Markets and Hierarchies*, 1983, 20

In the end, if we don't have drugs, people are going to die.
AIDS Activist Gregg Gonsalves, Interview, ACT UP Oral History Project,
19 July 2004

Markets are mechanisms for allocating goods and services. But what if some people are unhappy with the outcomes of market-based distributions? How can the allocation of goods and services be changed or transformed? Take, for example, the market for life-extending AIDS drugs, which provides our focal point. Ever since the appearance of these drugs in the 1980s, their very nature as economic goods has been hotly debated by stakeholders around the world. Are antiretroviral (ARV) drugs intrinsically private goods, like computers or cars? Or are they public goods that every member of society should have access to, like clean air or national security? Raising these questions suggests that the very nature of a good can be contested, its supply, demand, and price the subject of political debate.

This book is about a profound change that occurred in the allocation of life-extending ARV medications, from a model that was "high price, low volume" to one based on "universal access to treatment." We argue that advocates, including AIDS activists around the world, policy entrepreneurs in national governments and international institutions, and even some corporate executives who became devoted to this cause, challenged the market structure for these drugs, from one based on "ability to pay" to one based on "universal access." We show how social activists and their allies in government and business (we use the umbrella term "advocates" to refer to all those who made common cause in the campaign for universal access to AIDS treatment) helped *transform* ARVs from private goods into "merit goods," or private goods which everyone *should* have access to, regardless of their ability to pay for them. We then consider the lessons from the AIDS case for several other market arenas both within and outside public health.

1

The idea that a product's fundamental nature as a "private good" can be contested is of fundamental importance to the study of political economy. Whereas most economics textbooks assume that the division between different types of goods (i.e. public goods vs. private goods) is straightforward and "fixed" over time, we will see that advocacy movements have managed to "problematize" these markets in several different sectors. In some markets, like those for the ARV medications that combat HIV/AIDS, advocates have even succeeded in transforming what we call the "principle of access" to them, or the way these goods are allocated on a global basis. Issues of drug access are thus the real stuff of politics – of who gets what and why.

At the level of the international political economy, which is the arena that we examine in these pages, the issues of market structure and transformation are particularly compelling, since they are even more contentious and contestable. In the global economy, there is no ultimate arbiter of public opinion, no state with a monopoly on violence that can unilaterally set the rules of the game for all of the many players, including national governments and multinational corporations. In this arena, transnational social movements cannot make reference to "the constitution" or file all their grievances in courts of law, for these sorts of institutions are generally weak or altogether absent. Further, at the international level, advocates may not even have legal "standing" in those organizations where quasi-legal bodies are present (for example, the dispute resolution panels at the World Trade Organization (WTO)). Indeed, this is one reason why multinational corporations have become the object of transnational advocacy movements, since they can seek to change at least some aspects of how the global economy operates – how, for example, firms care for the health and safety of their workers in the developing world – by influencing the stroke of a chief executive's pen.

In this opening chapter, we introduce the topic of how advocacy movements can influence market structures and outcomes and outline the contribution we hope to make to the growing literature in this vibrant field. We attempt to extend this literature by generating some testable hypotheses concerning why certain movements are more successful than others in achieving a fundamental market transformation. To date, much of the literature on movement success has emphasized the *internal* resources and capabilities that advocates can muster as they launch their campaigns. Our emphasis, in contrast, is on the opportunities or openings generated by market and industry structures in particular economic sectors.

Why, for example, has it proved so difficult to transform the market for carbon by setting a firm price for that substance or by taxing it more aggressively? What are the barriers to change that the climate movement faces that the access to AIDS treatment campaign was able to overcome? Was it the immediacy of the AIDS threat, its choice of "life or death"? Is it simply easier to transform pharmaceutical vs. energy markets due to the respective structures of these industries? Or is it because the AIDS movement had a more targeted and coherent "ask"? By examining such questions in this book, we hope to shed light on what factors are most important in determining the likely success of a social advocacy movement as it engages in an effort at market restructuring.

Markets and market transformations

This is a book about the role of social movements in transforming the global marketplace for AIDS drugs. But what is a market? And what is a market transformation? Definitions of these concepts are surprisingly absent from many contemporary textbooks, so a brief overview will provide useful guidance for the discussion that follows.

In the simplest terms, markets may be viewed as arenas where economic agents meet to exchange goods and services. This interaction can be conducted in barter terms – as has often been the case throughout history (and still is today in various corners of the planet) – but it is more often than not shaped by money-based prices. These prices provide agents with signals about the conditions of supply for the things they crave, or the relative scarcity of the good. As the Scottish essayist Thomas Carlyle (who is also credited with describing economics as the "dismal science") famously put it: "Teach a parrot the terms 'supply and demand' and you've got an economist."

In most cases, the price of a good and the demand for it are, of course, inversely related, and markets are said to "clear," or to be in equilibrium, at the point where, at a given price, supply is equal to demand. Further, when markets are competitive, rents or extraordinary profits are driven away (since rents induce market entry) and prices reflect marginal cost, or the cost to the firm of producing the very last good. This leads to the normative view, broadly held by most economists, that competition should be encouraged by breaking down the barriers to entry that may exist in any given market (in fact, the introduction of competition solves many if not most economic ills, at least in theory). It should be emphasized that the competition norm has had important public policy implications for any number of industries, including pharmaceutical manufacturers, where entry by generic firms now plays a crucial role in bringing down the prices of drugs once patents have expired – and sometimes even beforehand, as we will see was the case with ARVs.

Economists have generally been less concerned, however, with the distributive effects of market transactions. The textbook view, usually implicit, is that consumers can purchase goods and services as they so choose and are only constrained by their budgets. The idea that the budgetary constraint may prevent some people from acquiring goods and services that are necessary for their survival or well-being is not one that is featured in most economic discussions. Instead, that problem has been largely left to the philosophers, like the late John Rawls, who famously argued that, if societies were organized from behind a "veil of ignorance," people would adopt a "maximin" principle, such that society would seek to maximize the life-chances of the most vulnerable among them (Rawls 1999).

It is the distributive consequences of market-based allocations that are often the root cause of anti-corporate campaigns. Anti-sweatshop campaigns, for example, dispute the division of rents between branded fashion companies (like Nike) and their (contract) workers (who often labor in the developing world, where wages and regulations are low by the standards of most industrialized nations). Patient advocacy campaigns, in contrast, often dispute the price of drugs, which places them out of reach for many consumers. For this reason, advocates often pursue what we call *market transformations*, or new principles of market access.[1] In the case of ARVs, they sought to transform the market from one based on the "ability to pay" to one grounded on the principle of "universal access to treatment." In the case of wages for "sweatshop" labor in the developing world, they sought to transform contract workers from being treated as mere commodities into employees who deserve decent salaries along with better health and safety standards.

Our main objective in this book is to examine the opportunities for market transformation that advocates face and the strategies they adopt in pursuit of that objective. We borrow the term "market transformation" from the energy policy literature, where such a transformation has been defined as a "strategic effort" by utility companies or other organizations to promote "increases in the adoption of energy-efficient products, services or practices." According to a group of energy policy specialists, "the fundamental goal of market transformation is to change markets and thereby save substantial amounts of energy in the long-term" (York 1999).

We are similarly interested in major long-term changes, *specifically in terms of fundamental shifts in the principle of access* to life-extending drugs.

---

[1] Here, we define access the way advocates do, in terms of the ability of people to gain access to the goods in question. Economists, for their part, define market access differently, in terms of market entry for producers.

Thus, a market (say, for drugs) is transformed when its principle of access or allocation shifts from "ability to pay" to "universal treatment," and our dependent variable in this case is the number of people on treatment (particularly people from developing countries). Naturally, the specific objectives that advocates set for market transformation (and thus the relevant dependent variable) will differ according to the particular issue-area at stake. In the case of climate change, for example, the principle might be to seek a level playing field between fossil fuels and alternative energy sources (e.g. through the imposition of a carbon tax), and the dependent variable could be adoption or take-up of new energy technologies.

Market transformations are difficult to achieve for many reasons, not the least of which is that markets may serve some interests at the expense of others, such as those of the dominant or incumbent firms versus those of potential new entrants. Regulations, for example, may serve as a barrier to entry for potential competitors. For this reason, it is often the underlying institutions or sets of rules that support or, to use Neil Fligstein's term, "stabilize" market structures that are the target of advocacy movements, no less than the firms themselves (Fligstein 2002). Since these rules are often written by governments, advocates in the domestic context have long pursued "contentious politics" aimed at changing legislation or judicial opinion, for example through lobbying and law suits, instead of "private politics" aimed at changing corporate behavior directly (Baron 2005); increasingly, however, they are deploying both strategies.

As noted above, many scholars have argued since at least the time of Karl Marx that markets do not necessarily level the playing field among economic agents, but instead represent and reproduce the underlying power configurations that shape socio-economic relations. To be sure, scholars differ with respect to who holds and reproduces power within markets; for Marx and his followers it was the "ruling class" or elites, while Fligstein focuses on incumbent or dominant firms. Both agree, however, that the market is hardly a "neutral" setting; it is tilted in the interests of some over others. Dani Rodrik of Harvard's Kennedy School of Government asserts that "economic rules are not written by Platonic rulers ... Those who have power get more out of the system than those who do not" (Rodrik 2002, 19). That makes markets and the institutions that support them a natural field for political contestation, since politics is ultimately about the distribution of power and authority.

More generally, Fligstein makes a functionalist argument that market institutions, like property rights, exist to *stabilize* the exchange process. These institutions are built by the dominant firms in a given market, as they seek to reproduce themselves over time; that is, they build institutions that they believe will enhance their own chances of long-run survival. These institutions, *inter alia*, serve to limit competition by creating barriers to entry of various kinds. At the same time, firms may try to build labor market institutions, such as the "cooperativist" social arrangements found in Northern Europe's social democracies, in order to stabilize relations between employers and workers. Firms also demand systems of property rights – e.g. patents, trademarks, copyrights, and the rule of law more generally – that fix their monopoly power for at least some period of time and provide them with the security or protection needed to conduct their operations (Fligstein 2002).

Economists now accept, at least implicitly, much of this sociological view of market structures. But an important normative gap still tends to separate the economists and sociologists. For their part, economists would hold, *ceteris paribus*, that monopolistic markets tend to be inefficient as compared to the competitive alternative. Sociologists as a group, in contrast, would probably hold that efficiency may be consistent with many different types of market structure, and that these structures are "sticky," being deeply embedded in local political and cultural configurations. Indeed, it is because there is no single way to achieve efficiency that the "varieties of capitalism" can co-exist without convergence, ranging from the Anglo-Saxon to the Scandinavian models of economic life (Granovetter 1985; Hall and Soskice 2001; Fligstein 2002). Still, the normative position held by most economists is that monopoly anywhere should be frowned upon (with the exception of "natural" monopolies like power plants, which then need to be regulated) and that steps should be taken, usually by governments, to undermine monopolistic positions in the interests of a more efficient economy.

That normative position, in turn, leads economists to assess markets in terms of their *contestability*, or the ability of competitors to threaten a monopolist with market entry, thus eroding its rents. It must be emphasized that it is the very *threat* of entry that drives down monopoly prices near the competitive level, without any regulatory actions on the part of policy-makers (Baumol 1982; Martin 2000). This observation implies that efficient outcomes can be approximated even in the absence of fully competitive markets.

The concept of market contestability is an intriguing one to build upon for students of market-oriented social movements, although it does not yet seem to have made much of an impact on the relevant social science literature. One powerful implication, however, is that action by "nonmarket" actors, like social movements, can be efficiency-enhancing to the extent that such actions erode the monopoly rents of dominant firms.

In this respect, these movements might be usefully conceptualized as, to use the jargon from welfare economics, "social planners," taking over the role once reserved for formal regulatory authorities within that literature. That social planning role of advocacy movements, or role as a public goods provider, is likely to be all the more prominent and contentious in the global political economy, where international regulatory authorities are often weak or absent. As Tim Bartley succinctly asserts, "The driving forces in this account [of market contestation] are conflicts among states, NGOs, social movements, and firms about the legitimacy of various ways of regulating global capitalism" (Bartley 2007, 310).

By encouraging generics manufacturers to enter the ARV market, for example, advocates helped to generate competition and lower prices for these drugs. The specific actions that advocates took included lobbying governments to adopt a public health exception to the international intellectual property regime and organizing developing countries into a pooled set of buyers, thereby creating a viable market. At the same time, they prodded industrialized world governments and the United Nations to create procurement mechanisms and to provide funding for the purchases of these medications. Advocates provided a host of other "services" to the market as well, including gathering crucial information about the price of ARV drugs that gave the market a transparency that it had previously lacked. Again we stress that these various market-oriented functions may be of particular importance in the setting of the global political economy, where international organizations do not always fill these institutional voids.

But it is also important to point out that the interactions between firms and social movements need not lead to more efficient economic outcomes. Instead, corporate executives and advocates could conspire to form a condominium, dividing the rents between them at the expense of consumers. Higher certification standards, for instance, could reward big firms at the expense of small ones, as they can more easily afford to adopt the new standards, and the non-governmental organizations that promote these standards can gain rents by providing firms with the specific certification (e.g. for "fair trade" coffee or for "sustainable" forest products) that they seek for labeling purposes. From this perspective, activists can be seen as rent-seekers rather than social planners (Kapstein 2001).

Advocacy movements that target the pharmaceutical sector might undermine consumer welfare in another, "inter-temporal" way as well. Let us suppose, for example, that social movements succeed in pressuring pharmaceutical manufacturers to reduce prices for "essential medicines." That may be good for consumers in the short-run, but in the longer run it may reduce the incentives of these firms to invest in research and development, undermining public health in future (Waning, Diedrichsen, and Moon 2010; Piot 2012, 308). These inter-temporal issues are of tremendous significance, and we will discuss them in more detail in the following chapters.

Global markets and transnational social movements

Market contention is a permanent feature of economic life. Whether the issue is the commodification of labor (as emphasized by Marx and Polanyi), property rights (as emphasized by de Soto), or the role of the private sector in society (as emphasized by Berle and Means), political and economic agents have contested market processes and outcomes (Berle and Means 1932; Polanyi 1944; Marx 1978; de Soto 2000). Traditionally, consumer movements and labor unions have been among the leaders in these struggles (Friedman 1999; Glickman 2009); more recently, however, advocacy groups that are issue-specific (e.g. those that target human rights or global poverty) have begun to attack firms directly as their preferred method for promoting social change (Soule 2009).

In recent decades, several of these social movements have matured and mimicked the globalization process in becoming "transnational," as exemplified by the geographic spread of such prominent groups as Oxfam, Doctors without Borders (hereinafter we will use the acronym MSF for its French name, *Médecins sans Frontières*), and Greenpeace. Of course, transnational groups like the Roman Catholic Church pre-date modern globalization by many centuries. This "transnational activism" has become the subject of an expanding literature in social science, as scholars have sought to analyze the role that these movements play in putting such issues as human rights and environmental causes on the agendas of governments and multinational corporations (Keck and Sikkink 1998; Tarrow 2005; King and Pearce 2010; Busby 2010a). Economists are also placing their distinctive stamp on this literature, developing formal models that, among other things, seek to clarify assumptions about the objective functions of social movements, illuminate the costs and benefits of different movement strategies, and outline the possibilities for regulation outside the public sphere, or what David Baron has called the emergence of "private politics" (Baron 2005).

This body of literature has taught us much about what Sidney Tarrow calls "contentious politics," or the ability of seemingly marginal groups or "outsiders" to upset the political and economic *status quo* (Tarrow 2005). It has emphasized the crucial importance of how activists "frame" and "scale" their issues, like "being green" or "fighting global poverty," for elites and the broader public in an effort to promote policy changes within governments and firms (within the social movements literature, contentious politics generally refers to advocacy which is targeted at governments, whereas "private politics" refers to advocacy targeted at firms (Baron 2005; Soule 2009). We use both terms in our discussion of the AIDS movement, since governments *and* firms were both targets and their engagement was needed to make the market transformation towards universal access possible).

Scholars have also described both the internal organizations of movements on the one hand and the "political opportunity structures" in the external environment on the other that are most conducive to movement "success" (Soule 2009). Research has further demonstrated through detailed process-tracing how the norms held by transnational social movements can "cascade" onto policy agendas by creating "shared meanings" or understandings for diverse stakeholders to a political debate. In the global context, finding shared meanings is especially challenging, given that societies around the world are characterized by very different normative commitments. In that regard, Keck and Sikkink find that defense against "bodily harm" and legal "equality of opportunity" are two norms that tend to resonate on a global basis (Keck and Sikkink 1998).

Naturally, there are significant differences between domestic and transnational social movements. For their part, domestic movements are usually able to capitalize on existing political and legal structures as the basis for their claims. Successive rights-based movements in the United States, for example, made claims based upon the nation's foundational document, the Constitution. Often making use of the courts, these movements challenged the laws of the land on a constitutional basis, forcing the judicial branch and ultimately legislatures to make fundamental determinations about the standing of claimants and their grievances. From this perspective, advocates for human rights, as with other social movements, face a particularly harsh climate in the international sphere, since few global bodies exist that possess anything like constitutional power.

This point is worth further emphasis. In "attacking" the international system, advocates have few lifelines to grab hold of; they lack the frameworks provided by domestic institutions like courts and legislatures. This relative weakness of advocacy groups helps to explain why multinational firms have become favored targets, since changes in such firms can be "made global" by unilateral decisions made in the corner office. It also helps to explain why the most quasi-constitutional body in the global economy, the WTO, has also been a focal point of activity, since its agreements are among the closest thing the international community has to a legally binding set of obligations (a point emphasized by Koppell 2010). In fact, one element in the pharmaceutical industry structure that was exploited by advocates for global public health in the 1990s was the fluid nature of the Agreement on Trade-Related Aspects of Intellectual Property Rights (TRIPS); controversy over TRIPS provided an "opening" for advocates to enter, and they shaped the TRIPS debate by providing information and advice, particularly to developing world governments.

How and when advocates choose to threaten firms and how such contestation is resolved is a topic of growing interest both within and outside the academy (Baron 2005; Bach and Allen 2010). As Brayden King and Nicholas Pearce note:

The focus of this research is on social movements and other change agents that bring contentiousness to markets ... [F]or markets to survive, they must be able to connect people and organizations, as well as satisfy the needs that each brings to the exchange; however, because markets tend to centralize resources and power, because not every member of society has equal access to all markets, and because markets sometimes produce harmful externalities, markets frequently become locations of contestation and disruption. (King and Pearce 2010, 250)

In order to contest the market, however, one must first "deconstruct" it in order to identify its moving parts and target its points of weakness. That exercise demonstrates the enormous challenges that advocates face in altering existing, and presumably "sticky," market arrangements. Again, as Fligstein has emphasized, market-oriented institutions – like property rights regimes – exist to *stabilize* market interactions and to eliminate "needless" or inefficient disputes over rules and outcomes (Fligstein 2002). If market structures are endogenous to underlying systems of power, it is unclear how and when and by whom these structures can be altered to reflect alternative sets of interests.

The same can be said, of course, about political opportunity structures (POS) or the underlying conditions within a given regime which enable citizens to make their voices heard and to exert real influence over outcomes (McAdam, McCarthy, and Zald 1996; Tarrow 2005). To take a dramatic example, the political opportunity structure available to social movements in Eastern Europe expanded greatly after the Soviet bloc collapsed and democratic regimes came to power. As a general proposition, scholars assert that the political opportunities available to advocates are greater in democracies than in authoritarian regimes.

Even within democratic regimes, we might add, political opportunities to express grievances and to make claims on government may ebb and flow. In the United States, for instance, the Vietnam War discredited the nation's elites, giving an opening to new voices in shaping political agendas and debates. Out of this opening an array of movements, including those pursuing rights for African-Americans, women, and the gay community, found new possibilities for advancing their respective causes (Hirshman 2012). The French experienced a similar opening in May 1968, which among other things set into motion profound changes in that country's approach to access to higher education (in this sense, May 1968 may have heralded a market transformation in that sector).

The POS concept has more recently been extended to the market realm as an "economic opportunity structure" (EOS) or "industry opportunity structure" (IOS) (Schurman 2004; King and Soule 2007). Just as the POS seeks to identify the political circumstances that are most amenable to social movements (e.g. democratic vs. authoritarian regimes), the EOS/IOS seeks to do the same from an economic perspective. It therefore identifies the economic conditions, market structures, and firm attributes that are most likely to provide an opening to social movement advocacy (in this book we will mainly refer instead to the "industry" or "market" structure, which we believe is somewhat more felicitous and also more recognizable to those readers from outside sociology. Further, we focus our attention at the micro- or industry level rather than at the macro- or global economy level, which some scholars use as their starting point for EOS analysis).

Drawing from the AIDS example, the campaign for universal treatment enjoyed several opportunities from a structural perspective. First, only a handful of companies initially produced the ARVs necessary for life, so if these few firms reduced their prices, as many of them did in response to advocacy pressure, such moves would dramatically change the global market and open the door to expanded access. Contrast this with other more fragmented sectors like education and water, where large numbers of providers would simultaneously have to change their behavior to yield a transformed market favoring access.

Second, the patent protection regime was only extended to drugs on a global basis in the 1990s, as part of the TRIPS process at the WTO, and aspects of that decision remained sharply contested. As a consequence, controversies over the TRIPS regime, particularly with respect to public health policy, left institutional "openings" that advocates could hope to influence (Devereaux, Lawrence, and Watkins 2006). As an example, South Africa's legal challenge to the TRIPS regime (discussed in more detail in Chapters 2 and 5) provided advocates with a prominent "focal point" which enabled them to win substantial media coverage for their "ask" of lower drug prices and, conversely, to deeply undermine the legitimacy of drug patents that seemingly denied drugs to those who needed them by keeping prices high.

Third, the 1990s was a period of turmoil for the pharmaceutical industry's structure and performance owing to a number of trends that all came to a head during this decade, including fading drug pipelines and the arrival of new entrants both on the demand (e.g. health maintenance organizations) and supply (e.g. biotechnology firms) sides of the equation. As a consequence, many firms engaged in global merger and acquisition (M&A) activity, disrupting existing corporate cultures and providing advocates with a space to help set the agendas of the new firms, particularly as many of these mergers required shareholder and/or regulatory approval. To take one example, Jean-Pierre Garnier, who became chairman of the newly created GlaxoSmithKline (GSK) in 2000, was very sensitive to activist critiques of the pharmaceutical industry, including shareholder activists who aimed to influence huge institutional investors like CalPERS, which managed pension assets for State of California employees (Liu and Lim 2003; Smith and Duncan 2005; King 2008).

Fourth, the pricing structure of the pharmaceutical industry was vulnerable to attack, in that many firms practiced "differential pricing," or selling the same drug to different consumers at different prices. Advocates saw this pricing structure as an opportunity, perceiving that wealthy consumers in the North might be persuaded to help subsidize the consumption of AIDS drugs by PWAs in the South.

Advocacy strategies that aimed to transform the market for ARVs used both "contentious" and "private" politics, a common thread in many market-targeted advocacy movements. The environmental movement in the United States, for example, has used the judicial branch to great effect over the past four decades in limiting the development of nuclear power plants, while the AIDS movement disputed the property rights validity of the initial ARV patent, which the firm Burroughs Wellcome received for the drug AZT (Arno and Feiden 1992).

But how do social movements go about influencing and changing the behavior of firms, households, or governments within specific markets, even given a favorable market structure or set of permissive underlying economic conditions (and we note that much of the relevant literature focuses on advocacy movements that target *firms* rather than *industries*; more on this below)? As King and Pearce note, "corporations generally provide few 'conventional access channels' to the non-shareholder public. *Lacking insider influence, social movements respond by using extrainstitutional tactics*" (King and Pearce 2010, 255, emphasis added). They argue that such tactics must be "both persuasive and disruptive. Persuasive tactics communicate a movement's message to a broad audience, make claims that politicize and vilify a practice, and convince third parties of the need for immediate change" (ibid.).

Disruptive tactics, in contrast, focus on bringing wide public attention – and particularly media attention – to a cause. Media coverage is particularly useful to advocates because it "also brings negative information about its target to light and potentially damages the public image of the target through 'naming and shaming'" (King and Pearce 2010; Busby 2010a). In the case of HIV/AIDS, the American group ACT UP made strategic use of the media, in part because its founder Larry Kramer had formerly been a Hollywood publicist who well understood the importance of staging media-friendly events (Kramer 2003). ACT UP's success in garnering media attention certainly spilled over to the global AIDS movement (Smith and Siplon 2006).

In attacking firm policies and activities, social movements tend to target corporate *reputations*, or the intangible goodwill that a firm holds as the difference between its stock price and its discounted cash flows (note, there are many definitions of corporate reputation; while one prominent focus is on stock price premiums, other researchers have examined the ability of firms to recruit top-notch workers or to charge higher prices for goods and services than its competitors. Most important, reputation is intangible and this is what makes it difficult for other firms to copy). As a case in point, pharmaceutical firms long garnered reputational capital for "doing good" through the development of innovative new medicines that greatly extended life; incredibly, treatment activists were able to tarnish that reputation, transforming these firms into ruthless monopolists. The AIDS treatment movement ACT UP, for example, held sit-ins at the New York Stock Exchange with banners accusing particular pharmaceutical firms of being complicit in the deaths of those with the HIV virus who could not afford expensive treatments. ACT UP likened AIDS deaths to the Holocaust and compared pharmaceutical executives to Nazis (Hirshman 2012). In short, it exploited well-known moral frames as a prism for its own campaign.

One tangible objective of "reputational campaigns" might be to lower the firm's share price; think of this as the "harm" an advocate can do to a firm. King and Soule (2007), for example, "demonstrate that protests against corporations cause its stock price to decline" and they use this as a proxy measure for damage to the firm's reputation. Yet one need not demonstrate a causal relationship between activist protests and stock price declines to argue that activism may be influential in changing corporate behavior. If one assumes that most monopolists wish to lead, in the words of John Hicks, a "quiet life," undisturbed by regulators, activists, consumers, or competitors, we can suppose that managers may take pre-emptive actions as necessary to head off disruptive forces before they become virulent. Evidence suggests, for example, that pharmaceutical firms have voluntarily resisted increasing the price of some of their drugs in the face of public pressures for price controls. During the early years of the Clinton administration, for example, as the president (and his wife, Hillary) tried to enact a national health care program, drug companies feared that price controls could be imposed upon them as part of that plan. In their effort to fight such controls, they voluntarily reduced prices on many of their products, especially those used most commonly by the elderly, which represented an important constituency for all sides in the health care battle (Ellison and Wolfram 2006).

Similarly, Bartley shows how "voluntary" certification programs for such goods as forest products and textiles represented an effort on the part of firms to derail any attempts at formal regulation of corporate activities (and this points to why activists normally target the leading firms in a sector that they know will be especially interested in preserving their dominant position and will thus be most likely to adopt preemptive, voluntary restrictions on their activities) (Bartley 2007). By targeting leading firms whose value proposition is bound up in their corporate reputation (think Johnson & Johnson or Coca-Cola), social movements may gain the leverage needed to alter firm strategy on particular issues. We note in passing here that this idea of possible preemptive strategic actions by the firm points to the utility of a case study approach to research, since scholars have yet to develop good proxy measures that isolate corporate reputation and, as a consequence, we cannot conduct large-N studies of such activity by managers.

If transnational social movements are to be successful in shaping the political and economic agendas of governments and firms, they must fuse both rational/analytical and emotional/normative appeals into a single "ask." In fact, earlier studies of the AIDS movement in the United States state that part of the movement's relative success in advancing its claims was due to this very fusion. As sociologist Steven Epstein put it regarding American treatment activists, "Few social movements are inclined to mix 'moral crusades' with 'practical crusades.' *Treatment activism in the late 1980s was distinctive for the powerful fusion of these two forms*" (Epstein 1996, 232, emphasis added).

Fusing different types of appeal into a single "ask" requires some serious attention not only to how movements "frame" their "messages," which has been the focus of much of the research on social activism to date (Keck and Sikkink 1998), but it also requires that close attention be paid to advocates' strategies for getting from point A to point B. As an example of a cause that has focused more on the message than on the strategy, take the modern anti-slave trade movement. Unlike the abolition movement of the nineteenth century, which had a message (slavery is immoral and corrupting) and a strategy (use the Royal Navy to stop the transatlantic slave trade), today's movement only has a message (mainly focusing on the cruelty of the sex trade) without any consensus on how to stop it (Kaufmann and Pape 1999; Kapstein 2006b). Some advocates focus on penalizing prostitution, while others focus on its legalization. Some focus on penalizing the slave traders, others on penalizing the client. While sex trafficking in particular has grabbed more attention in recent years, particularly on college campuses, the advocacy movement to stop it has yet to forge consensus on a single policy ask. Interestingly, however, it does seem to be learning from its traditional lack of strategy, in that the movement is increasingly cohering around a demand for tougher penalties against those convicted of human trafficking.

In contrast, think of the AIDS treatment advocates whom we examine in this book. They had a message – that it was fundamentally *unfair* for people in the South to be denied the very same life-extending drugs that people in the North had access to – and they also had a clear and seemingly *feasible* strategy: universal access to treatment on the basis of "cheap" ARVs. The strategy was feasible in this case because the industry's pricing structure permitted cross-subsidization of different consumer groups, while new entrants in the form of generics manufacturers could be encouraged to enter the ARV marketplace. Obviously, not every advocacy movement has the opportunity to pursue a market transformation strategy that can be made amenable to industry actors; in such cases, however, we would argue that the movement is less likely to achieve its objectives.

As this brief analysis of the AIDS movement suggests, missing from much of the previous work on social movements is a prominent question, namely, when do some movements succeed in transforming the market environment while others fail? What makes some anti-corporate campaigns more effective than others (O'Rourke 2005; Eesley and Lenox 2006; King and Pearce 2010)? To be sure, work has been done that looks at the outcomes of anti-corporate campaigns, most notably changes in the targeted firm's stock valuation and share price (Soule 2009). That approach, however, is problematic for several reasons; for one thing, as already noted, firms might respond *pro-actively* to an advocacy campaign, so that the share price doesn't reflect the underlying politics.

Why, we ask, was the AIDS movement so effective in creating a "universal access to treatment" regime while other contemporary movements, like those aimed at curbing climate change, have faltered at transforming the markets they critique? What, specifically, did the movement need to achieve in order to advance the access to treatment regime? In other words, what "moving parts" in market structures could activists latch onto and manipulate in support of their transformation agenda?

In raising these questions, we need to define with some precision what we mean by movement "success" or "effectiveness," and we will use the terms interchangeably, even though they are not, of course, necessarily the same thing. As Craig Smith has pointed out, a consumer boycott, for example, could be *effective* in reducing a firm's sales without *succeeding* in altering corporate strategy or government policy (Smith 1990). While we accept this distinction, our focus in this book is on the ability of social movements to change market structures in some fundamental way; this is what we mean by activist effectiveness or success. We also recognize that these concepts can have an important inter-temporal dimension, in that a failure one day can seemingly evolve into a success over time ("we lost the battle but won the war") and vice-versa. Indeed, much of the existing literature on social movements omits this inter-temporal dimension in making its assessments of movement success. Again, we try to assess the durability of the market transformations we analyze, and this motivates, in part, our focus on the institutional arrangements that treatment advocates have also put in place in order to "stabilize" the new market arrangements (Fligstein 2002).

It is popularly claimed in much of the relevant social science literature, for example, that activist pressure on the oil industry during the 1990s led companies like BP to become more "green," especially following the success of Greenpeace in forcing Shell to tow a dysfunctional rigging across the North Sea that it had planned to sink in 1995 (Spar and La Mure 2003; Baron 2005). BP even changed its corporate identity from *British* Petroleum to *Beyond* Petroleum to signify its alleged commitment to alternative energies like solar and wind power. As those living in the Gulf Coast of the United States in 2010 could attest, however, BP's commitment to "green" was not even skin-deep, and in fact, a previous series of spills in Alaska – not to mention a major explosion at a refinery in Texas in 2005 which killed 15 workers – suggested that the company had failed to adopt even minimal safety and environmental standards in many of its operations (PBS Frontline 2010). More to the point, advocates have yet to transform the market for fossil fuels in any fundamental way, for example, through the imposition of a hefty carbon tax that begins to place the "real" cost of using these fuels on consumers. Such a tax could be transformative to the extent it levels the playing field with alternative energy sources, and in this case the dependent variable would be uptake of such alternatives within an energy grid.

As this discussion indicates, one definition of success might be to see whether a movement transformed a firm's stated policies or procedures, whether it agreed, for example, to put environmental metrics into place. Many "socially responsible investment" funds judge firms by their policies and procedures, as opposed to their outcomes, and for them "success" is defined by the adoption of such policies. Yet another definition of success, as stated above, focuses on the *harm* that a movement did to a firm. Did its actions, for example, result in a lower share price, or in getting the firm to commit to an action (like towing a rig rather than sinking it) that it otherwise would not have done? Still another way to look at movement success is in terms of its spillover effects; did movement A catalyze the launch of movement B? (Soule 2009). Mukherjee, for example, argues that the AIDS movement has played a major role in catalyzing other disease advocates to stake their claims with government agencies and the pharmaceutical industry (Mukherjee 2010).

In the case of the movement aimed at achieving universal access to ARV drug treatment, one must be circumspect in defining, much less claiming "success," even in our sense of market transformation. After all, as of 2011, only 54 percent of those PWAs were receiving ARV treatment (UNAIDS 2012a), and it is unlikely that this number will ever reach anything close to 100 percent. Indeed, should the number of those infected with the HIV virus increase faster than the rollout of ARV treatment, this percentage will, of course, shrink further (WHO 2009a; Gudrais 2010; Over 2011). We will also provide some evidence suggesting that AIDS is confronting "donor exhaustion" and that funding pledges to buy ARV drugs have, at best, leveled off (McNeil Jr. 2010).

This book makes a unique empirical contribution to the social movements' literature by examining in detail the transformation of a highly contentious market, looking at the changes that occurred on both the demand and supply sides of the ARV equation, along with the institutional structures that were built to underpin and "stabilize" this new market structure (Fligstein 2002). On the demand side, stakeholders had to change their perception of whether ARVs would work in the developing world or "resource-constrained" setting, while on the supply side changes had to be made regarding pharmaceutical patents, pricing, and competition so that ample quantities of ARVs would be produced at prices that poor countries could afford.

This change in the market needed to be supported by institutions that made these changes credible, in particular, institutions that would ensure that funds would be made available for the purchase and uptake of high-quality ARV medications at the reduced prices. In essence, the social movement surrounding the access to treatment regime entailed changing the supply and demand for ARVs while contributing to institutional innovation aimed at ensuring the effectiveness of that regime, out to the distant future. It is this last, inter-temporal dimension that remains in question, however, leading us to raise the more general issue of the durability of the institutions that the AIDS movement has built (Shadlen 2007; Over 2008; Piot 2012).

Leaving aside these doubts about the long-term prospects of the ARV regime for the moment, contrast the success of AIDS activists with that of the movement that is seeking to counter global climate change. Despite the creation of "carbon markets" and various regulations aimed at curbing carbon emissions, it would be difficult to argue that the market for fossil fuels or for carbon has been altered in any major way since the onset of the climate change debate in the 1980s. Fossil fuels are still priced and traded more or less as they were before, and few public policies have made a major dent in either consumption patterns or the supply of clean energy. Carbon markets like the European emissions trading system do exist, but key countries like the United States have yet to price carbon, limiting market expansion. To be sure, wind farms and other alternative energy sources are on the rise, but even the most optimistic predictions suggest that these will make little impact on the global climate in any relevant time horizon. Indeed, a lively (and, at least in some eyes, somewhat nutty) political debate still exists, mainly in the United States, over the extent to which climate change is actually induced by human activities.

Within the arena of global health, contrast HIV with an issue like diarrheal diseases, which kill over 1.5 million children per year, mainly in sub-Saharan Africa (WHO 2009c). There are, in fact, cheap treatments for these diseases, and one might think that universal access to treatment is therefore well within the grasp of the international community. Yet there has been only weak political mobilization in that direction, and few resources are devoted to this scourge. A similar story might have been told for many decades regarding maternal mortality, which received little attention from the global public health community until quite recently (Shiffman and Smith 2007).

We should emphasize, however, that we do not speak of "success" in normative or ethical terms. That is, we do not assume that success, defined as movement-led market transformation, is necessarily "good" and that movement failure is "bad" in terms of social welfare or any other aggregate measure of a polity's aspirations. Too often in the social movements' literature, it is simply assumed or asserted that activists are "improvers" whose work benefits society as a whole. That may or may not be the case, and we leave deeper normative debate about the "best" allocation of scarce medical resources from an ethical standpoint largely to the side in this book (Pogge 2005; Dietrich 2007). Instead, we seek to make an analytical argument about what social activists do and how they advance their objectives; in this sense our exercise is closer to positive than normative political economy. This effort, in turn, will allow us to generate hypotheses that form the basis for the empirical research that is presented in subsequent chapters.

How transnational movements succeed: some hypotheses about market transformation

Thus far we have sketched some of the linkages between activists and markets, and in particular on how the social movements' literature has analyzed that interaction. Now we draw the threads together to advance several hypotheses that we will "test" in this book. We separate these into hypotheses about the market structure; framing and norms; movement coherence; advocacy strategy; and institutions. In a sense, these hypotheses can be viewed as sequential steps or elements in an advocacy campaign, and it should be noted that the substantive chapters that follow also address each element in turn in greater depth. Advocates thus need to ask whether they have identified the opportunities within the industry they are targeting (Chapter 2); whether they have framed the issue in a compelling way (Chapter 3); whether they have a coherent ask (Chapter 4); whether they have a feasible strategy that addresses concerns about costs by firms and governments (Chapter 5); and whether supporting institutions need to be built (Chapter 6). More generally, the hypotheses are concerned about the conditions that favor the likelihood of market transformation.

We draw these pieces together to offer a *theory of strategic moral action* (see Sell and Prakash 2004 for an argument that AIDS treatment activists were strategic actors not dissimilar from other interest groups). Our theory draws on diverse intellectual traditions, but broadly we attempt to synthesize constructivist and rationalist theories of world politics in making our claims. Constructivist theories help us to illuminate the role of frames in advancing advocacy agendas, but rationalist theories keep us attentive to the costs and benefits of alternative actions and strategies. We hope this synthesis will inspire others to escape from their academic pigeonholes in an effort to explain important global phenomena and outcomes.[2]

---

[2] We draw insights from a wide range of scholarly influences, from microeconomics to social psychology. We incorporate elements of structure and agency, and we bring together insights from ideational and institutional theory. On analytical eclecticism, see (Katzenstein and Okawara 2001). On bridging rationalism and constructivism, see (Fearon and Wendt 2003).

Hypotheses about market structure

As previously noted, much of the literature on "anti-" corporate movements focuses on attributes of particular firms that make them likely targets for advocacy pressures. Here we step back one level to consider the industry-level attributes that make entire sectors contestable from an advocacy standpoint. Although we discuss a variety of structural attributes that made the ARV market contestable, we focus on two structural issues here with respect to the industry's potential for market transformation.

H1: *The more concentrated the industry and the lower the access to its products, the more likely this market will be transformed.*

If there are only a few firms in a sector that control a large share of the market, then should these firms change their behavior, the market will be transformed quickly. Where there are large numbers of firms in a given industry with a wider distribution of sales across them, it will be harder to transform the market structure, as many firms will have to change their behavior. This is akin to the observation about the number of veto players and policy change. Where there are fewer veto players, policy, though potentially resistant to change depending on the attitudes of the main players, can change quickly if those actors capable of blocking policy lift their objections (Tsebelis 2002; Busby 2010a).

What this hypothesis suggests is that basic "mismatches" in a market structure will generate opportunities and/or demands for change in how that industry's products are delivered to consumers. Take, for example, the "universal access" provisions that government agencies have mandated with respect to public utilities. If electric utilities or telephone companies only served a few customers, they would face pressure from other consumers and regulators to extend that service. For this reason, many industries are characterized by cross-subsidization across different classes of consumers, enabling "universal access" to occur. However, some other industries – like pharmaceuticals – have not been subject to such provisions, making such industries targets for advocacy campaigns. At the same time, if a large number of people are not being served by a particular market structure, there will be incentives, all else being equal, for market entry in order to serve those consumers.

H2: *The more fluid the rules shaping the terms of market entry, the more likely the market will be transformed.*

Earlier in this chapter we spoke of the rules and institutions that shape market structures. These rules, however, are not "neutral," but may serve the interests of dominant firms. Further, the institutions that support these rules, like courts, may not provide a level playing field to claimants; in the United States, for example, it can prove very costly to sue a corporation, even if the claimant has a good chance at winning a favorable verdict. When rules are fluid, however, new entrants – like advocates – may have opportunities to influence how they are shaped. In the case of AIDS, for example, the shaping of the TRIPS regime during the 1990s provided an opening to influence its "public health" provisions. More generally, fluidity in market structures caused by internal or exogenous changes expands the opportunities for market transformation. We explore these issues of market structure in more detail in the following chapter.

Hypotheses about framing and norms

As Finnemore and Sikkink have written, "Arguments about which substantive normative claims will be more influential in world politics have varied widely" (1998, 907). Based on their review of several transnational activist movements, Sikkink and co-author Margaret Keck conclude that two sets of norms are likely to be most effective: "norms involving (1) bodily integrity and prevention of bodily harm for vulnerable or 'innocent' groups, especially when a short causal chain exists between cause and effect, and (2) legal equality of opportunity" (Keck and Sikkink 1998). With respect to the bodily harm norm, it is interesting to note that treatment activists gained much of their traction after equating people living with AIDS to Holocaust victims and, by extension, implying that the behavior of the pharmaceutical companies was as heinous as that of a Nazi regime that killed millions of innocents (Kramer 2003). When it was discovered that AIDS could be passed to babies *in vitro*, this argument about the death of the innocents because of an inability to acquire cheap drugs acquired even more moral suasion.

These arguments may be cast into the following "moral" hypothesis:

H3: *The greater the immediate bodily harm caused by existing market allocations (e.g. of pharmaceuticals), the more likely a social movement will succeed in generating a market transformation (e.g. towards universal access to medicines).*

As we explore in Chapter 3, another way to think about this is whether or not the good in question is essential for life. To the extent that the particular good is necessary for a person's survival, the more likely a campaign for access will be successful. We also unpack this idea in Chapter 3.

Hypotheses about movement coherence

To become a political force capable of transforming markets, a social movement must at some point evolve to possess unity or coherence around a common objective. The degree of "organization" can be temporary rather than permanent; it can be a coalition of actors brought together to achieve a specific purpose, which then disbands once its objective is achieved (Tarrow 2005). The organization can also be "informal" rather than formal, providing disparate groups with an umbrella for their joint activities and opposed to a single structure in which everyone must now work. What is most crucial to success is that the coalition achieve consensus on which goals are being pursued and which are being left dormant. To put this in strategic terms, movements need focal points (Schelling 1960).

Rather surprisingly, this essential point seems to have been lost on some activist movements. Tarrow, for example, has examined the inability of the global justice movement to have much influence over world politics. He argues that "the global justice frame lacks a clear directive toward a strategic repertoire of social justice" (2005, 75). Similarly, the Occupy Wall Street movement that emerged with much publicity in 2011 fizzled out in part because it was regarded as lacking a set of clear demands (Buckley 2011; Buckley and Moynihan 2011; Gitlin 2012). Likewise, climate change activists, after early convergence on legally binding targets and timetables for emissions reductions, have become increasingly divided on the appropriate strategy toward reduced carbon emissions. In contrast, AIDS treatment activists came to the conviction early in their campaign that access to treatment first depended on getting the prices of ARVs down. These points lead to our next hypothesis:

H4: *The more coherent or focused the social movement is on its shared objective or "ask," the more likely it is to succeed.*

This theme of movement coherence forms the basis for Chapter 4.

Hypotheses about strategy

Moral arguments that are diffuse do not succeed; they need focus and organization for collective action. But these are insufficient as well; they also need a feasible strategy that relates means and ends. What this suggests is that to be successful or effective, social movements also need a compelling business strategy, a feasible model of how to get from point A to point B. The precise elements of such a strategy, of course, will depend on the issue-area at stake, along with the associated parameters.

Here, we concentrate on two hypotheses concerning key elements in a successful strategy. The first focuses on lowering the costs of advocates' ask for both firms and government actors. The second focuses on raising the opportunity costs of inaction by target actors through reputational damage.

H5: *The higher (lower) the costs associated with market transformation, the less (more) likely that transformation will occur.*

As an example, Spar and La Mure cite the case of the Free Burma Coalition (FBC), which demanded the closure of Unocal's natural gas operations in Myanmar. Unocal refused to buckle in this case, given the high cost associated with developing alternative gas fields (Spar and La Mure 2003). Similarly, AIDS "treatment activism" could only credibly pursue "universal access" once generic drugs came on the scene which substantially lowered the costs of ARV medications (see York 1999). We discuss this hypothesis in Chapter 5 on movement strategy. In that chapter, we suggest that it is useful to think about the costs to firms and the costs to donors. In terms of firm-level costs, we distinguish between the costs to incumbent firms as well as the costs to potential new market entrants.

Actors who are targeted by advocates, whether firms or government agencies and officials, must take into account not just the costs associated with a given action, but the potential or opportunity costs associated with *inaction* as well. Advocates can raise the opportunity costs of inaction through a variety of strategies, including protests, boycotts, "naming and shaming" activities, and threatening corporate business models, e.g. by attacking patent rights regimes. A pharmaceutical firm, for example, might determine that while lowering the price on an ARV medication has real financial costs, the opportunity cost of not doing so could be even higher, if it leads to lawsuits aimed at their patent rights or to the mobilization of activist shareholders who create controversy and "bad" publicity for the firm and its management at annual meetings. These observations lead us to the following hypothesis:

H6: *The greater (lower) the opportunity costs of corporate or political inaction in the face of demands for market transformation, the more (less) likely that the transformation will occur.*

Taking H5 and H6 together, we see that *advocates can best advance their cause by lowering the financial costs of action and raising the opportunity costs of inaction.* To put this in other words, advocates advance their cause by changing the cost–benefit assessment of target firms regarding the best response to advocate demands.

Hypotheses about institutions

Even if activists succeed in building a coherent organization with a targeted message and credible strategy, what is to ensure that the movement will be successful over the long run? After all, any "wins" could be fleeting if market transformations are not somehow *institutionalized*. As Fligstein reminds us, capitalism rests upon institutions that stabilize the interactions of economic agents, lowering transactions costs and making it possible to engage in mutually beneficial exchange (Fligstein 2002). It is for this reason, for example, that AIDS activists rejected corporate *donation* schemes as the basis for a universal access to treatment regime; they feared that it was all-too-easy for firms, operating under this model, to turn off the spigot. This suggests our final hypothesis:

H7: *The more capable the institutions are of stabilizing a transformed market structure, for example by having enforcement or financial power, the more likely it is that the new principles on which the market is based will endure.*

To provide a concrete example, in market economies intellectual property rights (IPR) provide inventors with the incentive to make costly investments in product development; the combination of IPRs and legal enforcement thus provides necessary institutional underpinnings of an "innovation economy." As we noted earlier in this chapter, an array of institutions are needed to support markets, and in the case of the universal access to treatment regime these institutions had to provide such functions as financing, information gathering, and property rights protection. We discuss this hypothesis in Chapter 6 on the role of institutions.

In sum, in this book we advance several hypotheses and make a number of broader claims about what is required in order to cause a market transformation or to change a market in a fundamental way (e.g. in the terms of access to that market). We will show that even in the presence of a relatively open economic opportunity structure, advocates will still need to overcome numerous hurdles in order to succeed. At a minimum, they will need a compelling moral message, a coherent ask, a strategy to address cost concerns, and a set of supportive institutions. These points are suggestive of the immense challenges facing any advocacy movement that seeks to engage in the process of market transformation.

Conclusions

Markets are social institutions in which political and economic agents seek to advance their interests. While many market interactions are dominated by firms and households, others are contested by a host of other actors, including advocacy movements, all seeking to shape patterns of supply, demand, and price. That contention over who gets what is the very stuff of politics.

This is a book about a profound change that occurred in the allocation of life-extending ARV medications, from a model that was "high price, low volume" to one based on "universal access to treatment." Beyond that, however, it is about the conditions under which social movements are effective in influencing or transforming market structures. By using the ARV case as the basis for our analytical framework, and then expanding upon it by discussing other illustrative examples, we hope to say something of more general significance about the role of social movements in modern economic life. In the following chapters we thus address in some detail how a group of dedicated AIDS treatment activists, along with sympathetic policy entrepreneurs and corporate executives, managed to transform ARVs from private goods into merit goods.

Appendix A: A brief history of AIDS and the AIDS treatment movement

On June 5, 1981, the Mortality and Morbidity Weekly Report (MMWR) of the Centers for Disease Control (CDC) contained the following stark report: "In the period October 1980–May 1981, 5 young men, all active homosexuals, were treated for biopsy-confirmed Pneumocystis carinii pneumonia at 3 different hospitals in Los Angeles, California. Two of the patients died" (CDC 1981). Over the following weeks, more and more such cases were reported, with gay men suffering and dying not just from pneumonia but from a very rare form of cancer – Kaposi's sarcoma – as well. Based on the observation that it was only gay men who were affected by the disease, it was initially termed GRID (gay-related immune deficiency) in the United States. However, in July 1982, the CDC suggested the name Acquired Immune Deficiency Syndrome (AIDS). By 1984, researchers in France and the United States had identified the virus that causes AIDS.

In March 1986, the largely gay advocacy group ACT UP initiated its first action on Wall Street demanding access to treatment and an end to discrimination for those living with AIDS. That same year saw encouraging clinical trials of the first AIDS treatment drug, azidothymidine (AZT), originally developed as an anti-cancer medication in the 1960s. In March 1987, AZT was approved for use by the Food and Drug Administration (FDA). This drug, the sole of its kind at the time, was priced by its manufacturer, Burroughs Wellcome, at more than $10,000 per patient per year, which was well beyond the reach of many of those living with (and dying from) AIDS. These high prices spurred further protests, including at corporate headquarters.

By 1995, ample evidence had accumulated that people could become resistant to AZT on its own and that it might offer few benefits to people in the early phase of the disease. Further, it had strong side-effects in many cases. However, a so-called "combination therapy" (or "cocktail") with 3TC (lamuvidine) was found to be more effective and was approved for use in November 1995. These drugs attacked the disease in new ways and were called "antiretrovirals." A month later, saquinavir, the first of a new line of AIDS drugs called "protease inhibitors," was approved for use by the FDA.

This set the stage for the introduction of Highly Active Antiretroviral Therapy (HAART), where a combination of ARV drugs are taken to attack the virus in different ways. In 1996, wide-scale rollout of HAART would begin in the United States and other advanced industrialized countries, which would dramatically reduce the number of AIDS-related deaths and convert AIDS from a death sentence into a chronic condition. Again, these therapies all cost over $10,000 per patient per year, but by this time many patients in the industrialized world were covered by insurance. That, of course, was not the case with most developing countries, with the exception of Brazil, where low-cost generic substitutes were made available to the local AIDS community. Global health specialists thus began to turn their attention to how these drugs could be rolled out to poorer nations.

The mid 1990s were a time of flux in the international community's response to HIV/AIDS, with some movement in the direction of attacking the disease but paltry funding. Early in 1996, UNAIDS, a combined joint program by a number of United Nations (UN) agencies was launched. The following year, this new agency would begin a series of pilot projects to test the efficacy of ARV treatment in resource-poor settings through its "Drug Access Initiative" (DAI). Similar efforts were being sponsored by organizations like Partners in Health in Haiti.

But even as promising treatments were becoming available in the advanced industrialized countries, the high costs were preventing widespread rollout in the developing world. As a nascent global AIDS movement began to coalesce, it sought to understand the reasons for these high prices. One culprit that emerged was the so-called TRIPS Accord, negotiated as part of the new WTO in 1995. This accord would require all nations to issue patents on pharmaceutical products, though the agreement gave developing countries ten years to phase-in the rules. Still, the monopoly power conferred by patents seemingly provided one source for the high price of AIDS medications.

In 1998, AIDS advocates interested in access to treatment in the developing world had their cause bolstered by a singular, galvanizing event. In South Africa, the government of Nelson Mandela, having passed a Medicines Act intended to deal with the high cost of drugs in the fight against AIDS and other diseases, found itself in February 1998 on the receiving end of a lawsuit from a group of global pharmaceuticals companies, which charged that the Act violated companies' constitutional rights as well as South Africa's obligations under TRIPS. By year's end, South African AIDS activists would come together to form the Treatment Action Campaign (TAC), which would evolve into a globally influential group. Aided by such non-governmental organizations as MSF, the South African government would vigorously defend itself, generating terrible publicity for "big pharma," which eventually dropped the suit. Nonetheless, the reputational damage had been done and it likely spurred big pharma into actively seeking ways to help reduce AIDS drug prices.

Just as affected groups in countries like South Africa emerged to support access to treatment, activist groups in Europe and the United States also began to organize. In 1999, veterans of ACT UP, along with supporters from other organizations like CPTech, would come together in the United States to form the Health GAP coalition. In November 1999, MSF launched its own Access Campaign with the proceeds of the Nobel Prize the organization won earlier that year. At the end of the year, anti-globalization campaigners disrupted the meetings of the World Trade Organization in Seattle, Washington, prompting US President Bill Clinton to announce greater support for TRIPS flexibilities to support public health.

Growing awareness of the seriousness of the AIDS crisis led the UN Security Council to convene in January 2000 to discuss the problem, its first ever meeting on a health topic. Later that year UNAIDS, along with five branded pharmaceutical companies, launched the Accelerated Access Initiative (AAI) as a way of bringing down prices and providing wider treatment access to people in developing countries. In July, South Africa hosted the biennial International AIDS Society conference, during which time AIDS activists put treatment access squarely on the international agenda, in a series of public protests.

In September 2000, the Indian generic company Cipla, prompted by activists, would make a historic offer at a European Commission meeting to reduce the costs of ARV drugs to between $600 and $800 per patient per year. The following February, Cipla would go further and offer the same drug for less than a dollar a day, a move that garnered headlines around the world. The introduction of generic substitutes for ARV medications would prove to be an important moment in terms of access to treatment; still, the case had to be made that these drugs would prove effective in the developing world setting.

In June 2001, the UN General Assembly would further strengthen the international community's commitment to expanded access to ARV medications, declaring that universal treatment access should be a goal. And in the wake of the terrorist attacks of September 11, 2001, a meeting of the WTO was held in Doha in November to review the impact of the TRIPS accord on global health. At this meeting, countries agreed to the so-called health exception to TRIPS which re-affirmed governments' flexibilities to overcome drug patent laws in the midst of a health emergency. Delegates also extended the period for least-developed countries to comply with TRIPS provisions on pharmaceuticals until 2016.

With generic ARVs now available at low cost, donor nations were now more willing to fund access to these medications. In January of 2002, the Global Fund to Fight AIDS, Tuberculosis, and Malaria was formally created as an independent financing agency, with its secretariat in Geneva. In October of that year, the Clinton HIV/AIDS Initiative (CHAI) was initiated, and a year later, CHAI would announce its first agreements with generic drug companies for bulk-purchasing prices of ARVs.

In early 2003, US President George W. Bush announced the creation of the President's Emergency Plan for AIDS Relief (PEPFAR), pledging $15 billion over five years for the program. And in September 2006, UNITAID, another financing instrument in the fight against HIV/AIDS, was created. UNITAID's unique basis of support was a tax on airline flights, making it the world's first global tax scheme. As a result of these funding programs, coupled with the availability of generics, widespread rollout of AIDS drugs was in reach. By the end of 2008, more than 4 million people were on treatment in low- and middle-income countries.

By the beginning of the new millennium's second decade, AIDS advocates could look toward the future with mixed emotions. On the one hand were a series of concerns. First, while generic drugs had reduced the costs of the current generation of AIDS ARVs, it was unclear what would happen as new and more advanced drugs came on-line. Would these also be affordable? Second, with the financial crisis of 2008 and the economic slowdown that followed, it seemed unlikely that the resources to sustain a global treatment regime would be made available. Third, in 2011, the Global Fund confronted a management crisis after the media reported a small percentage of funds were misappropriated by recipients. The long-term effects of this crisis were uncertain as a new Executive Director, Dr. Mark Dybul of the United States, was appointed in November 2012, but it could reduce confidence in that organization.

On the other hand, it could not be forgotten that the net result of the global scale-up of treatment by the end of 2011 was that an estimated 8 million people in low- and middle-income countries had access to ARVs. That same year, the UN issued a political declaration to put 15 million on ARVs by 2015. Those numbers were reaffirmed in 2012, when Washington DC hosted the International AIDS Society meeting, the first time the United States had done so since finally lifting travel restrictions for those living with HIV in 2009. While the fight against AIDS had come a very long way in the three decades following its discovery, there was still no end in sight.

Appendix B: Key dates

1981–2
First cases of AIDS identified

1986
ACT UP begins actions in the United States

1987
First AIDS drug AZT approved for use

1995
TRIPS Agreement enters into force, 10-year phase-in for developing countries

1996
HAART introduced
Partners in Health pilots HAART in Haiti
January – UNAIDS created
July – Vancouver International AIDS Society meeting
December – Brazil begins universal ARV therapy

1997
November – DAI launched

1998
February – South African government sued over its "Medicines Act"
June–July – International AIDS Society meeting held in Geneva
December – South Africa's TAC formed

1999
MSF pilot projects
January – Health GAP formed
March – MSF, Health Action International (HAI), and the Consumer Project on Technology (CPTech) host Geneva meeting on compulsory licensing
November – MSF access campaign initiated
November – MSF, HAI, and CPTech host Amsterdam meeting on access to medicines
December – Seattle WTO meeting, Clinton announces will support TRIPS flexibilities

2000
January – UN Security Council meeting on AIDS
May – AAI announced
May – Clinton signs Executive Order stopping trade sanctions against countries with health emergencies
June–July – Presidential candidate Al Gore dogged by Health GAP on campaign trail
July – Durban AIDS meeting
September – Cipla offers $600–$800 price for generic AIDS drugs at European Commission meeting

2001
February – Cipla announces dollar a day triple cocktail
March – World Health Organization prequalification scheme created
April – South African lawsuit withdrawn
April – Abuja meeting, where Annan calls for Global Fund
June – UN General Assembly meeting on AIDS, political declaration supports universal treatment access
November – Doha health exception agreed

2002
January – Global Fund created
October – CHAI created

2003
January – PEPFAR announced
August – WTO enacts so-called "paragraph 6" decision on patent exceptions for importing countries
October – CHAI first agreements announced
December – World Health Organization/UNAIDS launch "3 by 5" initiative

2004
May – FDA fast-track approval process created

2005
India now must comply with TRIPS provisions

2006
September – UNITAID created

2008
July – PEPFAR re-authorized

2011
UN political declaration to put 15 million people with AIDS on ARVs by 2015

2 Industry structure and movement opportunities

> We don't want a black market. We want to make the real market work.
>
> ACT UP activist Jim Eigo on US AIDS treatment advocacy, interviewed in
> the documentary *How to Survive a Plague*

During the 1990s the pharmaceutical industry became among the most vilified sectors in the global economy. Rather than being associated with the development of essential medicines that save or extend human lives, it became the object of attack from disease advocacy movements that claimed the industry favored profits over access to treatment. What's more, some of these movements proved quite successful in promoting greater access, most notably in the case of HIV/AIDS.

The effectiveness of disease advocacy movements is surprising in some respects. After all, leading students of corporate social responsibility believed that the pharmaceutical industry presented a "hard case" for social advocates, given its monopoly power over certain drug classes and the inability of consumers to find substitutes (see Baron 2005). It was much easier, they believed, to rally consumers to an anti-corporate cause when the costs of switching to other products were low. What a product-level analysis overlooks, however, is the points of vulnerability that might exist within an industry's structure, making it amenable to advocacy pressure.

In this chapter we ask: what were the *structural features* of the pharmaceutical industry that provided the AIDS advocates with openings or points of leverage as they launched their campaign against it? To use the phrase employed in our hypothesis, how "contestable" was the pharmaceutical market from the perspective of the advocates? We emphasize that our focus here is on these structural or industry-level variables. In the next chapter, in contrast, we turn to the special "life or death" characteristics of access to pharmaceutical products and how AIDS advocates used that urgency in "framing" their movement for lower prices.

In addition to looking at products, students of private politics have also focused largely on the specific attributes of firms that make them particularly vulnerable to such actions as boycotts. Firms with the leading brand names in their industry, for example, seem to be targeted with greater frequency than firms with lesser brand recognition. As a case in point, the Rainforest Action Network (RAN), which focuses on preserving some of the world's most fragile and endangered ecosystems, "viewed companies with a public image and a strong brand as the most susceptible to its campaign tactics" (Yurday 2004, 4). In the case of AIDS drugs, the global pharmaceutical giant GSK was often targeted by the advocacy community for several reasons: first, because one of its predecessor firms, Burroughs Wellcome, held the patent on the first ARV, AZT; second, after several mergers, the company continued to play a major role in this market; and third, the chief executive officer of the newly created GSK, Jean-Pierre Garnier, had publicly stated his interest in increasing access to medicines in rich and poor countries through a variety of means (Abelson 2003). Further, after the merger that formed GSK in 2000, the company became an object of intense interest to antitrust regulators, shareholder activists, and advocates (and it is worth noting that groups like Oxfam, which targeted GSK in its own "cut the cost" campaign for lower prices, also held GSK stock in its pension fund, so it acted both as shareholder activist and as social advocate). Since advocates often target a firm's "reputation," those with prominent brands have the most to lose if they fall on the "wrong side" of a campaign.

Much of the advocates' activity, however, was focused on changing the behavior of the pharmaceutical industry as a whole rather than that of any particular company, and a deeper analysis of pharmaceutical industry structure reveals some of the "weaknesses" or points of leverage that advocates could exploit as they mounted their campaign for universal access to AIDS treatment. These points of leverage included targeting the reputation of individual firms, their reorganization plans, their patent portfolios, and their pricing strategies. Just as political opportunities for mobilization may differ across nations, so, too, do opportunities across industries. In fact, an analysis of industry or market structure would or should be an essential element in the advocates' calculus as they launch a campaign, since it can influence the movement's strategy and its allocation of scarce resources. All things being equal, more contestable industries present advocates with the greatest opportunities for changing the terms of market access.

We should emphasize that, whereas the economics literature speaks of contestability as the extent to which markets approach the competitive equilibrium, either due to actual or potential entry by newcomers, we adopt a somewhat broader perspective. By contestability, we mean that a market possesses features that allow both new market entrants and advocates to contest incumbents by challenging the existing patterns of production as well as the rules governing market access to consumers. While increasing access by generics manufacturers into the ARV market was one objective of the advocates, another goal was simply increased *responsiveness* by the branded pharmaceuticals to the plight of PWAs, especially in the developing world. Differential pricing of drugs for different markets, which did not necessarily represent the industry's competitive equilibrium, served to address, at least partly, advocates' concerns about "big pharma's" pricing policies.

In the economics literature, one of the major barriers to entry for new firms that seek to take market share from existing incumbents is the presence of upfront or sunk costs. Taking the case of the pharmaceutical industry, for example, the infrastructure and resources needed to engage in research, development, and clinical testing provide a major barrier to entry. The drugs that eventually emerge from this process are all covered by patents, and often multiple patents. One of the features that made the industry contestable, however, was the absence of this patent protection in certain foreign jurisdictions and the fluidity of the rules governing intellectual property rights globally. In essence, when certain countries refused to recognize strong pharmaceutical patents, the generics manu-facturers they enabled drove the costs of entry close to zero, and as a consequence the market became contestable, with ARV prices falling sharply towards marginal costs.[1]

We therefore emphasize two features of the ARV market that made it potentially contestable from the advocates' perspective: first, the presence of industry or market concentration in this therapeutic category (coupled with limited access to the industry's output by those who were most vulnerable), and second, the fluidity of the rules in many developing countries that shaped the industry's incentive system and ultimately its profits, namely, the IPR regime. To be sure, other features of the industry during the 1990s would also figure prominently in shaping opportunities to influence the pharmaceutical industry, including its growth during that decade into a "global oligopoly" (Galambos 2001), and we mention several of them in this chapter. Indeed, we would assert that students of social movements might profitably make use of the type of industrial analysis inspired by Michael Porter's "Five Forces" framework (which argues that industry profitability is a function of supplier power, buyer power, the threat of new entrants, the existence of substitutes, and the intensity of rivalry among the competitors) (Porter 1980, 2008). Our

[1] We thank Prof. Brad Jensen of Georgetown University for highlighting this point.

emphasis, however, is on the monopoly power the branded pharmaceuticals held over ARV drugs, a monopoly supported by the changing IP regime and the patents that countries issued to pharmaceutical firms.

We thus begin the chapter with some more description of what we mean by the terms "market concentration" and "fluid rules." We then examine pharmaceutical industry structure in order to understand why analysts have viewed it as difficult to influence, before turning to certain points of weakness, including pharmaceutical pricing policy and the role of IPRs, with a particular focus on the global harmonization of these rights through the TRIPS Agreement, which came into force in 1995. Overall, our purpose is to provide an analysis of how advocates came to view the pharmaceutical sector as one that was "ripe" for attack by the access to treatment movement.

Defining terms: market concentration and fluid rules

In stressing the role of advocates in making markets more contestable, we supplement the economics literature that focuses on the (potential or actual) role of new entrants in bringing competitive disciplines to an industry. We believe that two aspects of a market are of particular importance to advocates: first, industry concentration, coupled with access to the industry's output on the part of buyers; second, fluid rules.

Concentration means that within a given sector or product market, a limited number of firms are responsible for a large share of the market; the "Herfindahl" index provides one measure of such concentration that is widely used by economists. When this (monopoly) concentration yields a low degree of global access to an industry's output (or a large unmet demand for a good) through restricted supply (or high prices), incentives are created for new market entrants to seek opportunities to meet this demand (although aspects of the demand side, including its level of organization and purchasing power, can influence the attractiveness of these options, for better and for worse). For campaigners, this combination of high market concentration on the one hand and low access on the other creates an "injustice" or "unfairness" potential which can create incentives for advocates to seek changes in the principles by which access to the good is afforded.

Markets with high concentration are potentially resistant to change because a handful of producers have monopoly power and control the supply side, providing them few incentives to alter their profit-maximizing behavior. For this reason, some students of "private politics" argue that competitive industries are more likely to accept advocate demands. Yet, the presence of rents in an oligopolistic industry is what will attract potential new entrants (and advocates) in the first place to seek a piece of that particular action. At the same time, should incumbent firms decide to address advocates' concerns, the industry can change quickly, since only a few firms' behavior can alter market outcomes.

For about the first fifteen years of its existence, the ARV market had only a handful of suppliers producing a limited amount of high-priced goods. Indeed, for eight years beginning in 1987 with the introduction of the first ARV, AZT, Burroughs Wellcome had a monopoly on HIV therapies. Even when a variety of newer drugs came on the market starting in 1994, with the introduction of Starit (d4T) by Bristol Myers Squibb (BMS), the new offerings were dominated by a handful of firms. While countries like Brazil and Thailand made drugs sold at much lower prices for their local markets, the copycat drugs did not generally enter international trade. It was this market "gap" – the absence of low-priced ARVs on the global market – that advocates seized upon in the late 1990s as they sought to encourage generics manufacturers, primarily based in India, to offer this product.

On the other extreme, when markets are fragmented, with many different suppliers producing goods for disorganized consumers, advocates will face a more challenging task when it comes to transformation. In this context, think of another prominent universal access movement, the one targeting primary education. Educational services are delivered around the globe by numerous suppliers operating under a wide variety of conditions and constraints. The universal access to education movement must somehow confront these suppliers while organizing "buyers" of educational services who must demand these services. As a consequence, moving towards universal access to education (including the education of girls) is much more difficult from a *structural* perspective than promoting universal access to AIDS medications (even without considering the complicated economics and politics in each case) as it requires changing the incentives of many thousands of national and subnational educational authorities and providers, while organizing on the demand side a diverse group of "students" (or their parents) with differing needs and desires (again, unlike disease treatment advocates who presumably have a more or less coherent set of demands). In short, the organization of the market on the supply and demand sides will influence the ability of advocates to change the principles of access to an industry's output.

Another structural feature of the market that can facilitate or impede market transformation is the rules that shape the incentives of the participants. At the core of the AIDS movement's campaign for universal access to treatment was its contestation of the regulations that guide pharmaceutical industry investment and marketing, in particular with respect to IPRs.

These rules provided a focal point for the movement's ire and brought into sharp relief the key question of whether corporate profits should trump human lives. We hypothesize that if the rules of the market are fluid, then they can more readily be challenged by "outsiders" and, as a result, the market space can be contested. Newer rules of a more recent vintage are less likely to benefit from previous legal rulings and the presence of industry friendly regulatory structures. These moments of transition provide great opportunities to advocates who are prepared to seize them.

In the case of the ARV market, the WTO's TRIPS Agreement, which extended patent protection to pharmaceuticals in all member countries, came into force in 1995, although its implementation in developing countries was deferred for up to a decade and later extended for the least developing countries until 2016. Patent protection for pharmaceutical compounds is only recently available, if yet at all, in most developing countries. Because the TRIPS Agreement was so new and because its interpretation was ambiguous in critical issue-areas like public health, it became a focal point of advocacy attack. By contrast, other rules like those associated with the granting of most-favored nation status in the trade arena or the principles by which recognition is extended to new states, have longer established pedigrees. By their nature, rules that are long standing are more difficult to challenge and change than newer rules like the WTO's IPR rules or the highly contested rules of targets and timetables under the Kyoto Protocol, which was negotiated in 1997 but only came into force in 2005. (We should emphasize that it is not just an advocacy movement that can challenge new rules; firms and trade associations may do so as well.)

Analyzing industry structure: big pharma as a hard case

Among the lingering questions in the study of "anti-corporate" social movements are the related issues of which firms and industries are most likely to be targeted by advocacy campaigns and which of these campaigns are most likely to be successful in winning some fundamental changes in business strategy and policy. While making a ruckus may be an end in itself, we suppose that advocates get utility from running an effective campaign, meaning one that realizes their stated objectives (see Baron 2005). As a result of "winning" a fight against a major corporation, their organizations or movements may enjoy an increase in membership and funding, not to mention the immense personal satisfaction gained by movement partici-pants from advancing their cause. Running an effective campaign may therefore have both instrumental as well as intrinsic purposes.

Recent years have seen the emergence of the kind of structural analysis that we believe is useful to a fuller understanding of advocacy movement targets and their success. In her analysis of anti-biotech movements in Western Europe, for example, Rachel Schurman finds that the industry's structure and its value chain exposed the major firms in that sector to particular vulnerabilities that social activists could use to their advantage. Agro-business has to sell its products to supermarkets that, in turn, must attract customers to their stores. If "GMOs" could effectively be trans-formed into a bogeyman, raising the specter of coming environmental and health crises, and the end of rural culture, advocates could persuade consumers to stop purchasing certain products, which could in turn lead management to question and ultimately change what it stocks on the shelves. Schurman writes that anti-biotech activists were successful when they "strategically exploited certain key vulnerabilities of the industry" (Schurman 2004).

Schurman's focus on industry structure provides a promising avenue for further exploration. But finding the precise channels that relate indus-try structure to advocacy success remains an elusive enterprise. As noted above, Baron argues that pharmaceuticals companies were less suscep-tible to advocacy pressure because their products were of vital import-ance to their consumers and in many cases few substitutes were available (Baron 2005). For this reason alone, the pharmaceutical industry would seem an unpromising object of an advocacy movement. Below we explore other reasons why the pharmaceutical industry presents a "hard case" for advocacy movements.

In the pharmaceutical sector, consumers do not so much choose "brands" of drugs as they choose "types" of medications based on their expected efficacy; in this sense, pharmaceuticals are classic "experience" or "credence goods," whose value is only known based on actual use (Feddersen and Gilligan 2001). Targeting Merck is therefore not like targeting Coca-Cola; the greatest part of Coke's value is tied to its brand name, while the greatest part of Merck's (or Pfizer's) value is tied to the utility of its drugs, a value which has been vetted by governments through their market approval procedures, and by doctors who ultimately pre-scribe pharmaceuticals. The "reputation" of a pharmaceutical firm would thus not seem to offer an advocacy movement with a particularly easy target.

The pharmaceutical sector also differs in important respects from other industries in that consumers do not generally know or pay for the full cost of the products they consume, at least in the industrialized world, since prescription medicines are usually covered by public or private insurance schemes. Consumer mobilization is undermined because users are shielded from the real costs of the products they consume. The end consumer lacks the ability to meaningfully compare pharmaceutical prices against different classes of buyers. In some respects, drugs are like airline seats with each consumer paying something different depending on his or her insurance or payor policies. The issue of pharmaceutical pricing is so central to our discussion that it is detailed in a separate section below.

Consumers are also one step removed from the industry in that they rarely demand pharmaceutical products directly but instead are dependent upon agents, the doctors who make decisions for them about appropriate treatment and medication. The power of this agent, in turn, stems partly from his or her "authority" or professional training but also from the fact that he or she has monopoly power in most countries to write prescriptions for patented drugs. This structure means that patients face information asymmetries vis-à-vis their doctors regarding pharmaceutical compounds and treatments. Understanding treatment options takes a considerable investment of time and energy on the part of patients and yet again may work against advocacy efforts at mobilization. Indeed, AIDS advocates made it a point in their various national and, later, global campaigns to become quite expert in the science of HIV/AIDS, the pharmacology of AIDS drugs, and the regulatory process by which such drugs get approved.

The structure or industrial organization of the pharmaceutical sector is also difficult to penetrate, even for economists who specialize in its operations (see Comanor 1986; Scherer 1993). For example, while it does not appear to be a particularly concentrated industry compared to many other manufacturing sectors, at least according to the standard ratios used by government agencies, this statistic masks the great variability in concentration that exists with respect to particular disease categories and drug classes (Schweitzer 2006, 27). Drug companies may be fierce competitors in some "indications" (say, cancer drugs), but they may be much less so in others (say, ARVs), where a small number of firms may dominate that particular market. In any case, drug companies hold patents over the medications in their portfolios, giving them twenty years to block others from making, using or selling the compound, which usually translates into over a decade of monopoly power in the market (the initial years of patent protection are spent doing research, development and applying for regulatory approval). Industry concentration ratios, therefore, may mask the true power of a given firm in its therapeutic market.

Corporate power, of course, can be mitigated in several different ways, at least in theory. Government regulation, for example, could curb the industry's influence over its given markets (although the "Chicago School" famously claims that regulations are in the industry's interest, providing a costly barrier to entry). Because its products are so essential to health, in industrialized countries the pharmaceutical industry is highly regulated, in part to ensure the health and safety of consumers. As a consequence, companies must comply with a variety of rules that govern research, clinical trials, manufacturing, marketing, and reporting of post-market safety evaluations. Rules regarding the clinical testing and market approval of new drugs are set by agencies like the FDA in the United States and the European Medicines Agency (EMA) in Europe. To be sure, these regulations provide a barrier to entry to firms that would seek to enter the industry, as complying with these rules is extremely costly. Lowering these barriers to entry has been a major objective of advocates seeking to reduce the price of pharmaceuticals; in the United States, for example, the Hatch-Waxman Act of 1984 encouraged entry by generics suppliers, inter alia, by requiring them to show their product is pharmaceutically equivalent and bioequivalent to a patented drug. This allowed the generic manufacturer to rely on pre-existing safety and efficacy data for the drug product filed with the FDA and to gain market approval without having to go through a costly new drug approval process.

According to the Tufts Center for the Study of Drug Development, "less than 20 percent of the compounds that enter clinical testing eventually obtain marketing approval" (Tufts Center for the Study of Drug Development 2010). The reason for this attrition, as a Bayer executive put it, is that "drug development in the United States is time consuming, resource intensive, risky, and heavily regulated" (Stonebraker 2002). Given the stringent regulatory environment, pharmaceutical firms patent their drug candidates and will typically only pursue drug development for those products that are covered by one or more product or process patents. The monopoly-like protection a patent affords encourages firms to make investments in research and clinical development and thus to bring cutting-edge products to market.

As we will see below, the centrality of patents to the modern pharmaceutical business model was challenged by AIDS advocates who sought to lower ARV prices. While the industry believed that patent protection, coupled with "high" prices of drugs, was essential to its business model of creating "blockbuster" molecules, advocates argued that these patents kept some essential drugs out of the hands of patients who needed but could not afford them (Comanor 1986; Berndt 2002). We show how the extension of patent protection to new markets globally actually provided a lever for advocates as they sought to influence industry strategy.

For much of the postwar era, the pharmaceutical industry was a reliable generator of healthy profits based on the regular introduction of new, patented drugs, some of which became "blockbusters." During the 1990s, however, a number of changes began to strike the industry, constituting what some observers have called a "revolution," making its future profitability more uncertain; many of these changes are still playing out as of this writing (Somberg 2006). These changes gave disease or patient advocacy groups additional opportunities or openings to target the industry's practices, especially with regard to its prices.

While analysts continue to debate which among these new forces was the most significant driver of firm behavior, the faltering new product pipeline that faced many companies was undoubtedly a major contributor to industrial change beginning in the 1990s. Given fewer drugs in the pipeline and rising research and development costs, the industry sought to capture both new molecules and economic efficiencies through strategic alliances and M&A activity (US Federal Trade Commission 1999; Danzon and Towse 2003; Kesic 2011). During the decade 1990–2000 alone, for example, some 10,000 alliances among pharmaceutical companies were formed, while major examples of M&A activity included the following:

> 1995 Glaxo – Wellcome→GlaxoWellcome
> 1995 Pharmacia – Upjohn→Pharmacia & Upjohn
> 1995 Hoechst – MarrionMerrell Dow→HMR
> 1995 RPR – Fisons→RPR
> 1995 Ranbaxy – Ohm Laboratories→Ranbaxy
> 1995 BASF – Boots→BASF
> 1997 Ciba – Sandoz→Novartis
> 1997 Roche – Boehringer Mannheim→Roche
> 1998 Pharmacia & Upjohn – Sugen→Pharmacia & Upjohn
> 1998 Johnson & Johnson – Centocor →Johnson & Johnson
> 1999 Astra – Zeneca→AstraZeneca
> 1999 HMR-RPR→Aventis
> 1999 Sanofi – Synthelabo→Sanofi-Synthelabo
> 2000 Pharmacia & Upjohn – Monsanto (Searle)→Pharmacia
> 2000 GlaxoWellcome – SmithKlineBeecham→GlaxoSmithKline
> 2000 Pfizer –Warner Lambert→Pfizer
> 2000 Abbott – BASF Pharma – Knoll→Abbott
> 2000 Ranbaxy – Bayer Basics→Ranbaxy
> 2000 Elan – Dura Pharmaceuticals→Elan   (*Source*: Kesic 2011)

King has hypothesized that industries undergoing profound restructuring, as evidenced by M&A activities, are good candidates for "anti-corporate" movements, since their corporate cultures are changing (often including major shake-ups in management), while the M&A process itself often requires some combination of regulatory and shareholder approval (King 2008). Advocates can bring to the attention of regulators their concerns about the competitive effects of a given merger, while activist shareholders can raise tough questions about the effects of mergers on research and development and on prices in the context of annual meetings. These activists can also question executive pay packages, and executives may find corporate social responsibility programs useful in providing them with some "cover" as they seek higher levels of compensation.

Further, and of particular relevance to our concerns, many of these mergers involved cross-border activity, promoting globalization of the industry; in fact, historian Louis Galambos says that the 1990s witnessed the transformation of the pharmaceutical industry into a "global oligopoly" (Galambos 2001). This globalization process meant that while firms became ever more powerful on the one hand in terms of their assets, profits, and drug portfolios, on the other they had to deal with multiple regulatory bodies, disease burdens, income levels, and health care systems. It also meant that the industry took a heightened interest in the international protection of its property rights and, along with the software and movie industries, by the late 1980s had become one of the major lobbyists for a new international IPR regime (Devereaux, Lawrence, and Watkins 2006). Overall, then, the pharmaceutical industry was witnessing a profound shift from being a stable generator of rents to one that was being upended by such forces as globalization, rapid scientific development and technological change, new entrants, mergers and acquisitions, and new constellation of IP regulations internationally.

Advocacy opportunities to contest pricing and patents

What were the implications of these features of the industry's structure for disease advocates and specifically the AIDS treatment movement? Several points are worth emphasizing. First, given the new fluidity of corporate structures, advocates found openings to influence business policy that had not previously existed. As noted above, mergers and acquisitions required shareholder and regulatory approval, making that process a target for disease advocates who wished to put drug access policies on corporate and public policy agendas (Smith and Quelch 1996; Oxfam 2001; Liu and Lim 2003; King 2008). Indeed, some advocacy organizations, like Oxfam, were also shareholders in companies like GSK, giving them an active "voice" in its shareholder meetings (Oxfam 2001). Further, the legislative and regulatory changes (like the 1984 Hatch-Waxman Act) that were, in part, a response to growing global concentration in the industry, made it easier for generics manufacturers to enter pharmaceutical markets, putting pressure on drug prices in some therapeutic categories. These changes would prove instrumental for the AIDS movement. Industry turmoil provided openings to "new entrants" whether in the form of generics manufacturers, biotechnology companies, or even disease advocates, potentially increasing market contestability and decreasing the industry's pricing power.

Second, with the globalization of the industry, the 1990s saw the widespread introduction of "differential pricing" by the pharmaceutical industry for different classes of consumers; this differential pricing regime would also prove of critical importance for AIDS treatment advocates, and it will be a central focus of Chapter 5 (see US Federal Trade Commission 1999). The introduction of differential pricing models of drugs indicated to economists and to disease advocates that pharmaceutical companies were able and willing to subsidize some consumers at the expense of others. That ability to discriminate across consumers also demonstrated the industry's monopoly power in at least some market segments, since otherwise it would not be able to enforce such price differentiation across customers. This differential price structure would provide a crucial insight for global AIDS treatment advocates who wanted industrialized world consumers to subsidize ARV uptake by people with HIV in the developing world. As we will see in Chapter 5 on advocacy strategy, globalizing the differential pricing regime also had some unique challenges.

Third, as the pharmaceutical industry globalized during the 1980s and 1990s, it began to press developing country governments to adopt pharmaceutical patents. Those discussions between pharmaceutical firms (among those in other sectors) and governments led to the harmonization of IPR under the 1995 TRIPS Agreement regime under the WTO. AIDS advocates would make full use of the debate over TRIPS to press their arguments, pitting corporate patents and profits against human lives. In fact, a central pillar of the AIDS advocacy movement was its questioning of the extension of the WTO's trade disciplines to public health, and it made the argument that it was patents, above all else, that kept drug prices high. Given the centrality of this causal connection (patents lead to high prices which in turn erode global health) to the AIDS movement, we further elaborate the role of the advocacy movement in making those causal connections in the following section.

Unpacking market concentration: pharmaceutical pricing and the ARV market

Thus far we have examined the pharmaceutical industry in general, identifying certain structural characteristics of the industry and sectoral changes that gave potential openings to the AIDS movement to engage in market contestation. Beyond these broad structural characteristics, however, the specific market for ARVs had some additional aspects that deserve more detailed discussion if we are to understand the leverage points the AIDS advocates could exploit. In this section we examine the development and evolution of AIDS drugs and the emerging debate over greater access to them. The approval of the Burroughs Wellcome drug AZT in 1987 demonstrated that the AIDS virus could be attacked by the right medications. But the efficacy of AZT proved quite limited for most PWAs; some people quickly became resistant to it and, after a period of quietude, the disease would re-start its deadly progression. Nonetheless, AZT had shown that it was possible to produce AIDS-fighting drugs.

Still, several factors inhibited PWAs from getting "drugs into bodies," to use the phrase of AIDS activists at the time (Smith and Siplon 2006). First, when AZT was introduced, its price was exceedingly high – over $10,000 per patient per year. As *The New York Times* editorialized: "[T]here's a massive obstacle to wider use of this life-saving drug – its extraordinary cost ... AZT is said to be the most expensive prescription drug in history" (*The New York Times* 1989). The drug monopolized the AIDS market, and its manufacturer, Burroughs Wellcome, defended the high price by stating that it anticipated only 40,000 people per year would use it, making it a niche product, or one characterized by "high price, low volume." But AIDS activists, along with sympathetic media organs like *The Times*, retorted that the high price was also due to the patent that Burroughs held.

Indeed, soon after its introduction at $10,000, AIDS activists targeted the company with public protests at the New York Stock Exchange and at its North Carolina headquarters demanding that the price be lowered. They threatened the company with lawsuits over its patent rights and involved a wide range of sympathetic stakeholders in this fight, from members of Congress to scientists working at the US National Institutes of Health (NIH). The validity of the patent was challenged on the grounds that much of the underlying research had been conducted in government laboratories supported by NIH (Angell 2004, 24–7). They also targeted insurance schemes – both public and private – to lobby for the reimbursement of ARV treatment (Arno and Feiden 1992; Smith and Siplon 2006). By 1989, Burroughs had lowered the price to $8,000 per patient per year.

Nonetheless, the pharmaceutical companies were naturally reluctant to set or reduce their prices under political pressure. They claimed that drug prices reflected the high costs of research and development (R&D) and that these prices would be quickly driven down by competition from substitutes and generics. While most pharmas voluntarily offered some "access" programs to low-income patients, they believed that the financing of pharmaceutical purchases was generally a matter for other social agents, mainly public and private insurance schemes, to solve (Arno and Feiden 1992 remains the best account of the development of and debate surrounding AZT).

The AZT controversy mirrored long-standing public debates about the pricing of pharmaceuticals. Since at least the time of the Kefauver Committee investigations in the US Senate in the late 1950s, drug pricing has often arisen as a political issue in the United States and around the world (Comanor 1986). Critics have charged that big pharma used its "monopoly power" to extract substantial rents from consumers with inelastic demand for life-saving drugs, while "the industry replied that, on the contrary, prices were low relative to the value afforded customers" (Comanor 1986, 1178; Philipson and Jena 2005). Further, the industry has long argued that its business model demanded "high returns on successful products" in order to "balance the large number of unsuccessful ones" (Comanor 1986, 1178). Huge investments went into the R&D that generated the outputs of the drug industry, and only a small share of these investments ever paid dividends. Nonetheless, the drug industry in the United States has long lived under the "threat" of price regulation, while that, of course, has become a reality in many, if not most industrialized countries (Berndt 2002; Ellison and Wolfram 2006; OECD 2008).

The setting of pharmaceutical prices reflects a fairly straightforward economic problem. As the Organisation for Economic Cooperation and Development (OECD) puts it:

[M]aximizing profits translates into maximizing cash flows during the life of a product. In each market where sales would be expected to enhance a product's global profitability, pharmaceutical firms endeavor to launch products quickly at the price that maximizes prospective profits. Firms try to extend the period of market exclusivity and to engage in promotional activities that aim both to capture as large a market share as possible and to increase the potential market. By some estimates, pharmaceutical marketing expenditures account for a share of firms' outlays that exceeds that of R&D expenditures. (OECD 2008, 12)

Yet another way to look at the price of a pharmaceutical product is in terms of consumer vs. producer surplus (Philipson and Jena 2005). While the price of a given drug may seem to be "high," in fact it may be lower than a consumer's willingness to pay, an amount that reflects consumer surplus. Conversely, the price charged may be higher than the costs incurred, leading to producer surplus. Producer surplus, of course, provides the inducement for innovation, and prices that capture consumer surplus while reducing producer surplus may have inter-temporal effects that reduce future flows of new drugs.

Even in the case of a new drug, the market power of the firm is hardly unlimited. From an economic perspective, those bounds are set by a number of factors, including consumers' perceptions of the efficacy of the drug, the willingness to pay for it at a given price, along with the existence of competition from substitutes – either other drugs or therap-ies with similar treatment effects or, over time, from generics. Further, the threat of government regulation (e.g. through compulsory licensing) may, in and of itself, place an upper-bound on the prices charged (Ellison and Wolfram 2006).

Empirical studies of drug prices have, unsurprisingly, provided fodder for both proponents and opponents of more regulation of the allegedly monopolistic behavior of pharmaceutical firms. While drug prices overall have risen since the 1960s (as compared to the rate of inflation), Danzon emphasizes that, when quality improvements are introduced, then "hedonic prices" may in fact have fallen over time. Generally, the price of most individual drugs seems to fall over time as competition is intro-duced and the firm tries to maintain market share. Branded products, however, rarely fall to the price of generic substitutes; instead, brands try to maintain a higher price on the basis of consumer (or physician) loyalty to a particular mark (Danzon 1996).

The global pricing strategies of pharmaceutical firms have similarly challenged economists seeking to perform empirical research. While pharma prices differ considerably even among the industrialized coun-tries, it is difficult to understand the extent to which this is due to a profit-maximizing differential (or what is also called "Ramsey") pricing strategy on the part of the firms, or to the differing regulatory and tax structures and distribution networks that drugs confront when they cross borders (OECD 2008). A global profit-maximizing strategy would rely on the ability of drug firms to identify differing elasticities of demand for pharmaceutical products around the world, charging high prices to con-sumers with a high willingness to pay and reducing prices accordingly. As we will see in a later chapter, AIDS advocates would identify this profit-maximizing strategy as a point where they could essentially find common ground with the industry.

In the mid 1990s, when new, "second-generation" medications were introduced at seemingly high prices of more than $10,000, the price of AIDS drugs would again become a prominent issue. By 1996, scientists demonstrated that a combination of drugs, used as a "cocktail" or "triple therapy," could significantly hold HIV at bay. Indeed, these scientists began to claim that, with the introduction of new drugs used in new

Table 2.1: *Types and examples of ARV drugs*

Nucleoside Reverse Transcriptase Inhibitors (NRTIs)	Non-nucleoside Reverse Transcriptase Inhibitors (NNRTIs)	Protease Inhibitors (PIs)
Abacavir (Ziagen, ABC) Didanosine (Videx, dideoxyinosine, ddI) Emtricitabine (Emtriva, FTC) Lamivudine (Epivir, 3TC) Stavudine (Zerit, d4T) Tenofovir (Viread, TDF) Zalcitabine (Hivid, ddC) Zidovudine (Retrovir, ZDV or AZT)	Delvaridine (Rescriptor, DLV) Efravirenz (Sustiva, EFV) Nevirapine (Viramune, NVP)	Amprenavir (Agenerase, APV) Atazanavir (Reyataz, ATV) Fosamprenavir (Lexiva, FOS) Indinavir (Crixivan, IDV) Lopinavir (Kaletra, LPV/r) Ritonavir (Norvir, RIT) Saquinavir (Fortovase, Invirase, SQV)

Note: Drugs are listed by their brand name with other brand names/generic names and chemical compound names in parentheses.
Source: University of California San Francisco 2011.

ways, AIDS could be effectively transformed into a chronic condition for many PWAs. A report on these new ARV cocktails was the highlight of the 1996 International Aids Conference in Vancouver, and introduced the concept of "highly active antiretroviral therapy" (HAART). Soon, this became the regimen of choice throughout the industrialized world, even though it was a complicated protocol from a medical perspective. That complex protocol would, for some time, be held out as a reason why ARV therapy could not be extended to developing countries.

Doctors usually recommended an HAART cocktail of three or more different drugs, including both Nucleoside Reverse Transcriptase Inhibitors (NRTIs), which can block the virus from duplicating and therefore slow the spread of the disease (including AZT), and Non-Nucleoside Reverse Transcriptase Inhibitors (NNRTIs), which block the infection of new cells with HIV. The cocktail may also include protease inhibitors (PIs), which tend to be more expensive and stop reproduction of the HIV virus at a later stage in its life cycle. In the early naughts a fourth class of drugs entered the market – so-called fusion inhibitors – but they are less commonly used in developing countries (University of California San Francisco 2011). (See Table 2.1 for a list of AIDS drugs approved by the FDA by drug class.)

A number of different firms produced these drugs, including GSK, Gilead, BMS, and Pfizer. Interestingly, different companies tended to have a strong market share in different drug classes that made up the ARV cocktail. Thus, GSK held about 50 percent of the market for NRTIs (Griffin Securities 2005) sharing the market with Gilead, while BMS dominated the NNRTI part of the market; for its part, Pfizer's strength was in PIs. Overall, the market for these drugs was about $6 billion in 2003, making them a small share of the nearly $300 billion industry.

The industry's provision of ARVs was also split between these costly HAART cocktails that predominated in the industrialized world and the generic copies of "first line" drugs like AZT that continued to dominate developing world treatment regimens and that were purchased by donors like the United States through its "PEPFAR" program. These generics were largely produced by Indian companies like Cipla and Ranbaxy. The extension of HAART to the developing world would become a major "ask" of the advocacy community (but for a skeptical view of the long-run prospects of rolling out cutting-edge ARVs to the developing world, see Shadlen 2007).

The primary goal of ARV therapy for an HIV infection is the suppression of viral replication while limiting drug toxicity which can result in painful or even life-threatening side effects. Patients were generally selected for ARV therapy on the basis of their T-cell count (a proxy for the health of the immune system) and/or their "viral load," or the extent to which the HIV virus had replicated. The viral load was determined through expensive laboratory tests, and in the late 1990s patients whose viral loads were too high were deemed beyond the point at which ARVs would prove effective in holding the virus at bay. This view would change in 2001 when the *New England Journal of Medicine* reported that ARVs could increase the lifespan of patients, even those who were at an advanced stage of the disease (see Steinbrook and Drazen 2001). Further, the selection of the HAART cocktail by the prescribing doctor had to take into account the patient's prior history of ARV use, the side-effects of these agents, and drug–drug interactions that occurred between ARVs and other medications the PWA might be taking (Maenza and Flexner 1998; Institute of Medicine 2005). Overall, ARV protocols were complex and demanded significant doctor–patient interactions, along with considerable discipline on the part of patients who had to take their medications in precise doses and at specific times if treatment were to prove effective (Maenza and Flexner 1998; Institute of Medicine 2005). These ARVs, as already noted, were also exceedingly expensive. According to the *New England Journal of Medicine*, "Combination antiretroviral therapy typically cost $10,000 to $15,000 a year; this is a major barrier to increasing its availability" even in the United States (Steinbrook and Drazen 2001).

If ARVs were a complex and costly medication for the American medical system to handle, the situation was obviously much worse when it came to developing countries, and many, if not most, experts had little confidence that ARVs could be effectively deployed, for reasons not only of cost, but because of the severely limited medical infrastructure needed for AIDS diagnosis and testing. So long as "big pharma" and the broader global health community felt that introducing HAART into the developing world would be ineffective, then reduced prices alone would provide an insufficient foundation for a global access to treatment regime.

Understanding fluid rules: drug access and the TRIPS regime

What was the role of global pharmaceutical firms in promoting public health in the developing world? How could their products be made affordable for poor populations? In 1975, the World Health Organization (WHO) became deeply involved in these debates when it made "national drug policies" and "essential medicines" a "top priority for developing countries." According to the WHO, essential drugs were "those considered to be of the utmost importance and hence basic, indispensable, and necessary for the health needs of the population. They should be available at all times, in the proper dosage forms, to all segments of society" (cited in Reich 1987, 40). In 1998 the WHO Director-General, Gro Harlem Brundtland, made the argument for essential drugs even more strongly when she said essential medicines were "simply part of the *fundamental right to health care*" (Brundtland 1998, emphasis added).

The WHO was, for many years, ambiguous on the question of how these drugs would be provided, allocated, and purchased, and at what price. The Model List of Essential Medicines (EML) was first published in 1977 by the WHO and has been updated every two years. The EML is a guide for countries and organizations; it now identifies more than 300 safe, efficacious and cost-effective treatments for the majority of communicable and non-communicable diseases (WHO 2012a). While the model lists are primarily used by countries and organizations to set priorities for drug expenditures, over time, access to essential medicines, within and across countries, has become a measure of health equity.

In 1999, the year it won the Nobel Peace Prize, the non-governmental organization (NGO) MSF launched its Access Campaign, with a focus on increasing affordability of existing drugs and the availability of new drugs through an R&D agenda for diseases of the developing world. Dr. James Orbinski explained MSF's goals in the Nobel Prize address:

Some of the reasons that people die from diseases like AIDS, TB, Sleeping Sickness and other tropical diseases is that life saving essential medicines are either too expensive, are not available because they are not seen as financially viable, or because there is virtually no new research and development for priority tropical diseases. This market failure is our next challenge. The challenge however, is not ours alone. It is also for governments, International Government Institutions, the Pharmaceutical Industry and other NGOs to confront this injustice. What we as a civil society movement demand is change, not charity. (Orbinski 1999)

To the pharmaceutical industry, the idea of "access" to medicines was threatening because it suggested that the firms, as opposed to governments, had a major responsibility for making essential drugs universally available; it also signaled the growing role of the WHO in shaping global health policy, a concern that became more palpable after 1981 when the organization passed an "International Code of Marketing Breast-Milk Substitutes" in response to consumer outrage over Nestlé's aggressive sales of powdered milk in Africa (indeed, the Nestlé controversy also demonstrated the growing role of "civil society" in shaping international health agendas and debates) (Sikkink 1986; Reich 1987). As the WHO's Brundtland said in 1998, "Medicines are still unavailable or unaffordable for too many people – especially the poor and those most in need. Our aim must be to ensure equity of access to essential drugs" (Brundtland 1998). The lingering question was, "who was responsible for the lack of access?"

The answer was not self-evident. In an early case study of one "essential medicine," praziquantel (used in the treatment of the parasitic disease schistosomiasis), Harvard's Michael Reich and Ramesh Govindaraj of the World Bank found a myriad of reasons why the drug, despite its tremendous efficacy, was poorly distributed in a number of countries they surveyed, including in such West African countries as Nigeria and Ghana (Reich and Govindaraj 1998). They found that, initially, the high price of the patented drug was a major barrier to its international diffusion following its discovery during the late 1970s, but with the development of a cheaper manufacturing process by a South Korean manufacturer in the early 1980s, the molecule became much less expensive and more widely diffused.[2] Still, it failed to penetrate many

---

[2] It is notable that, prior to the introduction of the TRIPS Accord of the WTO, many countries found ways of circumventing product patents by developing new manufacturing processes and techniques; with TRIPS, both processes and products gained protection; more on this in the following section.

developing world markets despite its designation as an essential medicine. What explains this failure? Reich and Govindaraj found that:

The high price of praziquantel in the 1980s represented a major obstacle to its availability ... but it was not the only obstacle. Other factors included: low priority given to schistosomiasis control in some countries; organizational problems within schistosomiasis control programs; poorly functioning pharmaceutical distribution systems; and economic stagnation and political instability in many poor countries ... Our analysis suggests that an affordable price was a necessary, but not sufficient, condition to improve praziquantel's availability in poor countries. (1998, 10)

In another study, Attaran explored whether patents in fact impeded access in developing countries to the 2003 WHO EML (Attaran 2004). At the time, only 17 of the 319 items on the EML could have been covered by patents in developing countries; most products were either too old or the relevant countries did not yet grant pharmaceutical patents. Most of those patent-protected products were, indeed, AIDS drug-related, but Attaran further found that pharmaceutical firms actually forwent patent protection on those products in many developing countries. Therefore, patents could only be a factor impeding access to medicines for 1.4 percent of the essential medicines in the developing countries.

This debate about how to ensure universal access would be especially acrimonious in relation to AIDS treatment: was the lack of access to AIDS drugs in the developing world due to high prices, as the advocates asserted, or because of inadequate health institutions in those countries, as big pharma claimed? During the early 1990s, this question about "who was responsible" for the delivery of essential medicines emerged in sharp relief as ARV treatment came on-line. But unlike praziquantel, the dispute over diffusion of AIDS drugs was not limited to the small number of technical experts and philanthropists who followed tropical medicine at that time. Instead, the price of AIDS drugs would erupt onto the international agenda as a major political issue. It would do so within the context of an international trade negotiation that seemed far removed from the domain of global public health, but it was a negotiation that would come crashing into that seemingly alien sphere: namely, the ongoing talks over property rights being conducted within the context of the nascent WTO. These negotiations would bring into sharp relief, at least for many activists, the party responsible for high drug prices and, in turn, for the failure of essential medicines to reach the world's poorest populations: it was the pharmaceutical industry.

The conflict over the 1995 TRIPS Agreement of the WTO, which greatly extended the scope of patent protection across the developing world, was of tremendous political significance to the AIDS movement.

From its inception, TRIPS became the focal point of debate over whether the rights of companies should trump public health. The wording of the TRIPS Agreement would engender a lawsuit with South Africa in the late 1990s that cast pharmaceutical firms in a villainous light, even in the pages of business-friendly newspapers like *The Wall Street Journal*. More generally, the TRIPS controversy placed into sharp relief the question over whether "essential medicines" should be private goods or merit goods.

In the introduction to this chapter, we argued that one key variable in determining whether advocates can transform market structures is the fluidity of the rules which govern that market. Taking an institutionalist perspective, we claimed that markets depend on rules for their stable operation, but we further noted that these rules are generally written by the market's most powerful actors, such as the dominant or incumbent firms. A complicated set of government procurement rules, for example, may favor existing suppliers because the costs of meeting public agency regulations are simply too high for most new entrants, especially if they are small and medium-sized enterprises (SMEs). In the pharmaceutical arena, the FDA rules governing market access that require clinical trials for any new molecular entity or biologic make it exceedingly expensive for new drugs to enter the marketplace. Rules, in short, can provide a strong barrier to market contestability.

Of all the rules governing the pharmaceutical sector, perhaps none are as important as those relating to patents. At the very heart of the pharma business model is the promise of the twenty-year patent term, which grants a monopoly right to exclude others from making, using or selling the patented product (or process) during that period. Patents covering new drugs have become the main mechanism by which firms recoup investments necessary for drug development. We have already noted that this is an exceedingly expensive undertaking, and it is one that usually fails. Safe and effective treatments are hard to come by, and the economic motivation for trying to find them is the patent right.

For much of recent history, however, governments took very different attitudes towards the patenting of chemical and pharmaceutical products around the world. With the notable exception of the United States and United Kingdom (UK), most industrialized countries only introduced product patents for pharmaceuticals in the second half of the twentieth century, although those same countries often allowed patents on the process by which that pharmaceutical was created (Lanjouw 2003). France and Germany first allowed product patents for pharmaceuticals in the 1960s; in Japan no product patents for any type of invention were allowed until 1976; similarly, Italy, Sweden, and Switzerland extended product patents to pharmaceuticals in the late 1970s; Canada and Holland in the 1980s; while Spain, Greece, Norway, Portugal, and all Eastern Europe European Community (EC) accession countries in the 1990s. In the developing world, patents for pharmaceuticals were non-existent in many developing nations into the 2000s, even in some countries which actively sought to build the capability to develop generics or "copycat" drugs (most notably India). Clearly, as the pharmaceutical industry globalized, that patchwork of national patent rules could no longer stand.

When the idea of a global accord for property rights within the Global Agreement on Tariffs and Trade was first broached by the United States in the late 1980s – at the insistence of a coalition of firms representing the high-technology, media, and pharmaceutical industries – it was unclear whether IP would even get on the new Uruguay Round trade agenda, and if so, which technologies would be included (Lanjouw 2003). There were major, long-standing differences between "North" and "South" over the objectives of any international agreement on IP. But even among the United States, the European countries, and Japan, the structure of such an accord was initially unclear because each region had different approaches to patent policy. For example, patent term lengths varied, as did when patents were published or how they could be challenged. Equally important was what constituted patentable subject matter. Countries differed on whether patent protection extended to software, business methods, therapeutic and surgical methods, higher organisms, and what other exclusions might be allowed for reasons of public order or morality. Resolving these difficulties, even in the context of negotiations as protracted as those associated with international trade agreements, seemed unlikely to many who were active in planning and executing the Uruguay trade round that eventually created the WTO in 1994.

The TRIPS Agreement was a watershed moment for the international IPR regime. As one of the WTO's founding agreements, IP became formally linked to the multilateral trading system. All signatories to the WTO agreed to implement minimum standards for the protection of IPR. For patents, that included a twenty-year patent term and the requirement that "patents shall be available for *any* inventions, whether products or processes, *in all fields of technology*" (emphasis added). As Stanford law professor John Barton has written of TRIPS Article 27, "The clear intent was to prohibit exclusions of drug products such as those contained in the Indian law" (Barton 2004). Furthermore, TRIPS included a strong emphasis on enforcement of IP rights in Article 41 and cross-border protections. Furthermore, a mechanism for settling bilateral IP disputes was created with Article 64. All these elements of TRIPS made it a historic agreement that set an unprecedented high bar for the harmonization of IP regimes internationally. Advanced industrialized countries committed themselves to enforce the TRIPS Agreement as of 1995. Developing countries were given a five-year transition period, until 2000, and five additional years if they did not already provide patents for pharmaceuticals. The least developed countries (LDCs) were given a transition period that initially was to end in 2006 but, at the 2001 Doha meeting described below, was later pushed back to 2016.

TRIPS did leave a number of clauses worded in ways that left latitude for interpretation by countries, known as the "TRIPS flexibilities." First, while some countries, like the United States, prohibit parallel imports of medications (i.e. the import of products from abroad without the authorization of the domestic patent holder), in Article 6 TRIPS specifically does not address the issue of the exhaustion of IPR, recognizing these differing national doctrines. Second, Article 30 of TRIPS does allow countries to "provide limited exceptions to the exclusive rights conferred by a patent," which typically include the legal use of patented innovations for research, early working for regulatory reviews or private non-commercial uses (WTO undated).[3] Third, Article 31 states that countries may have laws for the compulsory licensing of patented products, which means that (with conditions) governments have the authority to license a patent to a third party without the consent of the patent owner (Thomas 2001). While, in general, there must first be an attempt to obtain a license from the patent holder, under certain circumstances, for example to meet national emergencies, that condition is waived. Thus, TRIPS left ambiguous a number of questions. For example, what counted as a national emergency? What did it mean that the compulsory license was to be "predominantly for the supply of the domestic market"? What happens if a country cannot grant a compulsory license to a domestic firm to respond to a national emergency?

Given the uncertainty over how these TRIPS flexibilities would in fact be interpreted, it was only a matter of time before they would be tested by member governments of the newly created WTO. The most prominent early tests occurred over the use of compulsory licenses for access to ARV medications, first by the South African and later by the Brazilian government. The South African government in 1997 proposed an amendment to its laws that would "allow the South African Health

---

[3] Primarily, these exceptions should not "unreasonably conflict with a normal exploitation of the patent" or "unreasonably prejudice the legitimate interests of the patent owner." See Article 30 of the TRIPS Agreement.

Minister to override patent rights to allow compulsory licensing and parallel importing" (Ford 2000). The South African law was challenged in court when the government was sued by a group of 39 pharmaceutical companies; and at the behest of the pharmaceutical industry, Washington placed South Africa on the United States Trade Representative (USTR) "Special 301 Watchlist" threatening sanctions. The dispute was closely watched internationally and did not reflect well on the pharmaceutical industry or the United States. In 2001 the case was dropped, and Washington and Pretoria came to a bilateral resolution.

Similarly, Brazil allows the issuance of compulsory licenses for national emergencies and situations of public interest. It began recognizing pharmaceutical patents in 1996, but also enacted legislation to restrict patentability and limit patent rights. It also linked its IP policies to health policy. Brazil has generous health policies which, starting in the late 1990s "guaranteed every AIDS patient state of the art treatment" in addition to the pre-existing obligation to provide free medicines (Rosenberg 2001). Since Brazil did not issue patents to medicines whose priority date internationally preceded 1996, it was able to begin producing domestic generic copies of brand name ARV drugs as soon as their effectiveness was documented (Shadlen 2009; for further discussion of these issues, see Shadlen *et al.* 2012). The United States challenged Brazil's laws under the Dispute Resolution Understanding of the WTO in 2001, in particular its compulsory licensing laws, but this case was also dropped.

In both the South Africa and Brazil cases the interests of developing countries were pitted against those of big pharma, and in each case public sympathy worldwide was decisively on the side of the "South." Advocates took full advantage of these cases, even serving as advisers, particularly to South Africa. Ultimately, the disputes would play a major role in shaping subsequent pharmaceutical sector actions and policies with respect to ARV access, as we will see in greater detail in Chapter 5 on advocacy strategy.

Advocates received a major fillip for their cause of delinking patents from public health from an unlikely source, the US government. Following the terrorist attacks of 11 September 2001, American officials became concerned by the possibility of a major anthrax attack, spurred by the finding that anthrax spores were being sent through the mail, where they had caused some highly publicized deaths. The only antibiotic for treating anthrax, Cipro, was produced by Bayer, which held the patent rights to that medication. As fears of an anthrax attack grew, "Human and Health Services Secretary Tommy Thompson threatened to override Bayer's patent unless . . . the company lowered the price of the drug. Bayer assented to a price of 95 cents a pill ... and no action was taken" (Devereaux, Lawrence, and Watkins 2006, 20).

AIDS advocates seized on the Thompson threat. In reference to his country's efforts to lower the price of ARVs, an adviser to Brazil's health minister said, "Thompson ... became our ally. He did what he thought was in the best interest of his country. Why can't others do the same?" *The Financial Times* editorialized that the Cipro incident "seriously weakened the industry's bargaining position" when it came to protecting patent rights in the face of health emergencies (cited in ibid., 21).

The tussle between industry and advocates over patents led in 2001 to an agreed interpretation of TRIPS, officially called the "WTO Declaration on the TRIPS Agreement and Public Health," but widely referred to as the Doha Declaration. This revision stated that "the TRIPS agreement does not and should not prevent Members from taking measures to protect public health." Explicitly, it granted each WTO member the right "to grant compulsory licenses," "to determine the grounds upon which such licenses are granted," and "to determine what constitutes a national emergency." It recognized that public health crises could constitute circumstances of extreme urgency (WTO 2001).

However, the Doha Declaration said nothing about parallel imports, or the import of generics to meet public health crises. Along these lines, all it could say was that "We recognize that WTO members with insufficient or no manufacturing capacities in the pharmaceutical sector could face difficulties in making effective use of compulsory licensing under the TRIPS Agreement." Thus, in many respects the Doha Declaration failed to resolve some of the fundamental tensions between patents and public health, and these would continue to play out in the AIDS arena, forcing advocates to look beyond the branded pharmaceutical companies to generics manufacturers as they sought lower prices for precious ARV.

Conclusions

This chapter has addressed some of the salient structural characteristics of the pharmaceutical industry and the market for ARVs. As we have seen, despite seemingly unpromising background conditions, the industry in fact presented advocates with points of leverage or openings that they could exploit, ultimately making the market more contestable. In IP regime were major targets for advocacy attack. To the extent that patents could be associated with high drug prices, and high prices with the inability of poor populations to acquire these medications, the pharmaceutical industry could be shown to favor profits over people.

The industry countered that it needed patents and high prices on its "winning" drugs to compensate for the high cost of pharmaceutical R&D, which most often led to a dead end. That incentive system, it argued, had motivated some of the greatest medical breakthroughs of the postwar era, including the introduction of ARV medications, only six years after the HIV virus was first identified. Stressing or breaking that model, the industry warned, could have severe consequences for the future of drug development and, in turn, global health.

In essence, the industry and the advocates would converge on the relationship between patents and prices as being the central issue in their conflict over how to extend access to ARV treatment, and this issue came to a head with the emergence of the TRIPS regime. Advocates were quick to recognize and seize upon the fluid nature of TRIPS rules that would play an increasing role in shaping the industry's incentive system, especially as it globalized and sought to develop new markets. Structural analysis reveals how a global industry requires some global rules, but given the weakness of international regulations, it also permits advocates a space to exercise their moral authority and to contest a given market structure. In the next chapter, we explore how advocates used their moral authority in framing the debate over drug access.

3   Drugs = life: framing access to AIDS drugs

> People With Aids Are Dying Because of Lack of Access to Life-Saving
> Drugs
> 1999 MSF Press Release
>
> MSF Calls on Davos Leaders to Stop People Dying of Market Failure
> 2000 MSF Press Release

Why do some appeals by advocates generate strong public support while other equally deserving issues fail to motivate a similar response? In a sense, this question animates our entire book. As we argued in the introductory chapter, advocates in support of market transformations need to identify and publicize a compelling frame. This statement begs the question of what counts as "compelling" and why it is important. In this chapter, building on the groundbreaking work of Margaret Keck and Kathryn Sikkink, we develop an empirically-informed account of what constitutes a compelling moral frame and why such a frame is a necessary but not sufficient factor in advocacy success.

We address these issues in reverse, starting with a short exposition of framing and why it is important. The second section explores what constitutes a "compelling" frame. The third section discusses what frames advocates and opponents used as they made the case for and against universal access to AIDS treatment. The final section draws on surveys that we conducted and which provide some empirical support for our view.

In brief, extending Keck and Sikkink's argument about the compelling nature of "bodily harm" as a universal frame, we argue that campaigns that promote access to goods necessary for life (like ARVs) are more likely to resonate internationally than goods that are less essential to survival. Thus, goods that extend or improve people's lives will receive some but perhaps not as much support as life-saving goods. We provide plausible support for this view from survey results that tested this proposition and others experimentally. The upshot of this evidence is that while HIV/AIDS advocates successfully generated cross-country resonance, the situation is hardly unique. Indeed, a host of other access campaigns for water, food, and other life-saving drugs like anti-cancer medications all have the potential to generate cross-national concern because they are necessary for life. As the rest of this book suggests, however, a successful frame alone will not generate movement effectiveness; still, campaigns for universal access that can generate cross-national appeal with a compelling frame, especially when combined with a feasible strategy (as we discuss in Chapter 5), are more likely to succeed in their objectives.

Framing: why is it important?

Frames and framing have become common subjects of inquiry in the academic world in many areas of study, including but not limited to the social movement literature in sociology. That literature has also inspired much of the scholarship in contemporary international relations theory. For scholars of social movements, frames are interpretive meanings that people ascribe to an issue, connecting cause and effect and linking possible solutions to that causal chain.[1] Frames are rhetorical messages that describe what kind of problem is being faced, and they can invoke different and sometimes multiple dimensions such as national security, morality, religion, law, efficiency, and human rights, in the effort to capture public attention. Frames help establish why the problem occurred, connecting facts in ways that also help us determine who the responsible parties are for addressing the issue.

The decision to frame HIV/AIDS treatment as an issue of justice and fairness was a conscious choice by advocates. It was simply unfair that developing world PWAs did not have access to the very same drugs that were available to people in industrialized nations and that were keeping them alive there. Creating a causal connection between the poor's lack of access to drug company pricing policies was another framing device. Asking drug companies to reduce their prices and allow generic competitors to enter the market was a third. Together, these elements shaped how the problem was viewed by the public (as one of fairness), who was responsible (drug companies), and what needed to be done (lower prices). As an alternative, one could imagine that the problem might

---

[1] The framing literature is extensive and has been more comprehensively discussed by one of us in previous work (see Busby 2010a, Ch. 2). Framing in the international relations literature is imported from the social movement literature in sociology pioneered by Mayer Zald, David Snow, Sidney Tarrow, and others. Snow defines framing as "the conscious strategic efforts by groups of people to fashion shared understandings of the world and of themselves that legitimate and motivate collective action" (McAdam, McCarthy, and Zald 1996, 6).

have been framed as one of discrimination (e.g. against Africans with AIDS), and that this was a modern manifestation of a neo-colonial heritage; thus the policy response that might have flowed from this frame was that industrialized countries were responsible (due to their colonial past and its contemporary vestiges) and they should simply buy ARVs from drug companies (which, in this case, would *not* have been conceptualized as the "guilty" party) and distribute them for free.

Some scholars look at framing in a different way, focusing on framing as a product of cognition on the part of the recipient rather than the sender. As Druckman notes, scholars of public opinion and political psychology focus on the interplay between the sender and the recipient to examine frame effects or how subtle shifts in the description of a problem may trigger different cognitive processes (framing choices as potential losses or gains, for example, can trigger radically different reactions in recipients, such as the choice between taking a 50 percent chance of winning $1 or receiving 50 cents immediately) (Druckman 2001).

Whereas scholars of social movements look to historical cases to see how different campaigns framed their arguments and seek to assess the relative efficacy of frames through comparative case study, a number of scholars of public opinion use survey evidence and experiments to assess how publics respond to individual frames. Our unique contribution bridges these two approaches, first by assessing the landscape of effective historical frames before providing survey evidence we collected on the micro-foundations of persuasive messages.

Why is a compelling frame important? In brief, advocates need to build public and elite support for their aims. A compelling frame, however defined, can help enlist the public to support the campaign's goals. For some, the frame will induce them to want to volunteer their time or money to support the campaign, to write letters, to buy or boycott certain products, etc. At the very least, a compelling message can generate a reservoir of public support signaling to elites that they too can side with activists without necessarily incurring political costs, or at least knowing that they will have the backing of some proportion of the public if the issue becomes contentious.

While advocates may seize on different dimensions of a problem for different audiences, they often have a dominant frame that receives the majority of their words in their messaging in press releases, public statements, website presence, etc. Frames have an important political function; successfully deployed, they can make it difficult for political opponents to have the rhetorical resources to respond by delegitimating certain policy positions (Krebs and Jackson 2007). Frames help fix meanings by focusing on a particular evaluative dimension and elevating its importance over other valued goals, such as prioritizing access to essential medicines over IPR. To use another example, calling an "inheritance tax" a "death tax" can help focus attention on the apparent injustice of taxing the dead rather than the broader goal of preventing an inherited aristocracy from forming.

Where frames and meanings are contested, what determines which frame dominates the public's imagination or "wins" is something the literature has struggled to answer and which forms a central question in this book (for one approach, see Chong and Druckman 2007). That issue is even more problematic in the international context, where a frame that resonates with one group may not do so with another (of course, that can be a problem *within* a given society as well). In the following section, we draw on Keck and Sikkink's work to address the issue of what makes a frame compelling. However, we reiterate our view that even powerful frames are unlikely on their own to make an advocacy campaign successful.

What frames are compelling?

In their foundational international relations work on transnational advocacy campaigns, Keck and Sikkink argue that activists need to think about the prospective universal resonance of their messages: "Norm entrepreneurs must speak to aspects of belief systems or life worlds that transcend a specific cultural or political context." They identify two characteristics that seem to have had the most historic effectiveness in mobilizing support: "(1) issues involving bodily harm to vulnerable individuals, especially when there is a short and clear causal chain (or story) assigning responsibility; and (2) issues involving legal equality of opportunity" (Keck and Sikkink 1998, 27).

In terms of the first "normative logic" based on bodily harm, Keck and Sikkink suggest campaigns against bodily harm have some universal appeal because they "avoid both the indifference resulting from cultural relativism and the arrogance of cultural imperialism" (ibid., 195). They assert that "[a]lthough issues of bodily harm resonate with the ideological traditions in Western liberal countries like the United States and Western Europe, they also resonate with basic ideas of human dignity common to most cultures" (ibid., 204–5). From this perspective, anti-slavery and women's suffrage campaigns had greater resonance than temperance movements (Finnemore and Sikkink 1998, 907). They elaborate by suggesting that "protecting the most vulnerable parts of the population – especially infants and children" also has transcultural appeal. They suggest that campaigns for infants like the Nestlé boycott over baby milk formula were more successful than anti-tobacco campaigns perhaps for this reason (Keck and Sikkink 1998, 205).

Moreover, the length of the causal chain for who bears responsibility for bodily harm is also important: "But the causal chain needs to be sufficiently short and clear to make the case convincing. The responsibility of a torturer who places an electric prod to a prisoner's genitals is quite clear" (ibid., 27). For this reason, they suggest that activists had more success holding the World Bank accountable for projects that had adverse environmental impact that the Bank directly funded, while the International Monetary Fund (IMF) has been a harder target to hold responsible for riots or hunger as a result of structural adjustment policies: "[T]he causal chain is longer, more complex, and much less visible" (ibid., 28).

Similarly, they argue that campaigns for legal equality of opportunity are amenable to transnational advocacy but for reasons that are not clear. They suggest that there does appear to be a process of expansion of liberal values around the world (ibid., 206), although such an observation runs the risk of "historical determinism." As Finnemore and Sikkink point out elsewhere, "Arguments that the substantive content of a norm determines whether it will be successful imply that norm evolution has a clear direction if not a final endpoint." Rather than a path-dependent product of historical choices, an argument that suggests the substance of certain frames is more effective than others implies a sort of "functional" efficiency (Finnemore and Sikkink 1998, 907–8).

Keck and Sikkink appear to reach these conclusions about the resonance of these kinds of claims based on inductive generalizations from their experience as largely qualitative scholars in the human rights arena: "As we look at the issues around which transnational advocacy networks have organized most effectively, we find two issue characteristics that appear most frequently: (1) issues involving bodily harm to vulnerable individuals ....; and (2) issues involving legal equality of opportunity" (Keck and Sikkink 1998, 27). However, this argument requires additional empirical support to know how valid the conclusions are. They are plausibly drawn from some important cases but would benefit from additional evidence from other cases and support from other methods such as surveys or experimental work. Moreover, despite being informed by some historical cases, the mechanisms of influence at the micro level need to be further developed. In short, their conjectures could usefully be reconceptualized as testable propositions. Moreover, the underlying premise in their work also seems to be based on the notion that somehow universal norm diffusion is a necessary condition for movement success. From this perspective, campaigns with narrowly parochial messages are unlikely to have sufficient appeal to generate transnational support. But how much universal buy-in is necessary for advocates to achieve their goals is underspecified. Not all states are created equal in terms of international politics, so it may not be as important for a campaign to have universal appeal as it is for the message to resonate in the "right" states, right being the states or targets that are necessary politically for the advocacy movement to succeed.

Since Keck and Sikkink wrote their hugely influential book on the subject of transnational advocacy groups, a number of scholars have further explored the issue of framing and resonance. Some, like Payne, dispute that this could be a profitable exercise, suggesting that frames that resonate in one case may not in another (Payne 2001). We are a bit more sanguine regarding the potential lessons one can learn about the properties of successful frames. Indeed, in the field of international relations, one of the chief theoretical and empirical moves in the decade since Keck and Sikkink wrote their book has been to focus on locally compelling frames rather than globally resonant ones. In this sense, frames that fit, match, or are congruent to the local cultural context are more likely to resonate (Entman 1993; Checkel 1999; Cortell and Davis 2000; Acharya 2004; Sundstrom 2005; Busby 2010a). Transnational campaigns are more likely to be successful either if they create nationally differentiated messages or if the publics in target states share a similar cultural outlook. Locally specific cultural messaging may be particularly important where just a few states are needed for policy change.

In terms of universal access campaigns, or campaigns with universal aspirations like human rights where most, if not all states are targets, it may be important, as Keck and Sikkink suggest, to identify a central frame that has broader appeal in many countries. As suggested above, Keck and Sikkink assert that there is something about bodily harm related to the dignity of the individual that gives issues framed in those terms more universal resonance. This response suggests a plausible social psychological mechanism that inheres in the human condition, as if human beings are able to engage in a kind of Rawlsian experiment behind the veil of ignorance to put themselves into the shoes of another. *I would not want to be tortured. Extending this idea to pharmaceuticals, I would want access to these life-saving drugs, so others should have access to them as well.*

Are there other reasons why campaigns might need to identify messages that are universally compelling? Here, the nature of decision-making in particular venues may be relevant. Some universal access campaigns may be discussed by bodies that have universal membership based on consensus rules. The WTO health exception that came out of the 2001 Doha meeting, discussed in the previous chapter, is one example. Because the decision was reached during the conference, advocates did not have the time to tailor country-specific arguments. For other issues, negotiators reach a decision and then have to submit the agreement to some domestic approval process, such as treaty ratification, or, as in the AIDS arena, appropriations of foreign assistance. For those kinds of decisions, advocates can employ locally compelling messages and serially lobby key countries.

Another reason for a broader, more universally appealing frame, is the potential for an issue to be brought up in multiple venues, requiring that it transcend the arguments invoked in a single organization. HIV/ AIDS, for example, had consequences for world trade (via IPR) and for international security, beyond its impact on health. This meant that it was discussed in several different venues including the WTO and UN Security Council beyond, say, the WHO. This provided advocates with incentives to develop arguments that would have broad support in different venues.[2]

Universally compelling messages may also be important in providing leverage to bureaucracies of international organizations vis-à-vis member governments or their governing boards. Some international bureaucracies, particularly technical bodies, are delegated authority by their principals to have independent powers to set agendas, take decisions, and implement policies.[3] For politically contentious issues, international bureaucrats can buttress their position by pointing to demand, or at least support from "the global public" for particular policies, such as essential medicines lists or drug certification guidelines.

The global dispersion of industry may also create incentives for more universally resonant messages. Since the large branded multinational firms have global reach and interests that transcend national borders, influencing their operations and therefore the broader market may

---

[2] We acknowledge that some movements still have strong incentives for advocates to tailor their messages to a particular audience (e.g. presenting AIDS as a security threat before the Security Council). In other cases, some international organizations may privilege certain kinds of arguments over others. For example, the Convention on the International Trade in Endangered Species (CITES) has norms that emphasize scientific arguments over material self-interests (Gehring and Ruffing 2008). The process creating the International Criminal Court (ICC) consisted largely of international lawyers for whom legalistic argumentation and global norms associated with human rights law were more accepted than arguments based on national interest (Deitelhoff 2008; 2009).

[3] (Abbott and Snidal 1998; Barnett and Finnemore 1999). Of course, whether or not international bureaucracies have such slack (or are merely the conduits for the interests of dominant states) is both contested in the literature (Mearsheimer 1994) and may vary by organization (Biermann and Siebenhüner 2009).

require appeals that have universal resonance.[4] Indeed, influencing these large firms may require a multinational campaign that simultaneously is able to generate media attention and support in multiple countries, again reinforcing the need for a frame with broader if not universal appeal. As we stress throughout this book, given the weakness or absence of international authorities to regulate these corporations, advocacy movements may play a special role here, bolstered by their claims to speak with a universal, moral voice.

What were the competing frames on access?

By the late 1990s, people in rich countries largely had access to ARVs, namely, the triple cocktail of HAART introduced in 1996, which immediately had a tremendous effect in staving off death for many people with HIV. Meanwhile, millions in poor countries lacked access to these medications, or even to older drugs like AZT. This inequality was deemed outrageous by campaigners, and they were able to frame the argument in terms of the moral responsibility of pharmaceutical companies to lower their prices in order to right that wrong. Framing the argument in those terms pitted the "intellectual property rights" of firms against the lives of millions of poor people who could be kept alive with these drugs. As Odell and Sell argued, "In the 1980s TRIPS advocates had framed it as an alternative to tolerating piracy of private property." Access activists, for their part, sought to re-frame the issue: "Now the NGOs compared TRIPS to a different reference point saving the lives of poor people suffering from HIV/AIDS" (Odell and Sell 2006, 93).

A few illustrative examples give some context to the arguments activists made. At the 1996 International AIDS Conference in Vancouver, Eric Sawyer of ACT UP gave a speech that represented an early, if strident, effort to re-cast the discussion in terms of greed versus life.

---

[4] We readily admit that locally compelling appeals will remain important for firms, targeting major seats of operations, including but not limited to headquarters. The pharmaceutical industry has strong traditional concentration in a few key countries like the United States, Germany, France, Switzerland, and the UK (although it is now growing in emerging markets like India, Brazil, and South Africa). The incumbent branded pharmaceuticals companies, despite having deep national roots based on their headquarters, also possess wide transnational ties based on the global reach of their marketing, the dispersion of manufacturing, and the accelerated processes of mergers and acquisitions where firms with roots in one country acquire or merge with firms with roots in another (think of GSK, which reflects the 2000 merger of GlaxoWellcome and SmithKlineBeecham, themselves products of earlier mergers of firms with roots in the UK, the United States, and New Zealand).

He invoked the word "genocide" (as American treatment activists had done earlier) to describe the pricing policies of pharmaceutical companies:

The truth is, genocide continues against poor people with AIDS, especially those from developing countries, by AIDS Profiteers who are more concerned about maximizing profits than saving lives. Drug Companies are killing people by charging excessive prices. This limits access to treatments. The greed of AIDS Profiteers is killing impoverished people with AIDS. (Sawyer 1996)

The theme that patent and drug prices policies were killing people became a dominant one of campaigners. In 2001, activists circulated a sign-on letter directed to the major pharmaceutical companies that were then suing the South African government for national legislation that would ostensibly have allowed the government to trump patent rights for AIDS drugs (this lawsuit is described in more detail in the following chapters). Activists wrote "You are receiving this letter because you are suing the government of South Africa in an effort to maintain high prices for patented pharmaceuticals, which will prevent millions of people from obtaining life extending treatment" (Health GAP Coalition 2001a). Elaborating further, the letter argued that firms were concerned with protecting profits in rich countries at the expense of people's lives in poor countries:

The Medicines Act, you claim, would unfairly infringe on the intellectual property rights of drug makers and would cost substantial profits. In fact, the entire continent of Africa generates less than 1.3 percent of global profits from drug sales. Clearly your concern lies not with the lives of the tens of millions of poor people who have no access to drugs, but with protecting your unfettered access to the few in the North who are willing to pay top dollar, no questions asked. (ibid.)

Though slightly less vociferous in tone, press releases from MSF capture a similar perspective, tying prevailing market dynamics to death, suggesting that "People with Aids are Dying Because of Lack of Access to Life-Saving Drugs" (MSF 1999) and "MSF Calls On Davos Leaders to Stop People Dying of Market Failure" (MSF 2000a).

Jamie Love of CPTech made a similar argument, suggesting that despite the complexity of the issue, communicating to policy-makers was, in the end, fairly straightforward:

I would put up some information about infection rates in African countries. How many pregnant women who were infected were going to die without access to treatment, how many people serving in the military were going to die because they were infected, how many fifteen year old kids were going to die because they were going to get AIDS without access to treatment, I just spent a little time on that, and then I put some information about the incomes . . . Then, I'd say, these people are really poor; they can't afford to pay very much money for drugs.

Our policy is to keep the price of the drugs high. That's wrong. . . . Believe me, it's not a very complicated story at that point. (Love 2003)

For their part, branded pharmaceutical companies emphasized the importance of patents in fostering innovation. They sought in turn to respond to these charges by emphasizing that they were in fact in favor of access and were, with respect to the court case in South Africa, merely pursuing their legal rights. As the International Federation of Pharmaceutical Manufacturers Associations (IFPMA) argued: "IFPMA finds it regrettable that the South African Constitutional Case is being used to portray the pharmaceutical industry as a barrier to sustainable access to medicines when in fact industry is a committed partner to finding solutions" (IFPMA 2001).

Defenders of the status quo in industry, like IFPMA president Harvey Bale, suggested that price was not such an important barrier to access compared to other issues like inadequate infrastructure: "[M]ore and more developing countries recognize the benefits of patents for pharmaceuticals and recognize that the significant issues of access to medicines lie elsewhere – in partnerships, financing, political and social commitment and infrastructure" (IFPMA 2002). A Merck spokesman made a similar claim: "There are issues associated with infrastructure, with providing proper care and treatment, distribution systems have to be in place – all these things are needed to ensure access to medicines" (Cooper, Zimmerman, and McGinley 2001).

Others focused on cultural and information barriers to extending treatment. Andrew Natsios, USAID administrator in the George W. Bush administration, famously said in 2001 that treatment was not possible because Africans could not tell time:

Many people in Africa have never seen a clock or a watch their entire lives. And if you say, 1 o'clock in the afternoon, they do not know what you are talking about. They know morning, they know noon, they know evening, they know the darkness at night. (quoted in Donnelly 2001)

As we discussed in Chapter 2, a number of observers, notably Amir Attaran, disputed that patents were a major barrier to access. In an influential 2001 study much touted by defenders of pharmaceutical patents, Attaran and Gillespie-White disputed that patents were a barrier to AIDS treatment access. They wrote: "The observed scarcity of patents cannot be simply explained by a lack of patent laws because most African countries have offered patent protection for pharmaceuticals for many years." They concluded that:

a variety of de facto barriers are more responsible for impeding access to antiretroviral treatment, including but not limited to the poverty of African countries, the high cost of antiretroviral treatment, national regulatory requirements for medicines, tariffs and sales taxes, and, above all, a lack of sufficient international financial aid to fund antiretroviral treatment. (Attaran and Gillespie-White 2001)

These claims were, of course, vigorously contested by advocates of access who sought to use more than moral logic to defend their claims; they buttressed their claims with a variety of arguments about the availability of cheaper generic alternatives, citing examples from Brazil and India (Love 2001b). MSF touted its experience using generic drugs in pilot projects (MSF 2000c). Critics of IPR, like James Love of CPTech, disputed Attaran's argument with a variety of examples of drugs or combination drugs that were patented (Love 2001a).

In announcing PEPFAR in his 2003 State of the Union address, President George W. Bush framed the issue as activists had by focusing on the immorality that so many people lacked access to life-saving drugs (see Chapter 6 for a discussion on the origins of PEPFAR; see also Busby 2010a, Ch. 5):

A doctor in rural South Africa describes his frustration. He says, "We have no medicines, many hospitals tell people, 'You've got AIDS. We can't help you. Go home and die'." In an age of miraculous medicines, no person should have to hear those words . . .. Anti-retroviral drugs can extend life for many years. And the cost of those drugs has dropped from $12,000 a year to under $300 a year, which places a tremendous possibility within our grasp. (Bush 2003)

Campaigners in this vein, rather than stressing the perfidy of the pharmaceutical companies, emphasized the unmet need in treatment. Indeed, in defense of the WHO's 3 by 5 initiative (the aspiration to get 3 million people on treatment by 2005), Jim Kim, who had been tapped to lead the effort, wrote:

AIDS is unusual in the history of epidemics because proven, effective ways of interrupting the course of the disease have existed since shortly after its emergence, yet those methods were foreclosed to most of the world's population. The announcement of 3 by 5 drew from a widespread sense that this inequality presented unacceptable economic, political, moral, and epidemiological consequences. (Kim and Ammann 2004)

We know in retrospect that these appeals helped contribute to a number of momentous changes. The Clinton administration issued an executive order suggesting that it would no longer pursue trade sanctions against countries that sought to prioritize access to medicines over IPR (this policy was extended during the Bush administration). Pharmaceutical companies, along with UNAIDS and WHO, launched the AAI in May 2000, and in April 2001 withdrew their lawsuit against the South African government. Soon thereafter, advocates would help generate an unprecedented shift in resources to support HIV/AIDS. The international community blessed the creation of the Global Fund, launched in 2002. In 2003, the Bush administration launched its own bilateral initiative with PEPFAR.

So, can we identify something about the frames advocates used or the nature of the issue that made HIV/AIDS different? Was HIV/AIDS a *sui generis* or unique case? As advocates of other health issues looked at successful mobilization on HIV/AIDS, they asked themselves the same question: what made AIDS special? As has been recounted elsewhere, there are a number of unique historically contingent aspects of the story that helped facilitate particular transformations along the way (Behrman 2004; d'Adesky 2004; d'Adesky and Rossetti 2005; Smith and Siplon 2006; Gartner 2009a; Geffen 2010; Timberg and Halperin 2012). For example, the decision by the Clinton administration to pursue trade sanctions against South Africa, in support of the pharmaceutical companies' lawsuit, ultimately created a public relations nightmare for both Al Gore as he launched his presidential campaign in 2000, and for branded drug companies as they tried to maintain their reputations. As *The Wall Street Journal* noted: "Can the pharmaceuticals industry inflict any more damage upon its ailing public image? Well, how about suing Nelson Mandela?" (Cooper, Zimmerman, and McGinley 2001).

By 2003, the AIDS crisis had become so severe that an American president looking to demonstrate his compassionate conservative bona fides was willing to put himself out on a limb and back an unprecedented degree of resources to support the fight against HIV/AIDS. However, if the mobilization on HIV/AIDS was not only historically contingent but also possessed distinctive attributes, then the story may be an important one but provide very little guidance for other campaigns that have aspirations for universal access.

We certainly do not dismiss the unique aspects of the AIDS case. Nonetheless, we believe that it presents useful lessons for advocates who would pursue market transformations in other issue-areas, both within and outside global health. Clearly, an essential step in gaining traction for any campaign is the development of a compelling frame.

The argument: access campaigns for life-saving goods are most compelling

While other research has recounted the history of key episodes in the modern history of AIDS (Behrman 2004; 't Hoen 2002; 2009), this book seeks to provide a plausible explanation for why the contests between treatment advocates and opponents were resolved in favor of expanded ARV access in poor countries. Sell and Prakash offered a preliminary account. In their 2004 landmark piece, they applied insights from the literature on framing and advocacy movements to explain the logic by which the access frame ("copy=life," or what we might think of as "generics=life") trumped the IPR frame ("patents = profits = research = cure)." In their view, advocates exploited external crises including the HIV/AIDS crisis and 9/11 and turned them into political opportunities to advance their agenda:

> In sum, the HIV/AIDS crisis presented an opportunity to NGOs (who extended the coalition to include eventually generic pharmaceutical companies, international organizations, foreign governments, and university law students) to temper industry dominance over the IPR agenda …. In the end, with its successful strategies of mobilizing a transnational coalition, framing policy problems, disseminating information, grafting its agenda as a solution to policy problems, and exploiting political opportunities that the 2000 presidential elections and the anthrax episode provided, the NGO network has clearly won some substantive victories and brought about normative change in the IPR debate. (Sell and Prakash 2004, 167)

They further suggest that by tying pharmaceutical company greed to unnecessary deaths, advocates invoked "a successful recipe" based on threats to bodily harm (ibid., 163).

Drezner, by contrast, provides an alternative explanation that downplays the role played by framing and social movement influence. He emphasizes concerns about state failure and security in AIDS-affected countries as well as security-related concerns about a failed Doha Round after 9/11 (Drezner 2007, 177). While security concerns certainly were invoked periodically by states and may have helped facilitate greater engagement by the international community, Drezner diminishes the importance of advocacy influence, particularly with respect to the public health frame, and unnecessarily elevates state-centric security motivations (for a critique, see Greenhill and Busby 2008).

While a compelling moral frame was only part of the reason advocates were so effective (subsequent chapters lay out additional pieces of our argument), it was an important piece. What is needed is a richer theoretical and empirical account of why appeals based on the injustice of limited access found so much support. This section provides such an argument.

There are a number of different possibilities, not mutually exclusive, to explain the resonance of the moral/justice frame for HIV. Different possibilities include the following: (1) because ARVs were essential for life, access appeals had a special moral resonance; (2) access to ARVs was framed in terms of human rights, and rights-based claims have special power; (3) the scale of the epidemic was so large that it elicited a powerful response; (4) advocates were able to transform the perception that people living with AIDS were personally responsible for their own condition, triggering a broader empathetic response; (5) the universality of AIDS, that it affected people in both rich and poor countries, provided an opportunity for global mobilization that other endemic diseases confined to developing countries lack; and relatedly, (6) drawing attention to the inequality of access between those who had access in the North and those who lacked access in the South brought the injustice into stark relief. We discuss each of these possibilities in turn, emphasizing the importance of the power of ARVs as essential for life.

Goods essential for life

Campaigns for universal access can vary in what goods or services advocates believe are worthy of being made available to everyone. They range from a variety of goods that are needed for survival to those that are luxury goods that perhaps enhance life. In between, there are goods that may be needed for a successful life but are not necessary for survival. Life-saving goods would include food, water, shelter, sanitation, clean air, vaccines, maternal mortality services, ARVs, anti-cancer drugs, seeds, and a host of other drugs used to treat life-threatening ailments. Luxury goods would include such things as plastic surgery, sexual impotence drugs, entertainment, and alcohol. Life-enhancing goods necessary for a successful life but not for survival include information/media, education, broadband, energy, insurance, credit, family planning, mental health services, fertilizer, irrigation, transportation, and software/hardware (see continuum in Figure 3.1).

ARVs are clearly on the left side of goods necessary for survival. We believe that successful advocacy around ARVs succeeded in part because they were necessary for survival. By contrast, we would expect that a campaign for universal access for luxury goods like sexual impotence drugs such as Viagra would fail miserably. This is perhaps an extreme contrast, but we might expect that universal access campaigns for education or broadband or one laptop per child might not be as directly related to an individual's survival and therefore be less compelling than the set of goods that are clearly necessary for survival. Within the domain of drugs, we might think that access campaigns for essential medicines like ARVs would be more compelling than access campaigns for Viagra. In between, access campaigns for cholesterol or hypertension drugs might have more mixed support. This is a plausible hypothesis and one that we seek to test experimentally.

Jamie Love, a long-time advocate for more flexibility in IPR rules, makes a similar argument about why access campaigns for life-saving medicines are so compelling:

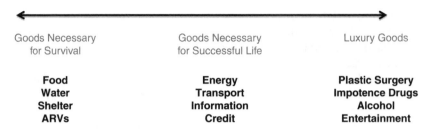

Figure 3.1: Continuum of necessity of different goods
Source: E. Kapstein and J. Busby.

If you have a problem of access to medicine, it's a moral and ethical issue in a way that access to, say, music CDs or Hollywood movies is not. You're not going to get people to protest in Washington, DC because the US wants people to pay for Mickey Mouse or Walt Disney films. A lot of people feel that's not an essential good. They don't care if people have to pay for popular music or for movies …. But the medicine is quite different, it's whether people suffer or whether people die, it's pretty dramatic stuff. (Love 2003)

Access to treatment is a human right

When the world first became aware of HIV and AIDS, fears about the disease led to discriminatory practices against those who were infected with the virus, from the murder of Gugu Diamini in December 1998 in Durban, South Africa after she disclosed her HIV status, to Cuba's efforts to quarantine HIV+ individuals, to bans on travel for those living with the virus, to a host of other measures by both governments and broader societies that stigmatized vulnerable communities heavily affected by the AIDS virus. Jonathan Mann, who led the WHO's early efforts to address HIV/AIDS, was a vigorous champion of human rights for those living with HIV. He, perhaps more than any other public official, was identified as the major champion who connected health and human rights, drawing attention to the social determinants of poor health (Mann 1999; Marks 2001; Gostin 2001).[5]

In 1996, in the *British Medical Journal*, Mann suggested that a human rights frame would be particularly effective: "The current health and human rights movement is based on a working hypothesis: that the human rights framework provides a more useful approach for analysing

---

[5] Paul Hunt, the UN's Special Rapporteur on the Right to Health from 2002 to 2008 would take on some of this mantle (Boseley 2007; Backman *et al.* 2008).

and responding to modern public health challenges than any framework thus far available within the biomedical tradition" (Mann 1996, 924). Even earlier, in launching the journal *Health and Human Rights* in 1994, Mann and his co-authors suggested that human rights language might offer a way forward to improve health outcomes, noting that "[w]hile there are few legal sanctions to compel states to meet their human rights obligations, states are increasingly monitored for their compliance with human rights norms by other states, nongovernmental organizations, the media and private individuals" (Mann *et al.* 1994, 11).

Gostin has argued that human rights rhetoric has a particular power because "[w]hen 'rights' language is invoked, it is intended to convey the fundamental importance of the claim … 'Human rights' when it is invoked in reasoning or argument, commands reverence and respect" (Gostin 2001, 128). Two authors with the WHO wrote of the political utility offered by human rights language in the fight for access to medicines, contrasting IPR and human rights: "While intellectual property rights can be allocated, traded, amended, forfeited and are basically limited in time and scope, human rights are timeless expressions of fundamental entitlements of the human person" (Nguyen-Krug and Hogerzeil 2006).

Indeed, human rights language became more commonplace as part of the vocabulary advocates used to address the AIDS crisis as well as broader efforts to support access to essential medicines (Seuba 2006). As Peter Piot noted in his memoir: "Human rights issues were never far away when working on AIDS. They were not just part of our values, but we learned that discrimination and stigma were major impediments for both prevention and access to treatment. Therefore AIDS-related human rights promotion was an essential part of our work" (Piot 2012, Kindle location 6279). Indeed, Lieberman argues that "the framing of HIV/AIDS as a human rights issue has pervaded the other components of the Geneva Consensus [his term for best practices in AIDS policy]" (Lieberman 2009, 102).

In terms of access to treatment, the argument might go as follows: given the power of human rights language, framing treatment access as a human right was particularly potent both in terms of triggering public and elite support. The problem from this point of view is that while civil and political rights have come to have near universal acceptance, social and economic rights have a much more contentious place in international politics. As Hawkins concluded in his study of human rights mobilization in Chile, "it is significant that the network focused on rights related to personal integrity and civil liberties, which are more established internationally than other kinds of rights. In particular, it is difficult to imagine that a network focusing on economic and social rights would have had the same level of success as the Chilean network" (Hawkins 2002, 68). Indicative of this perspective is the edited volume by Risse, Ropp, and Sikkink, *The Power of Human Rights*, in which the authors explicitly note:

> We chose a central core of rights – the right to life (which we define as the right to be free from extrajudicial execution and disappearance) and the freedom from torture and arbitrary arrest and detention. By choosing to focus on these rights we do not suggest that other rights in the Declaration [of Human Rights] are unimportant. But these basic "rights of the person" have been most accepted as universal rights, and not simply rights associated with a particular political ideology or system. (Risse, Ropp, and Sikkink 1999, 2)

As Keck and Sikkink noted, rights-based framing in their view historically worked best for issues involving bodily harm and denial of equal opportunity. For some issues, human rights frames might not work as well. For example, they note that framing women's issues in terms of "rights," with a focus on violence against women, "supplemented," if not supplanted, earlier "discrimination" and "development" frames. This frame addressed some aspects of women's status but did not address inequalities unrelated to violence. Despite their potential power, some within the movement questioned the appropriateness of a human rights frame: "Other activists, especially from the developed world, believe that the rights frame privileges certain political and civil rights to the exclusion of economic, social, and cultural rights" (Keck and Sikkink 1998, 184).

Nonetheless, given their putative political power, human rights frames became very popular as different campaigns sought to cast or recast their issues including landmines (Price), women's issues (Keck and Sikkink, Joachim), environmental destruction (Keck and Sikkink), core labor standards (Payne), labor rights (Hertel), apartheid (Klotz), among numerous others (Keck and Sikkink 1998; Klotz 1999; Payne 2001; Hertel 2006; Joachim 2007). However, the proliferation of rights-based claims potentially upends their power if every issue can be re-cast in terms of fundamental rights. If all desirable human ends can be rights that trump other human goals, then what specific power can rights-based language ultimately have?

Even as advocates like Mann sought to extend an appreciation for a right to health, the concept may lack analytical clarity. Gostin in 2001 wrote the following just as treatment activists were making their push:

> Considerable disagreement exists, however, as to whether "health" is a meaningful, identifiable, operational, and enforceable right, or whether it is

merely aspirational or rhetorical. A right to health that is too broadly defined lacks clear content and is less likely to have meaningful effect. (Gostin 2001, 128)

To be sure, there have been attempts by prominent ethicists like Thomas Pogge to flesh out a political, moral, and legal rationale for why lack of access to medicines constitutes a human rights violation, but the timing and tenor of this work suggests much remains to be done to inculcate a near universal embrace of access to health as a human right (Pogge 2005). Youde argues that the previous Health for All initiative in the late 1970s failed precisely because it was framed as a human rights issue "at a time when the right to health was highly contested" (Youde 2008). Though Youde suggests the international normative context has become more favorable to health as a human right, it remains unclear how much further we have come in this regard; we revisit this issue in particular in the book's concluding chapter.

Even if health as a human right continues to face challenges conceptually in elite circles, framing health issues as human rights still might resonate with mass audiences and be effective as a mobilizing argument. Moreover, while a right to health may be vague, a right to ARV treatment is much more specific. That said, it is difficult to imagine that a specific right to a particular health intervention could exist in the absence of a broader acceptance of global rights to health. Moreover, rights-based claims may also be more difficult to impose on private actors, as Johnson notes in her study on human rights mobilization in South Africa:

While a human rights approach has often and perhaps appropriately been used to shame governments for their conduct or inaction, in the era of neoliberalism, rights discourse has been much less effective at shaming powerful economic interests who may be at least as culpable of violating human rights. (Johnson 2006, 668–9)

Since AIDS treatment advocates mobilized, they may have created near-universal acceptance that AIDS treatment is something people ought to have access to wherever they live (which is akin to elevating it to the status of a human right) (Youde 2008). However, the diffusion of support for universal treatment access is a product of the mobilization, not, in our view, what fundamentally explains the success of the campaign.

Even if the human rights frame cannot fully explain the success treatment activists had in advancing their agenda, they were clearly inspired by human rights campaigners in a number of respects. AIDS treatment advocates have emulated the success of human rights campaigners by linking high prices of AIDS drugs to active efforts by pharmaceutical companies to deny access. Such actions to defend patents and profits in turn are blamed for the deaths of millions. Like the activists associated with the Health GAP Coalition discussed in the next chapter, a 2012 documentary, *Fire in the Blood*, makes that explicit connection, tightening the causal chain of responsibility (Gray 2012).

What is more, human rights and rights language did have national significance in a number of country contexts. Certainly, in countries like Brazil and South Africa, where constitutional provisions (in the case of Brazil) and court cases (in the case of South Africa) established the legal rights to treatment of affected populations (Johnson 2006; Nunn 2008; Matthews 2011). Here, rights-based claims had particular effectiveness, given the legal backing such claims could command. Internationally, aspects of the AIDS crisis such as discriminatory policies that limited the freedom of movement and physical safety of people living with AIDS, could be and were framed in terms of traditional understandings of human rights. Treatment access, however, was more akin to contested social and economic rights, except in countries where rights to health were more enshrined in the legal fabric of the country.

The scale of the epidemic

There are other plausible hypotheses that are worth mentioning. For one, the death total from AIDS is staggering. Cumulatively, by the late 2000s, more than 25 million had died from AIDS, and more than 30 million were living with HIV (UNAIDS 2008). Annually, more than two-and-a-half million people a year were dying from the disease. One could argue that the unprecedented scale of the pandemic triggered a different sort of response than other health issues.

The difficulty with this interpretation is that other equally deserving health problems kill large numbers of people. Even in low- and middle-income countries, HIV is not the leading cause of death. In low-income countries, the WHO estimated that, in 2008, lower respiratory infections and diarrheal disease killed an estimated 1.05 million and 760,000, respectively, compared to 720,000 who died of AIDS. In middle-income countries, heart disease killed an estimated 5.72 million, followed by stroke (4.91m), chronic pulmonary disease (2.79m), lower respiratory infections (2.07m), diarrheal disease (1.68m), with AIDS sixth at 1.03 million (WHO 2008).

Indeed, one of the findings in psychology bears out the unfortunate maxim often attributed to Soviet dictator Joseph Stalin that "[a] single death is a tragedy; a million is a statistic." Experimental evidence suggests that people find stories of single individuals going through a difficult experience far more compelling than large numbers of people experiencing the same phenomenon. Keith Payne and Daryl Cameron ran an experiment where in one condition a single individual, a girl named Rokia, experienced tragedy in Darfur. Accompanying the article was a picture of the girl. In another condition, respondents read about and saw pictures of eight individuals who were victims of similar ethnic violence. They found that people had less sympathy for the larger group. Where earlier studies had also found similar evidence of declining sympathy for large numbers of sufferers, Payne and Cameron's new study provided additional nuance, only finding the phenomenon in the group that was able to control their emotions. The researchers developed other experiments that affirmed their finding that people try to keep their emotions in check as the number of victims increases:

We found evidence that as the number of victims goes up, so does the motivation to squelch our feelings of sympathy. In other words, when people see multiple victims, they turn the volume down on their emotions for fear of being overwhelmed. (Payne 2010; Cameron and Payne 2011)

These findings make the HIV/AIDS case an anomaly for this work that suggests large numbers of people suffering may turn off the empathy of others.

Personal responsibility for the disease

Another alternative explanation that also poses some challenges for why HIV/AIDS was able to elicit such support is the perceived responsibility of the person for their own problems. One of the findings in the health politics literature is that diseases vary in the perceived responsibility of the sufferer for their own health condition. Oliver and Lee find, for example, that "[m]ost Americans viewed obesity primarily as a case of individual moral failure rather than the result of the food environment or genetics" (Oliver and Lee 2005, 925). What this means politically is that "[i]f obesity is understood to result from individual moral failure, then there should be little support for obesity target policies, particularly those that would come at the expense of the general population" (ibid., 929). Their findings generally support this hypothesis, but they suggest a pathway by which obesity policies could ultimately gain public support: "If the public embraces dominant opinion among experts and agrees that obesity is the result of environmental and genetic factors, we would predict greater support for obesity-related policies in the coming years" (ibid., 947).

In the AIDS arena, this is precisely the sort of problem that historically was seen as a product of the moral failure of individuals by those who opposed action on HIV/AIDS. Indeed, it was Senator Jesse Helms, later a convert to the cause of HIV/AIDS treatment, who suggested those suffering from AIDS brought the disease on themselves for "deliberately engaging in unnatural acts" and "disgusting, revolting conduct" (Dunlap 1995). HIV/AIDS was identified with what were perceived to be risky and, by some, morally repellant behavior including homosexuality, IV drug use, and prostitution. In Western countries, the status of some of these groups has changed dramatically in terms of their broader acceptance in society, and the stigma in Western countries for those living with HIV/AIDS declined significantly beginning in the 1990s (Herek, Capitanio, and Widaman 2002). In countries like, but not limited to the United States, homosexuals have gone from being perceived as a morally suspect minority to being worthy of having more equal rights. Rising tolerance for homosexuality, one of the communities most strongly affected by HIV/AIDS, has increased dramatically in recent decades in the United States and other advanced industrialized countries (Pew Research Center 2012). Even as the status of communities affected by HIV has changed, the face of the epidemic changed, as heterosexual populations in Africa became seen as the epicenter of the crisis. By 2000, 70 percent of Americans recognized Africa as the region of the world most affected by HIV/AIDS (WorldPublicOpinion.org undated).

As the appreciation of Africa's particular vulnerability to HIV/AIDS increased in countries like the United States, so, too, did the understanding that infants and married women, communities seen as more innocent of blame, were among those affected by it. At the same time, polls in the United States showed a change in the extent to which people blamed individuals for bringing HIV/AIDS on themselves. The proportion of people who agreed with the statement, "In general, it's people's own fault if they get AIDS," declined from 51 percent in 1987 to 29 percent in 2011. Similarly, the percentage of people who agreed with the statement, "I sometimes think that AIDS is a punishment for the decline in moral standards" declined from 43 percent in 1987 to 16 percent in 2011 (Kaiser Family Foundation 2012a, 8).

Still, in 2012, with respect to the global AIDS crisis, despite sustained support for US assistance to fight AIDS, a lingering sense that individuals still bear responsibility for the crisis remained. The highest percentage of Americans – 85 percent – identified as a "major reason" the "unwillingness of people in developing countries to change their unsafe sexual practices" as the most important factor impeding progress in controlling the spread of AIDS in developing countries. Compare this result to poverty (76%), developing countries' governments not doing enough (74%), corruption (71%), and not enough support from the United States and other developed countries (31%) (*Washington Post*-Kaiser Family Foundation 2012).

Together, these results suggest a concern that universal access campaigns to address health issues deemed the personal responsibility of individuals are less likely to resonate. HIV/AIDS on some level may be an anomaly or, more likely, HIV/AIDS may now be viewed differently. What this means is that campaigners may have to change attitudes about the degree to which individuals are responsible for their problems before, or at least alongside messages that promote expanded access.

The universality of the problem

HIV/AIDS is a problem that affects both rich and poor countries, which has practical benefits as well as ones that potentially affected the degree to which international concern could be generated for access. In practical terms, people living with HIV/AIDS in the developed world have helped catalyze the creation of pharmaceutical products that first became available in rich countries but offered the promise (and increasingly the reality) of helping people in poor countries. In terms of attitudes, the familiarity of HIV/AIDS potentially creates communities of affinity, both among those living with HIV/AIDS as well as among the wider public.

In contrast, for orphan diseases that almost exclusively affect people in developing countries, like river blindness, the broader public in non-tropical countries may have little familiarity or awareness of these problems. Even problems like diarrheal disease that ostensibly could be known in rich countries may be so rare due to good sanitation and hygiene standards, or when they do occur are regarded as nuisances rather than fatal diseases. Such problems that lack transmission potential from developing to developed countries may not trigger transnational concern in the same way as pandemic flu. That said, publics may misperceive the transmission potential of disease and think a problem represents a more serious or less serious transmission risk than it actually possesses.

Even where we have survey evidence that suggests the public regards a problem as serious, such surveys may not allow us to distinguish whether the public's perception is based on concern about contagion and/or motivated by empathy for the suffering. For example, a 2007 US poll found that 82 percent thought HIV/AIDS was a very serious problem around the world, followed by cancer (79%), poor nutrition (75%), with tuberculosis (TB) (24%) and malaria (24%) trailing substantially. A plausible reason here, aside from differential media attention which has often driven concern about public health problems (Ho, Brossard, and Scheufele 2007), is the extent to which malaria and TB are perceived as other countries' problems (Gallup 2007). Here, responsiveness to an appeal could have both empathetic and self-interested qualities: "I care because I have some familiarity with the problem and the horrendous consequences that go with it. I care because I worry that left unattended the problem could spread here." HIV/AIDS initially had qualities of the latter, but not the former. It was seen as a disease of quasi-alien "at-risk" groups, but people became worried that the disease could spread to the wider public.

With the wider mainstreaming of gay populations in countries like the United States, however, people came to know friends or family who were affected by HIV, or at least became aware of the problem through increasing public and media attention. By 2012, 45 percent of those surveyed in the United States said they know someone who has AIDS, died of AIDS, or has tested positive for HIV, up from 2 percent in 1983 (*Washington Post*–Kaiser Family Foundation 2012).[6] But that trend towards greater visibility may be reversing. Whereas in 2004 some 34 percent of Americans reported that they personally had seen, read, or heard "a lot" about AIDS in the United States, by 2012 that percentage had declined to 14. At the same time, awareness of the epidemic in Africa also declined from a high of 51 percent in 2004 to 22 percent in 2012 (Kaiser Family Foundation 2012a, 9).

Public support for AIDS spending was also relatively high after the millennium. For example, even after the rollout of increased funding for HIV/AIDS, a 2005 poll of citizens in G7 advanced industrialized countries found that large majorities thought that their countries were either not spending enough or were spending about the right amount on actions to address HIV/AIDS. Only Japan, which has lagged behind other donors, showed low awareness of their own country's contribution levels (Kaiser Family Foundation 2005).

Unequal access is what matters

From this related perspective, the universality of the problem may only partially explain the willingness by people in the advanced industrialized world to support access to a particular good by people in the developing world. If people in the developed world lack access themselves, it may be difficult for them to imagine extension of access to others. As the next chapter on movement coherence suggests, it was not until HAART treatment had dramatically reduced death rates in the United States that American AIDS treatment activists coalesced around supporting global

---

[6] There were some racial differences here, with African-Americans more likely to say they knew someone affected by HIV/AIDS.

ARV treatment access. Before then, even within the community most likely to understand the horrors of AIDS, there was reticence about supporting global treatment, that domestic problems still took precedence, that antagonizing pharmaceutical companies could undermine the pipeline of new innovations which might be needed if drug resistance to first-line therapies developed.

Assessing these disparate explanations through surveys

We sought to assess the validity of these six explanations – the centrality of the good for life, the importance of human rights, the scale of the epidemic, personal responsibility, the universality of the problem, and inequality among countries – through a variety of surveys, including survey experiments. The aim of the surveys was to surface the microfoundations by which publics might be prepared to take political action in support of campaigns for universal access.

We emphasize that we see these results as suggestive. While we were able to conduct three experiments with subjects in both the United States and India with some consistency in results across surveys, the experiments undoubtedly raise almost as many questions as they answered. For example, in some of our experiments, we were able to generate statistically significant differences in the willingness by subjects to support campaigns for universal access just by altering a few words. The real world is obviously much more complex. Despite their limitations, surveys help surface how publics, who are among the people advocacy groups hope to enlist in support of their cause, think about the issues we explore in this book.

Survey 1: first access experiment

In our first experiment of 200 respondents, we focused on our central framing argument that access campaigns are more likely to resonate when the goods in question are essential for life. The sample was drawn from Amazon's Mechanical Turk, a web-based service that allows researchers to ask people to perform small tasks for a fee. In this case, we paid respondents $0.50 to answer the survey which was hosted on a survey platform from SurveyGizmo. Mechanical Turk subjects tend to be a little more liberal and educated on average than a national sample, but as Adam Berinsky *et al.* found, it has proven reliable as a means of replicating major findings in political psychology and has the advantage of being much less expensive than survey market research firms (Berinsky, Huber, and Lenz 2012). This sample was 39.5% Democrat,

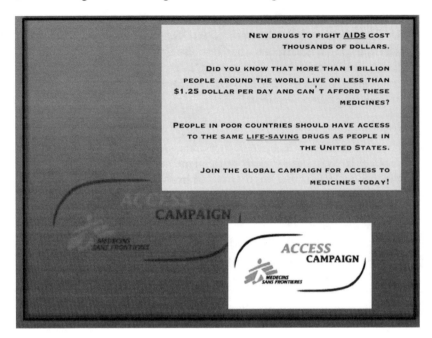

NEW DRUGS TO FIGHT <u>AIDS</u> COST
THOUSANDS OF DOLLARS.

DID YOU KNOW THAT MORE THAN 1 BILLION
PEOPLE AROUND THE WORLD LIVE ON LESS THAN
$1.25 DOLLAR PER DAY AND CAN'T AFFORD THESE
MEDICINES?

PEOPLE IN POOR COUNTRIES SHOULD HAVE ACCESS
TO THE SAME <u>LIFE-SAVING</u> DRUGS AS PEOPLE IN
THE UNITED STATES.

JOIN THE GLOBAL CAMPAIGN FOR ACCESS TO
MEDICINES TODAY!

CAMPAIGN

ACCESS CAMPAIGN

MEDECINS SANS FRONTIERES

Figure 3.2: Mock ad on AIDS drug access

37% Independent, and 19% Republican, with 4.5% signaling Other. The sample was 57% female: 39.5% had a college degree, with another 14.5% having an M.A. or higher; 31% had some college education, only 15% had high school alone. Nonetheless, the sample is large and diverse enough to generate statistically significant differences with minimal changes in the framing of a political ad to which different groups were exposed.

We tested three experimental conditions and a control condition. In the experimental conditions, respondents saw a mock ad from MSF asking them to support their campaign for Access to Medicines. One group saw a print ad about HIV/AIDS, another saw an ad on hypertension drug access, and a third saw an ad about sexual impotence. In the control condition, respondents did not see an ad from an advocacy group.

In the first experimental condition, respondents were asked to support a campaign with information that new drugs to fight *AIDS* cost thousands of dollars and that people in poor countries should have access to *life-saving* drugs (see Figure 3.2). In the second experimental condition, the word AIDS was replaced with *hypertension* and life-saving was changed to *life-extending*. In the third experimental condition, the word AIDS was replaced with *sexual impotence* and *life-enhancing* replaced life-saving. Respondents were then asked whether or not they would be willing to carry out a variety of actions in support of the campaign – sign a petition, write to a member of Congress, write a letter to the editor, talk to friends and family, donate money to the campaign, or join a group in support of the campaign.

The results of this preliminary experiment show strong differences in people's willingness to support access campaigns for AIDS and hypertension compared to an access campaign to address sexual impotence. While the level of support for AIDS and hypertension are not statistically distinguishable, respondents in the experimental condition with the sexual impotence ad were much less supportive of actions to support access. The answers ranged from "not at all likely" to "not very likely" to "somewhat likely" to "very likely." If we assign each of these a number (from 1 for "not at all likely" to 4 for "very likely") we observe that the average willingness to sign a petition was 2.72 by those who saw an AIDS ad compared to 2.85 for the hypertension ad, somewhere between "not very likely" and "somewhat likely." By contrast, those who read the sexual impotence ad averaged 1.71, somewhere between "not at all likely" and "not very likely."

Similar results are found for talking to friends and family and donating money. For more costly actions like writing a letter to a member of Congress or the local paper, differences remained between those who saw the AIDS and hypertension ads and those who saw the sexual impotence ad, but the willingness by all groups to take action dropped further. Interestingly, people in the control condition who read no ad at all were much more willing to signal their willingness to sign a petition in support of access to AIDS and hypertension medicines than in any of the experimental conditions (3.43 for AIDS and 3.24 for hypertension), while nearly equally unwilling to support access to sexual impotence medicines (1.92) (see Figure 3.3).[7]

From this experiment, we conclude that there is some preliminary evidence to support the claim that drugs necessary for life are much more likely to generate political support than luxury, convenience, or lifestyle drugs. While hypertension drugs were assumed to be less necessary for saving someone's life than ARVs, this experiment suggests that respondents might view them as equally important or plausible drugs to save people's lives. We did not ask for more information in this survey to

---

[7] Contact the authors for full statistical results.

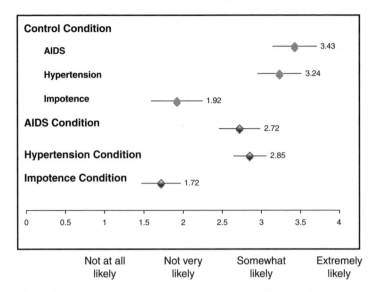

Figure 3.3: Willingness to sign a petition – first US experiment
Source: E. Kapstein and J. Busby.

ascertain their understanding of the essential contribution of these drugs to life, nor did we seek to elicit information about other potential explanations like human rights, the scale of the disease, personal responsibility for their condition, the universality of the problem, or inequality of access between North and South.[8]

Survey 2: pre-test of attitudes toward diseases

As a consequence, we sought to develop another experiment that might do a better job addressing people's underlying attitudes toward the necessity of certain medications for life, as well as to address some of the other alternative explanations explored in this chapter. To identify the health problems to include in a revised survey, we first conducted a pre-test of 100 respondents via Mechanical Turk. Like the first survey, the sample was majority female, highly educated, and more liberal than the general public.

---

[8] One issue that we observe is lower levels of support for those who see an ad compared to the control condition, an anomaly we have observed in other experiments that we worry suggests a disconcerting sign that people are turned off by active political or policy appeals, even on topics they otherwise might support if presented with a petition without efforts to package or frame a problem by an advocacy group.

We first asked these respondents questions about what they thought the main consequences of specific health problems were for people who suffered from them. Health conditions included: allergies, alcoholism, Alzheimer's, cancer, cholera, diarrhea, diabetes, eczema, flu, guinea worm, high cholesterol, HIV/AIDS, hypertension, malaria, obesity, sexual impotence, shingles, and TB. The aim was to include a variety of health problems, some more serious than others, some affecting far greater numbers, some more universal, others regional, and some more strongly associated with lifestyle choices than others.

The consequences ranged from the least serious (inconvenience) to the most serious (death). Intermediate categories ranged from lost days at work, to emotional impact, to disability. AIDS and cancer were the two diseases identified most strongly with death, more than 90 percent in both cases. Sexual impotence, allergies, and eczema were among the least identified with death – 0%, 1%, and 2%, respectively. Interestingly, diarrhea and flu were identified with death as the main consequence by only 1% and 3%, respectively; 64% said diarrhea's main consequence was an inconvenience, suggesting that advocates seeking to address diarrheal disease as a leading cause of death in the developing world have much work to do. Other health problems like diabetes (23%), hypertension (36%), high cholesterol (41%), and obesity (30%), were less strongly associated with death, with disability frequently another major consequence, although inconvenience was also often cited (24% and 33% for hypertension and high cholesterol, respectively). Here, our initial presumption that hypertension should have commanded less support than HIV/AIDS based solely on its association with death is borne out in this sample, albeit small.

We then asked respondents about the numbers of people who were affected by these problems, ranging from less than 1,000 to millions. Only a few diseases like guinea worm were regarded by few respondents as affecting millions. Interestingly, both TB and cholera were only thought by 16% and 15%, respectively, to affect millions, suggesting that there is little awareness in the United States about the scale of these problems in the developing world. While not as large as some other health problems like the flu, majorities of respondents suggested AIDS and cancer affected millions.

When asked about who is affected by these problems, the options ranged from "everyone" to "mostly people in developed countries" to "mostly people in developing countries" to "don't know." Again, large majorities – 70% and 80% – for HIV/AIDS and cancer suggested the problem was universal, affecting everyone. Other diseases like malaria, TB, cholera, and guinea worm were identified as overwhelmingly developing world problems while high cholesterol, hypertension, and obesity were seen as primarily developed world problems. Here, the familiarity of hypertension might cut both ways, in the sense that appeals for access might command less support if people in developed countries don't think this is a problem that affects the developing world. However, because hypertension is something they are likely much more familiar with from their own lived experience than HIV/AIDS, they might be more willing to support actions to address it.

In terms of personal responsibility, some problems were more clearly identified as being entirely or mostly driven by lifestyle choices, including HIV/AIDS, alcoholism, hypertension, high cholesterol, and obesity: 23% and 57%, respectively, said lifestyle choices were "entirely" or "mostly" responsible for HIV/AIDS. Cancer, by contrast, was identified as mostly (59%) or entirely (20%) a product of factors unrelated to lifestyle. These figures suggest that appeals to treatment access for cancer might be even more potent than HIV/AIDS. Like HIV/AIDS, cancer is identified with death, thought to affect millions, and is a universal disease. However, HIV/AIDS and hypertension have in common that people see lifestyle reasons as their main driver.

When asked about who had access to health care in the United States and then in the developing world, respondents suggested for nearly all health problems that Americans generally get access to treatment. Only for certain problems identified as lifestyle issues, like alcoholism and hypertension, were majorities lower. In developing countries, most respondents thought people lacked access to treatment for all these health problems.

Interestingly, when asked whether access to health care is a right, 72 percent said it was a right, regardless of nationality, 2 percent said health care was a right for Americans only, with 22 percent saying health care, while desirable, was not a right. These figures support the suggestion that access to health as a right still might be a potent frame, its contested legal and moral status among elites notwithstanding.

We also asked respondents about a number of non-health-related problems where campaigns for universal access might be initiated. We asked them to rank problems from least important to most important on a scale of 1 (having the least impact on life) to 5 (having the most impact on life). Problems included: lack of education, lack of credit, lack of clean drinking water, lack of insurance, unemployment, lack of access to seeds, lack of food, lack of shelter, lack of transport, lack of information, and lack of energy. Not surprisingly, lack of food and clean drinking water were deemed the most important for life (in excess of 90% ranked them a 5). Lack of shelter was a distant third, with more than 60% giving it a ranking of 5. No other problem achieved more than 40%, with unemployment and education at 35% and 30%, respectively receiving a ranking of 5. This finding suggests that universal access campaigns for food, water, and shelter may resonate quite broadly, but other campaigns – for education, for example – may have more difficulty generating as much support.

In the subsequent experiment of 200 respondents (discussed in the next section below), these results were confirmed. Subjects identified HIV/AIDS and cancer with death, other problems like hypertension and high cholesterol less so. Millions everywhere were seen as affected by HIV/AIDS and cancer. Some diseases like cancer were seen as primarily driven by factors other than lifestyle, while HIV/AIDS, hypertension, and high cholesterol were seen as especially driven by lifestyle choices. As before, respondents overwhelmingly regarded access to health care as a human right. Moreover, respondents also ranked non-health problems in a similar fashion, highlighting the centrality of food, water, and shelter to life, with other problems ranking quite far behind.

Survey 3: second United States access experiment

Based on the pre-test, we conducted a third sample of convenience with 200 US subjects using Mechanical Turk. This sample was more evenly split by gender (47% male, 52% female), still tended to be over-educated (41% with a college degree and another 17% with a professional degree), and more liberal (43% Democratic, 37% Independent, and 17% Republican) than the general public.

The aim was to identify a health condition that shared in common a number of characteristics with HIV/AIDS to see if a different disease might engender strong support for a universal access campaign. Keeping the experimental conditions for hypertension and sexual impotence the same, this experiment substituted cancer instead of HIV/AIDS. Like HIV/AIDS, cancer is strongly identified with death (and by implication, anti-cancer drugs are identified with saving lives). In addition, cancer, like HIV/AIDS, is thought to affect millions and is present everywhere with the sense that people in advanced industrialized countries have access to medications while those in developing countries do not. However, cancer, unlike HIV/AIDS, is not thought to be driven by lifestyle choices and therefore an access campaign for cancer drugs ought to resonate even more strongly among members of the public.

As suggested in the previous section, we also asked all respondents in this survey the same battery of questions about the consequences of different health problems, the numbers affected, the universality of the

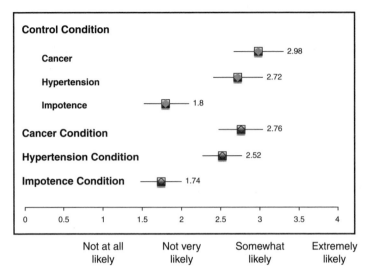

Figure 3.4: Willingness to sign a petition
Source: E. Kapstein and J. Busby.

problem, the degree of access in the United States and developing countries, and the importance of human rights. The results largely support the conclusions in the first experimental study and the expected effects of substituting cancer for the HIV/AIDS condition. Where respondents saw no political ads, their baseline level of support for signing a cancer petition was "somewhat likely." Important for our purposes, they were more willing to sign a petition for cancer drug access than hypertension. The baseline level of support was much higher for both than it was for a petition for universal access to sexual impotence drugs, which hovered below "not very likely." In the experimental condition, again we find the same pattern; those who saw just the cancer ad were willing to support signing a petition at an average level of 2.76, between "not very likely" and "somewhat likely." Again, these results were higher than those who just read the hypertension ad who were willing to support access to hypertension drugs at an average level of 2.52. Again, in both conditions, respondents were much more willing to sign a petition for cancer and hypertension drug access than they were for access to sexual impotence drugs, consistent with our hypothesis that goods necessary for life will resonate more than luxury items (see Figure 3.4).

The differences between the baseline level of support for signing petitions was only marginally higher than the experimental conditions where respondents saw only one ad for one of the medicines. In theory, one would hope that political ads actually persuade people to support policies even more than the baseline condition, but this could be a product of the quality of the print ad. In any case, when we asked people in each experimental condition about their willingness to carry out other measures in support of the campaign (write letters, donate money, join, etc.), we find similar results. In all but one instance (writing a letter to the local paper), people's willingness to carry out actions was higher for those who saw the cancer ad than hypertension, and both were much higher than those who saw the impotence ad. Differences between cancer and hypertension were not always statistically significant, perhaps suggesting that Americans may regard hypertension as a serious health issue where drugs could have life-saving qualities, like for cancer. In general, people were more supportive of talking to friends and family or donating money than they were of writing letters or joining a group, suggesting that more costly behavior like writing letters or joining groups for global access causes may only be a concern among a small number of Americans more generally. Motivating that sliver of the American population to support global campaigns for justice may be tricky and require more selective microtargeting, including messaging that comes from trusted interlocutors, than a single print ad from an advocacy group on its own can achieve.

We also asked these respondents, as well as approximately 120 other subjects, the battery of questions from the pre-test about their attitudes toward the seriousness of health problems, how many and who are affected, the comparative access in the United States and the developing world, and people's personal responsibility for various health problems. Here, again we find cancer and AIDS overwhelmingly identified with death by more than 92% and 83%, respectively. Though less identified with death, hypertension is seen as a serious condition, with a majority identifying disability or death as the major consequence. As we found in the pre-test, diarrhea was identified by most American respondents with inconvenience, suggesting that those concerned about diarrheal disease would need to inform the public about the deadly consequences in developing countries. Interestingly, majorities identified malaria and TB with death, although respondents estimated that the number of people affected by these problems was quite small. For example, between 15% and 20% of respondents thought that fewer than 10,000 people around the world were affected by malaria and TB, respectively. Nearly another 30 percent thought the numbers were in the tens of thousands. The correct figure is in the millions for both. Given that large majorities believed both problems primarily affect developing countries, the lack of awareness of the scale of these problems is somewhat understandable. Interestingly, a number of problems like hypertension, obesity, and diabetes were more strongly identified as developed world problems, suggesting access campaigns may need to inform publics that these problems are more widely dispersed. That said, large majorities saw these problems, as well as HIV/AIDS, as primarily driven by lifestyle choices, suggesting further challenges of mobilizing support. By contrast, large majorities attributed other problems, including cancer, but also TB and malaria to non-lifestyle reasons.

As in the pre-test, we find that large majorities believed most Americans have access to treatment for most of the health problems identified here, save for those like alcoholism and obesity, which were seen by most to be lifestyle choices. Again, consistent with earlier results, large majorities believed that most people in developing countries lacked access to treatment for all of these health problems. As before, we find that a large majority (68%) regarded access to health care as a human right, regardless of nationality, suggesting that these inequalities of access might be salient, particularly for problems deemed as especially serious.

Finally, when asked to rank the importance of other non-health-related problems, respondents in this survey again identified access to food and water as most critical; in excess of 80% rated these issues as a 5, as most important for life. Shelter as before was rated the third most important need for life, ranked as a 5 by nearly 60% of respondents, suggesting that a universal housing campaign might have some salience. Education and employment were again distant followers, with nearly 30% rating them as a 5 in importance for life. Other issues like access to seeds, energy, and insurance followed further behind, identified by about 20% as especially important, with credit, transport, and entertainment deemed the least important by these respondents.

Survey 4: India experiment

We sought to demonstrate the generalizability of these findings by conducting another experiment via Mechanical Turk in a different country context. We selected India, in part because Indians are highly responsive to Mechanical Turk work requests but also because, as an emerging economy with a large population, health access issues are especially salient. India's generic pharmaceuticals industry is the dominant provider of HIV/AIDS drugs worldwide as well as other generic formulations, and issues surrounding the disease and the generics industry are widely reported in the Indian press. Problems like hypertension and

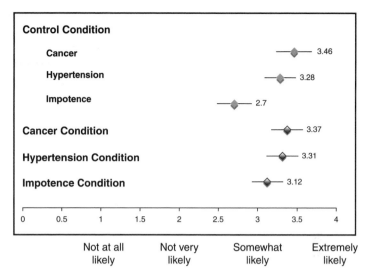

Figure 3.5: Willingness to sign a petition – India experiment
Source: E. Kapstein and J. Busby.

cancer are becoming more common as India becomes richer and its population lives longer.

As in the previous experiments, we find strong differences in the control condition between people's willingness to support signing a petition for access to cancer and hypertension medications compared to impotence drugs. Again, as we have seen in other experiments, the political ads themselves do no better than the control condition. Here, the patterns are largely similar to the cancer experimental condition; the mean willingness to sign a petition was 3.37, compared to 3.31 for the hypertension condition and 3.12 for the impotence condition (see Figure 3.5). The differences are statistically significant between the cancer and impotence conditions, but not between cancer and hypertension or between hypertension and impotence. Interestingly, the access ad does appear to motivate respondents in the experimental condition to support a campaign for universal access to impotence drugs. Part of these stronger results for impotence may result from a sample that is disproportionately male (61%).

The results for the other questions – about the willingness to send a letter to a member of Parliament, write a letter or email to a newspaper, tell friends and family, donate time, or join a group – generally show similar patterns, cancer receiving more support than hypertension and impotence, with statistically significant differences between cancer and impotence.[9]

In this experiment, we also asked respondents about the battery of questions from the pre-test. Here, the results showed some similarities, but also some distinct differences. As in other surveys, AIDS and cancer were strongly identified with death by more than 70% of the respondents. TB and alcoholism were the next two health problems most identified with death, by more than 30% in both cases. Interestingly, hypertension is not strongly identified with death. Rather, 51% of respondents saw its major consequence as emotional. Malaria and diarrhea were mostly identified with lost days at work, more than 40% in both cases. Few diseases were identified strongly with developing or developed countries. Responses were more evenly spread across the categories. Allergies – by 50% of the respondents – was seen as the problem most affecting everyone followed by diarrhea, diabetes, flu, alcoholism, cancer, and hypertension, all of which exceeded 40%. Malaria was the only health problem seen by a narrow majority – by 50.2% – as primarily affecting developing countries.

In terms of access, a majority of the respondents thought most people in the United States had access to medications for all the health problems. Interestingly, a majority of respondents thought people in developing countries had access to medication for hypertension, malaria, flu, diabetes, allergies, and high cholesterol. Majorities thought people lacked access for health problems like cancer and HIV/AIDS. As in previous surveys, a number of problems were strongly identified as entirely or primarily driven by lifestyle choices, including HIV/AIDS, high cholesterol, alcoholism, diabetes, and hypertension. However, for these problems, non-lifestyle reasons loomed larger for Indian respondents. Whereas less than 25% of respondents in the US surveys tended to identify problems like HIV/AIDS, obesity, and high cholesterol as driven by non-lifestyle reasons, more than 30–35% of respondents in the Indian sample emphasized such reasons. As in previous surveys, 85% identified health as a human right regardless of nationality. In terms of other issues, Indian respondents identified lack of food and water as centrally important to life (63% and 59% ranking them a 5), followed closely by education (56%) and then shelter and unemployment (47%). This result suggests that education access might be more salient in developing countries.

---

[9] On "send a letter to Parliament" and "donations," differences are not statistically significant. On "talk to friends and family" and "joining groups," differences between hypertension and impotence were statistically significant.

Survey 5: third United States access experiment

We prepared a third US-based experiment with Pacific Market Research, a survey market research firm, to see if our results with US subjects held up outside the context of Mechanical Turk. Our sample was 204 subjects, split nearly equally between men and women (48% men and 52% women). The sample was 42% Democratic, 33% Independent, 19% Republican, with 5 plus percent Other. In terms of education, this group was more like the nation as a whole, with 29% having completed college and about 8% with a master's degree or higher. We repeated the US experiment with this group, where a control group was asked about its willingness to sign a petition for people in poor countries to have access to anti-cancer drugs, hypertension drugs, and impotence drugs. The three experimental conditions were as before, one for cancer drug access, one for hypertension, and one for impotence. We then asked all respondents the same questions about a variety of health conditions, personal responsibility, comparative access, human rights, etc.

As in previous surveys, we found that in the control condition, respondents were more supportive of cancer drug access than hypertension and preferred both over impotence drugs. In the experimental conditions, we found no statistically significant difference, however, between support for signing a petition for cancer and hypertension drug access, but with both preferred over impotence drugs. In the experimental conditions, people were slightly less than "somewhat likely" on average to support signing a petition for cancer and hypertension drug access, while they were closer to "not very likely" for impotence drugs (see Figure 3.6). As for the other political actions like joining groups, donating money and writing letters to Congress or the local newspaper, we found similar patterns with access for cancer and hypertension drugs indistinguishable, but both were more supported than impotence drugs.[10]

The difference between the cancer/hypertension and impotence conditions supports our main argument about the nature of the underlying medical condition and the resonance of a universal access appeal. The similar levels supporting political actions for both the cancer and hypertension conditions, however, raise challenging questions for future research. Respondents overwhelmingly identified cancer with death (72%) compared to only 27% for hypertension. Respondents also were more likely to identify hypertension with lifestyle choices than cancer.

---

[10] While the coefficient for hypertension sometimes is larger than for the cancer condition, the differences are not statistically significant.

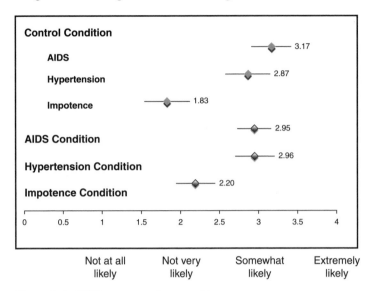

Figure 3.6: Willingness to sign a petition
Source: E. Kapstein and J. Busby.

While this issue bears further scrutiny in subsequent work, the results of this survey reinforce those from Mechanical Turk: 68% of respondents saw health as a human right, regardless of nationality. AIDS was identified with death and was seen as a problem affecting millions, with lifestyle reasons identified as the leading cause of the problem, and with those in the developing world largely lacking access to treatment. Indeed, a majority of the respondents, as in the other US surveys, thought most people in developing countries lacked access to treatment for all the health problems in the survey. As for other problems outside the health arena, clean water and food were the two issues most strongly identified with survival; shelter, education, and employment were distantly behind.

From this diverse set of surveys, our takeaways are that differences in underlying health conditions can help us understand the appeal of access campaigns, but the broad appeal of health as a human right and the recognition of widespread inequalities in access can help create broader support for health access for problems like hypertension, which was perceived as less serious than cancer and HIV/AIDS. That said, the baseline level of willingness by respondents to engage in political activity of any kind in either the control or experimental conditions was fairly low, on average just below or above "somewhat likely," even for issues like cancer and HIV/AIDS. Mobilization of likely activists might require more targeted messages to affinity groups of patients affected by the same ailment, to faith groups, to people with shared background like ethnicity, and other characteristics that may move away from resonant universal messages to more locally persuasive ones.

Conclusions

From this diverse survey evidence, we find suggestive support that goods deemed essential for life command the most public support for universal access campaigns, while campaigns promoting access to what are deemed "luxury" goods are least likely to resonate. At the same time, we also found some support for some of the alternative explanations we identified in the previous section. Across the two US surveys and the Indian survey, health was widely regarded as a human right. From the vantage of people in the United States, developing countries were viewed as lacking access to most areas of health care. Indian respondents were more likely to support all kinds of access campaigns, including for sexual impotence drugs, and, at the same time, their views about access in the developing world were more nuanced, with most people perceived as having access to treatment for "minor" problems like flu. In sum, while we are convinced that the core frame of access to treatment based on the centrality of ARVs to survival holds up, other dimensions of the problem – including human rights and inequality – also are potentially important.

In this chapter, we explored the logic by which advocates were able to mobilize broad international support for extending access to ARV therapy, drawing from the larger framing literature as well as unique survey evidence. Although mobilization in support of HIV/AIDS access was historic, looking at the panoply of other goods that are also essential for life (such as water and drugs to fight non-communicable diseases), many other causes from a framing perspective have the potential to resonate transnationally. In some respects, this is "good news" from the advocacy perspective, suggesting that HIV/AIDS is not a unique case, but one from which other social movements can learn.

4   Movement coherence and mobilization

> If people are getting the same ask from everybody, they obviously have to take you seriously. If you have ten different groups asking for ten different things, nothing happens.
>
> Mark Milano, ACT UP activist, 2012

In this chapter, we provide a theoretically informed account of why movement coherence around a common "ask" – global treatment access based on lower drug prices – was a necessary albeit insufficient condition contributing to the AIDS treatment campaign's overall or relative success. The chapter elucidates the importance and mechanisms of influence of movement coherence contrasted with other less successful campaigns, namely, those addressing climate change and maternal mortality. We also examine within-case variation in the AIDS advocacy movement, including differences between treatment and prevention, the effects of splintering among national level AIDS advocates in the United States, and changes in unity over time in support for the global treatment agenda.

Using interviews, archival material, and other narratives, we provide a historically contingent account of how the movement cohered around global access to treatment. The main contribution of this chapter is thus conceptual, clarifying why movements that lack coherence or unity tend to fail. While a number of other important foundational pieces have told the chronological history of treatment advocacy (Sawyer 2002; Behrman 2004; d'Adesky 2004; 't Hoen 2009; Geffen 2010), these pieces by their nature are more descriptive than analytical, making it difficult to identify generalizable aspects of the campaign's organization. Even more theoretically inclined accounts (such as Smith and Siplon 2006; Grebe 2008; 2011; Messac 2008; Gartner 2009a) tend to use existing scholarship instrumentally (such as McAdam, McCarthy, and Zald 1996; Zald 1996; Keck and Sikkink 1998) rather than make their own theoretical contributions or systematically test their arguments.

The first section of this chapter defines movement coherence, while the second examines two mechanisms by which movement coherence exercises influence, one pressure-based and the second informational.

The third section examines the effects of incoherence on other movements – climate change and maternal mortality – before examining disunity among AIDS advocates. The final section unpacks the emergence of unity among global treatment advocates and how this helped set the stage for expanded access.

Defining movement coherence

Movement coherence broadly means that movement actors share similar principles and concrete objectives for what they hope to achieve. Coherence means that the advocates share a similar diagnosis regarding the barriers to access and what the movement's "ask" should be of target actors. An "ask" is, unsurprisingly, what advocates are seeking from their targets in terms of specific actions, whether it be governments or firms.[1] In the case of treatment access, high drug prices were seen as the principal barrier to access, and therefore, lowering drug prices was the general means to extend access to more people.

Coherence does not necessarily imply agreement among actors about the specific *means* to attain their objective, at least in the initial phases of a campaign. AIDS advocates, for example, did not all agree that compulsory licensing of drugs by developing countries was the appropriate solution to high ARV prices. Other means, such as voluntary licensing of patented drugs by branded pharmaceutical companies to generic companies, could have been employed. As discussed below in the section on movement coherence and global treatment access, some advocates were more wedded to compulsory licensing as a solution than others. Despite some differences of opinion about the appropriate strategy, however, all of the actors agreed that universal treatment access was desirable and that pressure on branded drug companies and governments should be brought to bear to bring prices down.

While coherence is important, we should emphasize that it may be the product of temporary, somewhat ephemeral coalitions between groups with quite disparate approaches and attitudes in other spheres, just as military alliances may bring together otherwise strange bedfellows. Taking issue with the notion that a "shared identity" is necessary for a successful social movement, Eduard Grebe in his analysis of treatment advocacy makes a similar point about social movements as "networks of influence" that may serve as transitory "alignments of purpose" for groups with different perspectives:

---

[1] http://dp.continuousprogress.org/node/22.

Rather, it points to the many ways in which seemingly insurmountable differences and divergent interests are overcome by means of temporary and strategic alliances mobilised through networks that are capable of accommodating diversity precisely because they do not necessarily imply closely-knit integration between all participants. (Grebe 2008, 9)

While these groups may have some differences in perspective, what characterizes members of the movement or broader network is that they are, as Jennifer Hadden recognizes, all "on the same side." How can we recognize members of the same team from counter-movements? They cannot be diametrically opposed in principle and still be on the same side (for example, climate skeptics and environmentalists are rivals). Hadden notes that even in a divided network, there ought to be scope for some overlap so that members of one network might also be participants in another network. Finally, she suggests that one can look back in time and see the origins of the divisions that splinter a once unified network (Hadden 2012, 5–6).

Operationally, she argues one can recognize relatively more coherent networks by the extent of connectivity within the network, often forged by "brokers" who bridge different organizations. The presence of few brokers or bridges is reflective of a more divided network. Another way to observe declining coherence is whether the coalition's "main hub" – its "central" or "peak" organization or association – encompasses over time a *smaller* share of the organizations working in that space. For example, by the mid 2000s, the Climate Action Network (CAN) was coordinating fewer and fewer of the groups working on climate change as the number of civil society players grew dramatically (ibid., 18).

How else can we recognize coherence and incoherence? First, public statements (traced, for example, through content analysis) by different individuals and organizations should be roughly similar in terms of their characterization of the problem and potential solutions. If different actors join a coalition and endorse a common agenda, this is a sign of coherence. A more limited indicator of coherence would be the range of endorsement signatures of support for a one-off solidarity letter or manifesto. Incoherence, by contrast, is observable in terms of open conflict between rival coalitions or groups. Media reports of conflict among groups can provide yet another indicator of divisions (see Table 4.1 for a set of questions to assess movement coherence).

Mechanisms of influence

Movement coherence or unity serves to project a clear message to target actors about the movement's principles and more concrete objectives. Coherence has two dimensions, one *pressure-based* and the other

Table 4.1: *Questions to assess movement coherence*

(1) Is there an overarching umbrella organization to coordinate the network?
(2) Have member organizations signed on to a common platform?
(3) Are there petitions or solidarity appeals that members have signed on to?
(4) Has the movement experienced a rupture into rival factions with breakaway organizations?
(5) What percent of the organizations or individuals belong to competing networks?
(6) Has the media reported conflict between groups within the movement?

Source: E. Kapstein and J. Busby.

informational. In their landmark study, Keck and Sikkink identify four mechanisms by which transnational activists seek to influence target actors – information, accountability, leverage, and symbolic politics (Keck and Sikkink 1998). However, we can think of these more broadly as two kinds of movement actions, one to make it more costly for target actors to fail to heed campaigners' demands (by using leverage and holding targets to account for broken promises) and another to inform policymakers about a problem. Part of that information function necessarily involves getting the attention of decision-makers (hence the importance of symbolic actions like civil disobedience, die-ins, and other forms of protest activity) and part of it involves advocates communicating substantive information to targets about the issues at hand. Symbolic actions, of course, are not distinct from pressure. The power of advocates to mobilize supporters for protest action – to disrupt meetings and name and shame targets for failure to live up to campaigners' expectations or previous commitments – is all part and parcel of raising the costs of inaction.

Advocates for universal access to drugs (among other goods and services, like education) are able to draw on both their expertise and their perceived standing as principled champions acting on behalf of the aggrieved group. Together, these attributes give movement actors credibility to speak up for greater access (Keck and Sikkink 1998, 19, 23, 29). Many Northern NGOs, by virtue of their professionalism, funds, and tighter ties to their governments, have historically enjoyed the privilege of speaking for Southern actors to target audiences (Bob 2005; Carpenter 2011). To the extent that this community is united, both within Northern countries and between North and South, they are more likely to speak with authority to their targets.

We can understand the effect of coherence by way of contrast with its mirror image: incoherence. Incoherence, what we might also call disunity, dissipates the limited influence campaigners possess, diminishing the pressures on firms and political actors who might have the capacity to rewrite rules in favor of access. One way to think of the role of movement unity is in terms of principal–agent (P–A) theory. However, in this context, advocates are the principals and the target actors in governments and firms are the agents. One of the central findings of P–A theory is that where the principals are divided, agents have more free rein to pursue their preferences (Avant 1994; Brenner 2003; Hawkins *et al.* 2006).

Disunity confuses the message that busy decision-makers are expected to hear. With advocates openly disagreeing among themselves about the right course of action, policy-makers cannot discern what it is they are expected to do. With incoherence, the "signal-to-noise" ratio becomes smaller, more unfavorable to receipt of the message. As long-time ACT UP New York activist Mark Milano noted: "If people are getting the same ask from everybody, they obviously have to take you seriously. If you have ten different groups asking for ten different things, nothing happens." He elaborated why. If one group is asking for 15 million people on treatment by 2015 and somebody else is asking for some other number, then the people in Congress who work on hundreds of issues and don't have the expertise "don't know who to listen to" (Milano 2012).

Legro offers a similar perspective on ideational changes in grand strategy. Recognizing the importance of one single unifying idea, he writes: "In cases where a single alternative idea exists, a more natural focal point of opposition is available and it is easier for those disenchanted with the old ideas to coordinate and effect change" (Legro 2005, 35). The contrast he suggests is where there are many ideas competing to replace the old grand strategy. In this situation, he notes "Each replacement camp will compete with others for backing and it will be harder to gather the necessary momentum to debunk the old one and avoid a divisive conflict over what will replace it" (ibid., 36).

Another way to approach this question is offered by the literature on public opinion. John Zaller's landmark study of persuasive messages and public opinion finds that politically aware publics are most likely to be persuaded by elites where they are united. Where elites are divided, mass publics are more likely to respond to partisan cues (Zaller 1992). Unless they are specialists, target actors are likely to receive very little information from campaigners, unless it breaks through the din and receives coverage in the mainstream media or is somehow brought to their attention through acts like civil disobedience.

Where campaigners have incoherent messages, their aims are less likely to receive attention, or the attention they receive may report on division within the movement so that the movement's internal conflict becomes the story rather than their substantive goals (for a similar perspective on movement fragmentation, see Odell and Sell 2006). Even in areas where there is seemingly epistemic consensus, sowing dissent can be extremely effective. For example, although scientists almost universally agree that human beings have dramatically changed the earth's climate system, climate skeptics have been extremely effective in undermining public support for action and in softening the elite consensus that the problem is real, particularly in the United States (Cohen and Bell 2007; Dunlap 2008; Saad 2009; McCright and Dunlap 2011).

Case studies of incoherence

Where movements are not united, their ability to mobilize pressure and signal a clear ask to target actors is compromised, undermining their potential effectiveness. We can observe the effects of movement incoherence and division through a series of case studies, including an analysis of advocacy around climate change and maternal mortality. We also provide examples within the AIDS arena, namely, disagreements over the global AIDS prevention agenda as well as the senescence and fissures in domestic AIDS advocacy in the United States.

Climate change – increasing division

In the lead-up to the 1997 Kyoto Protocol, advocates rallied around a compelling idea modeled on the legal accords related to the hole in the ozone layer, namely, legally binding targets and timetables for reducing emissions. As the issue became politically salient, politicians who wanted to be green found their options constrained by what was perceived to be politically acceptable. While decision-makers departed from the orthodoxy preferred by environmental campaigners, chiefly, by designing flexibility mechanisms that would make meeting these targets and timetables cheaper, political leaders nonetheless committed themselves to a process largely in keeping with this template. For political leaders who sought green credentials, environmental groups would only praise and provide reputational benefits if decision-makers hewed near to the path. It was, it must be remembered, Vice President Al Gore who arrived at the end of the Kyoto negotiations to save the day, by committing his nation to a deeper emissions target. Collectively, rich countries at Kyoto committed to reduce their emissions by 5 percent below 1990 levels by 2008–12 (Busby 2008; 2010a).

Flash forward to 2008. By then, global emissions of greenhouse gases had increased by nearly 30 percent above 1990 levels.[2] Although the Kyoto Protocol entered into force, a number of key states, principally the

---

[2] In 1990, the world produced an estimated 36,405 metric tons of CO_2 equivalent. By 2008, the total had increased to 46,917 metric tons for CO_2 and five other greenhouse gases (Netherlands Environmental Assessment Agency 2012).

United States, did not ratify the agreement, undermining its effectiveness. Other countries like China and India that lacked legal commitments under Kyoto had emerged as some of the world's largest emitters of greenhouse gases. By then, George W. Bush was concluding his second term in office during which environmentalists were largely shut out from having any influence. Among his first acts as president, Bush repudiated the Kyoto Protocol that his predecessor had signed but not submitted to the Senate for advice and consent (La Guardia and Hamden 2001; Pianin 2001).

As we discuss in later chapters, while the European emissions trading scheme that was launched in 2005 started to create market-transforming effects by virtue of tradable emissions permits, the lack of participation by the United States, and the absence of commitments for countries like China and India, meant that these effects only partially transformed the market. Given the way permits were generously handed out in Europe and in the face of economic crisis, the price of permits remained so low that a number of critics suggested the scheme was no longer living up to its transformative potential (Hoag 2011; Van Noorden 2011).

In this context of Kyoto's ratification but implementation failure, the environmental movement fractured into different factions. Hadden uses network analysis to document this landscape of division. At the 2009 Copenhagen climate negotiations, she suggests that the climate change advocacy movement had fissured into mainstream advocacy organizations and those taking a "climate justice" approach. She concludes that "[a]s a result of these divisions it was more difficult for the network to facilitate coordination of collective action, communicate a coherent advocacy message, and participate effectively in international negotiations" (Hadden 2012). While CAN was the lead coalition coordinator throughout the 1990s and early 2000s in support of targets and timetables, by 2007, a rival network, Climate Justice Now!, had emerged. Where the CAN network of mainstream environmental organizations emphasized science-based framing of the issue and relied on information, Climate Justice Now! focused more on morality and justice approaches to climate change with a wider embrace of civil disobedience tactics. Hadden suggests that there were few binding connections – less than 1 percent of the total ties – between these two coalitions (as well as two coalitions that largely mirrored this divide) (ibid., 23). She notes that groups like Friends of the Earth (which had withdrawn from CAN) could potentially have brokered connections between the coalitions but did not.

From this evidence, she concludes that a hand already stacked against advocates, given the structural difficulties of dramatically reducing greenhouse gas emissions, became even harder to play. She argues that the lack of coherence of the movement undermined its coordination capacity and information provision. She notes that "difficulties managing tensions *within* coalitions detracted from the ability to negotiate divides *between* coalitions." Moreover, the absence of a common message and in-fighting itself became part of the story that the media picked up. The different interpretative frames also led the different factions to support different policy prescriptions. Finally, she argues that the two factions worked at cross-purposes, undermining their political influence, as the CAN group favored "the best deal possible," while the justice group favored a process that was inclusive. These differences led to some fragmentation among environmentally minded states that rallied behind each faction, which in turn produced different outcomes from the negotiations (Hadden 2012, 26–30).

Maternal mortality: an issue in search of movement unity

In 2010, nearly 300,000 women died during and after childbirth. Most of these were preventable deaths. In 2000, the UN initiated the Millennium Development Goals (MDGs), by which countries of the world committed to reducing maternal mortality 75 percent below 1990 levels by 2015 (WHO 2012c). While maternal deaths had dropped by more than 30 percent, from roughly 409,100 in 1990 to 273,500 in 2011, only 31 countries were poised to meet the MDG goal 4 for maternal mortality (Lozano et al. 2011; for an earlier study, see Hogan et al. 2010).

Maternal mortality has not traditionally commanded significant resources or attention from the global health community. Despite the launch of a safe motherhood initiative in 1987, this issue languished in relative obscurity until the mid 2000s. Unlike HIV/AIDS, maternal mortality did not experience a huge increase in resources in the early 2000s. Scholars cite insufficient cohesion and consensus among advocates as one of the major reasons contributing to this lack of profile and support.

In a 2007 piece, Shiffman and Smith note the problems advocates had in finding a resonant frame around which to mobilize and influence policy outcomes. Advocates struggled to find a common message other than "maternal mortality is a neglected tragedy that demands redress." The problem with this formulation is that "beyond this core point of agreement, the policy community until recently has had difficulty identifying common ideas" (Shiffman and Smith 2007, 1375).

The framing around "safe motherhood," which was thought to be politically neutral, ended up turning off some feminist groups and was regarded by some movement supporters as just not that compelling to

men, many of whom were in positions of influence and were not interested in women's issues. As one respondent to their research notes,
"maternal health does involve sex and sexuality; it is bloody and messy;
and I think many men (not all, of course) have a visceral antipathy for
dealing with it" (quoted in ibid., 1375).

The authors note that advocates were divided about the appropriate
policy response: "Throughout the 1970–80s antenatal risk screening and
the training of traditional birth attendants formed the core strategies for
maternal survival." However, an influential article in *The Lancet* in 1985
suggests that many maternal deaths were not preventable, particularly
without emergency obstetric care in times of need, suggesting that community care would not be sufficient. Advocates of community care
countered, and these debates increasingly took on a personal, combative
tone. These divisions led one observer to describe the situation as "one of
competing camps" (Shiffman and Smith 2007, 1374).

To make progress, they suggested that the community needed to figure
out if the focus were going to be maternal mortality or maternal health
more broadly, how to measure progress, what specific strategies would be
needed to address the problem, and how concerns about maternal mortality relate to issues like family planning, reproductive health, and health
systems development (ibid., 1376). While Shiffman and Smith identify a
host of other barriers to why advocates for maternal health had failed, they
recommend a number of remedies, beginning with fostering movement
coherence around a common platform: "First is building on the growing
cohesion in the policy community so that it can speak with authority and
unity to international and national political leaders" (ibid., 1378).

By 2006, it appears that advocates started to coalesce around a
common strategy. *The Lancet* presented a series of articles that suggested
the importance of births attended by midwives with access to more
skilled professionals if necessary. Shiffman and Smith conclude that
many of their respondents "noted a substantial decrease in tension in
the policy community, partly because of this emerging consensus." They
hesitate not to overstate this consensus, noting that there were still a
number of advocates worried about what to do in the interim while more
expansive services were unavailable for emergency situations (ibid.,
1374). Despite these concerns, the more optimistic assessment of practitioners about the issue's increasing profile has been (at least partially)
supported by analysis of funding. Between 2003 and 2008, funding for
maternal and child health increased, by one assessment, from $563
million to $1.2275 billion (in constant 2008 dollars). While this increase
was important, the authors note that this was in line with the broader
trend of increasing resources for global health (Pitt *et al.* 2010, 1488).

Climate change and maternal mortality offer just two examples of how movement incoherence can impede political influence. They suggest the utility of a comparative approach to advocacy movements, providing clues about the drivers behind success and failure. Within the AIDS arena itself, however, two episodes – first, the "failure" of global AIDS prevention and second, the decline in the domestic AIDS movement in the United States – demonstrate how one can use "within-case" variation to explore a movement's fortunes. We turn to these cases in the following sections.

Global AIDS advocacy prevention: mired in ideological spats

As many observers have noted, with the introduction of more powerful AIDS treatments in the late 1990s and early 2000s, and even the promise of a vaccine, AIDS prevention took a backseat on global health agendas. By 2008, Laurie Garrett documented how far the treatment agenda had come to displace prevention: "The slogan of the first 15 years of the pandemic was, 'Until there is a cure!' Today it seems the global health leadership of the world is satisfied with, 'Until there is lifelong drug therapy for everybody, and no prevention strategy!'" (Garrett 2008). How did treatment come to sideline prevention? Grepin observes that part of the problem was insufficient attention to which prevention strategies are most effective. AIDS treatment, in her view, was easier to measure and quantify, making it politically more attractive than prevention, whose outcomes were more opaque. Writing in 2009, she said, "There is not even agreement that prevention efforts have worked, and a lot of skepticism if they have worked at all" (Grepin 2009).

Beyond programmatic issues associated with measuring and monitoring prevention, division among AIDS advocates over prevention was one of the major reasons contributing to insufficient attention to this aspect of the AIDS crisis.[3] Where treatment united a broad coalition in support, prevention, particularly in the United States, was mired in ideological spats between advocates of abstinence and advocates of condoms. As Burkhalter notes, one of the reasons for this prevention failure was the division between AIDS advocates:

The future of U.S. global AIDS policy will be complicated, however, because the conservative groups interested in the issue have different tactical priorities than their liberal counterparts and the broader medical establishment. They have traditionally been hostile to some important AIDS-prevention strategies such as

[3] For critiques of the West's approach to prevention, see Epstein 2007; Timberg and Halperin 2012.

comprehensive sex education and condom distribution, and they are much more enthusiastic than others about policies such as the promotion of abstinence. (Burkhalter 2004)

These views were echoed by Member of Congress Jim Kolbe of Arizona, who said that "treatment had to be the centerpiece" of the US response to the global AIDS epidemic, because you "could not have built that kind of consensus on prevention, condoms vs. abstinence, couldn't have done it" (quoted in Gartner 2009a, 95, 126). By contrast, treatment was the area where consensus was possible; as one Democratic staffer on the House Foreign Affairs Committee put it: "Treatment was a different driving factor each time. The first time [2003 legislation] it allowed us to come up with a coalition. The second time, it was our rationale as to why $50 billion made sense" (quoted in ibid., 126).

The rift on prevention is evident in the rhetoric between US groups on opposing sides of the abstinence vs. condoms divide. Conservative religious organizations like Focus on the Family were opposed to condoms, arguing that "[c]ondoms promote promiscuity" and sexually transmitted diseases and suggested that abstinence-based policies form the cornerstone of the prevention agenda (Charity Wire 2003; Behrman 2004, 286; Sealy 2005). Paul Zeitz, head of the liberal Global AIDS Alliance, took the Bush administration's prevention policies to task for following the lead of conservative groups like Focus on the Family:

There are some very right wing social conservatives that are promoting a primacy of abstinence as the solution. This is not a consensus view in the Administration. The Administration is focused on best practices and scientifically proven strategies. There is NO scientific evidence anywhere that I know of that shows that abstinence only programs work.[4] (quoted in Levey 2003)

What is important here is that in other respects, groups on the left and the right were supportive of the treatment agenda. Rick Warren, conservative pastor of Saddleback Church, awarded President George W. Bush an "International Medal of PEACE" in 2008 for his service on global health and AIDS treatment in particular (Rick Warren News 2008).

Division over prevention was not purely an American problem. In his memoir, Peter Piot, the first director of UNAIDS, bemoans the Catholic Church's stance on condoms (Piot 2012, Kindle Location 4678).

---

[4] Even by 2009 and 2010, these tensions remained salient as left-leaning campaigners from ACRAA (AIDS Community Research Agenda of America) and GMHC (formerly Gay Men's Health Crisis) penned an essay called "The Christian Right: Wrong on AIDS" (Cahill and Urbano 2009).

He writes of the challenges of coming up with a prevention agenda in the UN system as late as mid 2005:

> I found I could no longer hold off the pressure from UNAIDS board members who wanted an official strategy statement on HIV prevention, as this would then not only be official policy for the whole UN system but also provide authoritative guidance for countries. I had been for years ducking this task, because I feared that what would emerge in a board made up of member states with highly divergent positions would be a more or less meaningless and diluted document. (Piot 2012, Kindle Location 6263)

The consequence of division on prevention was strategic drift and inadequate attention to prevention, particularly by the world's leaders in efforts to fight the pandemic. In 2006, the Government Accountability Office (GAO) issued a critical report on US prevention strategies, noting that Congress recommended 20 percent of the PEPFAR funds be dedicated to prevention, of which one-third should be spent on abstinence policies. These policies were to become a requirement in 2006. The GAO concludes that the spending requirement on abstinence was problematic, as it limited the ability of teams on the ground, some waiver provisions notwithstanding, "to design prevention programs that are integrated and responsive to local prevention needs" (GAO 2006). The economist Mead Over, in a Working Paper for the Center for Global Development, argues that the prevention agenda had been a failure. Over documented declining percentages of funds dedicated to prevention between 2004 and 2006 and estimated that 9 of 15 focus countries actually experienced absolute declines in prevention budgets. With, at the time, 1.4 million new infections of HIV holding steady, he concludes that "US assistance has made little measurable progress on prevention" (Over 2008, 12–13).

US domestic AIDS advocacy after the fissure of ACT UP

The absence of movement coherence and its effects can be observed in other spheres of AIDS advocacy. In the early 1990s, the domestic AIDS advocacy movement in the United States began to decline and splinter (Gould 2009). Chapters of ACT UP began to lose members and gradually wither away, though ACT UP NYC and Philadelphia remained hotspots of activity, particularly in the turn toward global treatment later in the decade. Larry Kramer, founder of ACT UP, trenchantly summarizes what happened to the organization and the broader movement in a 2012 opinion piece: "ACT UP self-destructed. For a variety of reasons, men and women who had worked so lovingly and courageously hand in hand in the kind of cooperation I have never ever seen before turned upon each other and effectively put paid to the organization's usefulness" (Kramer 2012).

Smith and Siplon catalogue a number of reasons for the movement's decline. First, government drug assistance programs became available, making the battle over domestic prices of therapies less acute and therefore less of a rallying cry. Second, with the movement's relative success in putting AIDS on the public agenda, some activists left to move on to other issues. Third, and most tragically, some of the movement's leaders died of AIDS (Smith and Siplon 2006, 35).

Of even greater importance, perhaps, some ACT UP members abandoned the organization's confrontational techniques and embraced more "cooperative" or "insider" tactics with government agencies and pharmaceutical firms. These members, led by Mark Harrington, broke off to form the Treatment Action Group (TAG) in 1992. The less-militant TAG, unlike ACT UP, hired paid staff and became more of a "conventional" NGO, providing information to its members and working closely with the public and private sectors to support funding for AIDS research and the rapid rollout of the best medicines available (Harrington 2003).

Still other AIDS activists turned their attention to other issues like Housing Works and the HIV Law Project, both of which sought to overcome discrimination in "mainstream" society. Yet another rupture occurred when ACT UP San Francisco was infiltrated by AIDS "denialists" who essentially seized the group and repurposed it to challenge the science behind AIDS. Because of the anarchic ethos of ACT UP, there were no legal or institutional means to prevent the appropriation of the group's name. The thuggish tactics of this denialist group, which sought to excoriate and intimidate movement leaders and scientists, embarrassed other ACT UP advocates and confused and tarnished the brand. As a consequence, a number of other treatment-oriented AIDS groups emerged on the San Francisco scene (Szymanski 2000; Shiffman and Smith 2007, 36). This sense of a movement adrift was captured in a 1993 *New York Times Magazine* cover story. The author, himself HIV+, wrote two days before his death: "the AIDS movement was built on grassroots efforts. Now those efforts are in disarray" (quoted in Smith and Siplon 2006, 37).

Though some might suggest that success helped kill the movement, one of the animating ideas for advocacy – finding a cure – has still not been found. Moreover, while the domestic AIDS advocacy movement in the United States had done much to speed up and usher along new treatment technologies, ACT UP and the broader movement declined before protease inhibitors and HAART were introduced in 1995 and 1996. Gould notes that in the years of "ACT UP's decline many in the movement reached a point of despair about the AIDS crisis" (Gould 2009, 269).

Gould suggests that divisions within the movement were both tactical and political, a result of different priorities and strategies for fighting AIDS. Gould notes that one of the points of contention was whether the movement's sole focus should be on fighting for AIDS drugs or addressing the wider set of issues impeding access to health care for people with AIDS, including issues of discrimination and poverty (ibid., 337). These same tensions, between the "treatment activists" who wanted to get "drugs into bodies" and the "social activists" who wanted to address issues like racism and sexism, had been around in the early days but had not led to the movement's decline. Later, these divisions would contribute to more polarized factions, roughly between HIV+ gay men and women (many of whom were HIV-negative lesbians) along with people of color, though this certainly does violence to the complexity of the splits that occurred, which were not purely based on identity-based divisions, but reflected a mix of personality clashes and divisions over strategic direction and tactics (Harrington 2003, 45–6; Saunders 2003, 27; Eigo 2004, 38–40; Gonsalves 2004, 43–5; Wolfe 2004, 96; Barr 2007, 82; Dorow 2007, 55–6; Franke-Ruta 2007, 33–4; Gould 2009, 340). One specific source of division sprang from growing distrust of the members of the "Treatment and Data Committee" of ACT UP NYC, who had gained direct access to AIDS scientists and FDA officials and were thus allegedly able to obtain new (and even experimental) treatments before others in the movement (Gould 2009, 339); indeed, it was the members of this group who were behind TAG's founding (some of these divisions are documented in the film *How to Survive a Plague*).

With the decline of the domestic movement, one might have expected deterioration in the status of people living with AIDS, but other developments helped staunch the tide of AIDS-related deaths. First, a Democratic administration more responsive to the concerns of gays and lesbians came into power. Second, the development of new, effective drug therapies, coupled with state programs to support their purchase, helped transform AIDS from a death sentence into a chronic condition in Western countries. Buoyant economic times made it possible to extend these drugs to most people living with HIV/AIDS in the United States and other advanced industrialized countries by the end of the decade. AIDS-related deaths in the United States (and other Western countries) began to decline dramatically by the end of the 1990s despite the decline of the movement.

However, the absence of a vibrant domestic advocacy movement was felt in other ways in the 2000s. Several negative developments might have been resisted or turned around had the domestic advocacy movement been as strong as it once was. First, a few American cities like Washington DC suffered shockingly high prevalence levels of HIV infection, higher than a number of countries in Africa (PBS Frontline 2012a; b). Second, while the deaths from AIDS have remained flat at around 40,000 per year since the late 1990s, new infections in the African-American community have remained high since the mid 2000s, at about 1.5 times higher than the rates of whites (CDC 2010). Moreover, with the economic crisis that began in 2008, budget restrictions in many states led to a rise in the number of people on waiting lists for ARVs, swelling to more than 9,000 people in late 2011 before emergency measures from the Obama administration reduced these to slightly more than 2,000 in mid 2012 (Sack 2010; Kulkarni 2011; NASTAD 2011; 2012). A unified advocacy movement might not have been capable to shift policies in ways to remedy all these problems (and some of them like the ARV waiting lists were addressed despite the movement's relative weakness). However, the decline of ACT UP and the lack of an aggressive domestic AIDS advocacy movement dampened the pressure on and urgency of policymakers to confront the persistent problems associated with HIV, including the lack of a cure and continued high rates of incidence and mortality, particularly in the black community.

Movement coherence and global treatment access

As we demonstrated in the previous section, incoherent, divided movements are unable to channel and coordinate their activities and information in a way that yields effective influence on target actors. Although not a sufficient condition for advocacy success, coherent movements can be more effective. Here, we assess the emergence of global treatment advocacy as the unifying objective of AIDS advocates. While we believe that coherence around this goal was essential to its progress, we also note (and more fully elaborate in the concluding chapter of this book) ongoing problems with the treatment agenda that also lead us to question how firmly institutionalized it is in the global health arena.

Anatomy of the movement

In order to address the issue of movement coherence, we first have to ask, what do we mean by the AIDS treatment advocacy movement? Do we mean exclusively activist organizations like ACT UP, the Treatment

Action Campaign (TAC), or Health GAP? Or, did the movement include sympathetic allies inside the formal governmental sector of national governments and intergovernmental organizations as well as private sector entities and individuals like foundations, for-profit companies, and health professionals? What about conservative groups like Samaritan's Purse or Rick Warren's Saddleback Church? Were they part of the global treatment advocacy movement?

If we define the realm of the movement narrowly, then understanding the roots and sources of coherence around treatment revolves around the handful of activist organizations in the United States, Europe, and countries with a large HIV/AIDS disease burden like South Africa, Brazil, and Thailand. However, seen through the prism of a wider advocacy network, the movement was much broader and included allies inside governments and international organizations, as well as within pharmaceutical firms, both branded and generic. Indeed, in Keck and Sikkink's foundational work on the topic, individuals from international organizations as well as sympathetic elites inside the executive branch and legislature can also be part of the wider network (Keck and Sikkink 1998, 9).

As former UNAIDS director Peter Piot documents in his memoir, the "broad coalition" supporting treatment access included people like himself inside the architecture of global organizations and national governments (Piot 2012). Indeed, for activists to succeed, they needed a large number of "Piots" inside governments and international organizations as allies. Moreover, the Piots were not merely the passive recipients of civil society ministrations about what was to be done. They were advocates in their own right, with agendas and perceptions not always in keeping with what activist organizations on the outside wanted. Piot described himself, among other things, as "a stubborn campaigner reaching out to the powerful of this world and bringing AIDS awareness to unexpected places ... an activist from the beginning" (Piot 2012, Kindle Location 102).

Moreover, many individuals in the official governmental sector would go on to create their own foundations and civil society organizations that became powerful change agents, most notably the Clinton Foundation's work through CHAI. Also influential were vehicles such as the Global Business Coalition against AIDS founded by the US diplomat Richard Holbrooke, who played a prominent role in prodding the UN Security Council to host a special session on AIDS as a threat to international peace and security in January 2000.

In this sense, the portrait of transnational advocacy networks in Keck and Sikkink's work may have much in common with the networks of government officials described in Anne-Marie Slaughter's book, *A New*

World Order (Slaughter 2004). Both capture transnational processes of like-minded people finding each other across borders to form webs of common purpose and expertise, with Keck and Sikkink having a wider aperture to encompass non-governmental actors.

The government and intergovernmental officials who supported changes in IP rules that facilitated access as well as the drug quality and procurement policies that opened the door to generic competition also can be considered part of the broader advocacy network. Certainly, Kofi Annan was the most prominent intergovernmental proponent of access, "the world's chief AIDS advocate" in Piot's description (Piot 2012, Kindle Location 4265). In April 2001, Annan made the keynote address at a summit in Abuja, Nigeria, where he called for the creation of a $7–$10 billion fund to fight HIV/AIDS and other infectious diseases (Annan 2001). In June 2001, the UN General Assembly had a special session on HIV/AIDS, which set as one of its top priorities "treatment to all those infected" (UN 2001).

To build support for this initiative inside the UN, Annan relied on a network of allies in it, including his deputy, Louise Frechette, his senior adviser on HIV/AIDS, R.P. Eddy, as well as Piot at UNAIDS, Mark Malloch Brown at UNDP, and Gro Harlem Brundtland, and her successor, Jong Wook Lee, at the WHO. Once the Global Fund was created in 2002, its first executive director, Richard Feachem, was responsible for helping create an important funding platform that facilitated generic access. Less prominent officials include Lembit Rago and Andre Van Zyl at the WHO, who led the efforts to create the prequalification for medicines program, discussed in Chapter 6.

One of the interesting features of AIDS advocacy is how outsiders become insiders, as movements mature and their aims become institutionalized in policy. For example, in 2009 MSF advocate Ellen 't Hoen joined UNITAID to lead the MPP.[5] Other prominent examples include Partners in Health co-founder Jim Kim, who would go on to lead the WHO's 3 by 5 initiative to extend ARV treatment to 3 million people by 2005 (and later the World Bank), as well as Christoph Benn, a German AIDS campaigner who became Director of External Relations at the Global Fund. Less prominent examples include the MSF pharmacist Carmen Perez Casas, who would go on to work at the Global Fund and UNAIDS, and American campaigner Eric Sawyer, who became the UNAIDS Civil Society Partnership Advisor.

---

[5] UNITAID is an innovative financing mechanism hosted by the WHO, with the Medicines Patent Pool, before spinning off as an independent entity in 2010, beginning as an internal project to fund new drug developments.

Aside from international organizations, government officials in key countries had an important role as advocates for market transformation. Brazilian officials such as former health minister José Serra, and Paolo Teixiera, then head of the agency's AIDS program, played a particularly prominent role in this regard. Nunn described Serra's relationship with the Brazilian AIDS movement as "symbiotic" (Nunn 2008, 140–1). Having adopted national legislation in 1996 that made free, universal HIV/AIDS treatment a right, the Brazilian government was committed to driving the costs of ARVs down. The state-run drug company Far-Manguinhos, under the leadership of Eloan Pinheiro from 1994 to 2002, procured raw materials from generic drug producers in India to bring down the costs of ARVs (Flynn 2008). Moreover, Brazil, through its negotiator Francisco Cannabrava, led efforts in 2001 at Doha to defend the rights of poor nations to use TRIPS flexibilities during health emergencies (Nunn 2008, 138–42).

One way to think about the movement is in terms of different constellations or nodes. A study depicting the US advocacy landscape identified four somewhat overlapping constituencies: (1) one including the Global AIDS Roundtable (a network of 100 organizations staffed by the Global Health Council, that included groups like CARE as well as the AFL-CIO); (2) another around more left-leaning advocacy-oriented organizations including the Global AIDS Alliance (launched in 2001), MSF, Health GAP, the Advocacy Network for Africa, and the RESULTS Alliance; (3) another of evangelical Christians; and, finally, (4) the last centered on Bono's more centrist advocacy outfits DATA and the ONE Campaign that were created in January 2002 and May 2004, respectively (and which merged in 2007) (McDonnell 2007).

This portrait, of course, largely captures the civil society actors but does not pick up on the change agents inside the US government who supported treatment access, notably the president and his then National Security Advisor, Condoleezza Rice, as well as others who supported or helped create PEPFAR, such as Anthony Fauci of the NIH, Mark Dybul (at the time also at NIH), then Deputy Chief of Staff Josh Bolten, Senior Policy Advisor Jay Lefkowitz, Robin Cleveland from the Office of Management and Budget, Deputy National Security Advisor Gary Edson, speechwriter Michael Gerson, as well as Congressional allies like Senator Bill Frist (Behrman 2004, 293; Lefkowitz 2009).

Including conservative activists and organizations in the United States as part of the broader treatment movement is potentially more problematic, since groups like Samaritan's Purse, Empower America, and the Family Research Council had views antithetical to groups like ACT UP and Health GAP on a number of issues, both those specifically related to AIDS prevention, but also wider social issues like treatment of gays and lesbians. However, ignoring their presence as supporters of the treatment movement would do violence to the historical record, since such groups are often mentioned as being especially influential in shaping the Bush administration's awareness of and approach to the problem (Behrman 2004, 270; Burkhalter 2004; Chawla 2005, 26; Lefkowitz 2009; Busby 2010a).

Moreover, describing networks as passing constellations of common purpose, as Grebe does, captures the way in which diverse groups can come together. Such an approach makes intelligible Piot's depiction of just some of the diverse actors that supported a common agenda:

> What could the South African Chamber of Mines, Anglican Church, Community Party, and trades unions have in common with the Treatment Action Campaign, Médecins Sans Frontières, and UNAIDS? A common goal: defeating the AIDS epidemic and caring for its victims. A powerful joint desire to be a force for change. (Piot 2012, Kindle Location 4757)

Grebe provides a portrait of the network in South Africa (TAC) at the center with organizations and individual activists radiating around the leaders of TAC (which included Zackie Achmat, Mark Heywood, and Nathan Geffen) and the AIDS Law Project (which included Jonathan Berger). In his depiction, Grebe shows TAC being orbited by allies in South African civil society organizations like trade unions, churches, and NGOs, as well as those inside state institutions and the South African scientific community.

TAC was also supported by a variety of international actors, including allies in UNAIDS and the WHO (including Peter Piot, Stephen Lewis, Kalle Almedal, and Kevin De Cock). In addition to support by international NGOs including MSF and Oxfam, TAC was supported by other international organizations like the International Treatment Preparedness Coalition (ITPC), a coalition of national organizations dedicated to treatment access that was formed in 2003. In particular, Grebe noted that TAC received support from several US civil society groups, including the ACT UP NYC/Treatment Action Group (with Gregg Gonsalves and Mark Harrington as key individuals), ACT UP Philadelphia/Health GAP (with Alan Berkman, Asia Russell, and Paul Davis as key individuals), and CPTech (with Jamie Love and Thiru Balasubramaniam the main points of contact) (Grebe 2008, 28). Although Grebe does not mention them, we know that Bernard Pécoul and Ellen 't Hoen at MSF were key individuals as well.

In Grebe's analysis, South African scientists are included as part of an "epistemic community" of experts who supported access on the basis of their professional analysis of the AIDS pandemic and the best means to address it. Internationally, there were a number of physicians and scholars from various disciplines who were prominent in supporting treatment access, notably Paul Farmer, co-founder of Partners in Health, whose treatments projects in Haiti featured as an exemplar of what could be done in resource-poor settings. Farmer was consulted by the Bush administration in the lead-up to the creation of PEPFAR, and a number of other experts also had a hand in shaping PEPFAR. The health expert and head of the Global Health Council, Nils Daulaire, the Cornell doctor, Jean William Pape (who, along with Farmer, had done pioneering work in Haiti), the physician and former Clinton official Eric Goosby, and the Ugandan doctor Peter Mugyenyi, are also credited as being especially influential in helping shape Bush administration thinking on HIV/AIDS (Behrman 2004, 293; Lefkowitz 2009).

Beyond these doctors and scientists, the economist Jeffrey Sachs is often credited for helping Kofi Annan and the UN with estimates of the billions that would be needed to support treatment access. Nine months before Kofi Annan would call for a multi-billion fund to support AIDS treatment in Nigeria, Sachs made such a call at the July 2000 Durban International AIDS Conference (Attaran and Sachs 2002; Behrman 2004, 254).[6] Sachs was also prominent in linking economic performance and health more generally.

Largely missing from this universe, however, are private sector supporters of access, foremost among them leaders of the Indian generics industry. The Indian generic drug maker Cipla, led by Yusuf Hamied, was the leading generics company whose collaborations with activists at MSF and CPTech helped transform the ARV market with the offer to sell a low-cost triple ARV cocktail in September 2000. However, even before Hamied and Cipla's entry into the ARV market, other Indian generic drug makers had been selling Active Pharmaceutical Ingredients (APIs) to Brazil, beginning with Ranbaxy, later overshadowed by Hetero, and joined later still by Aurobindo (d'Adesky 2004, 54).

Some members of the branded pharmaceutical community took up the cause of treatment access as well. Indeed, this community worked closely with UNAIDS in creating the first major initiatives to promote global treatment rollout, namely, the DAI and AAI; these are described in more detail in Chapter 5. While some members of the treatment movement clearly demonized the branded pharmaceutical firms and believed that their property rights were the main barrier to universal drug access, others like

---

[6] In Piot's memoir, Bernard Schwartländer of UNAIDS and other colleagues are credited for working up such a figure (Piot 2012, Kindle Locations 5052–69).

Peter Piot tried to provide a bridge that brought these actors into the same big tent, with the common objective of getting "drugs into bodies."

Beyond describing the landscape of organizations and individuals involved in treatment advocacy, identifying their different functions offers useful details that suggest advocates can play far more varied roles than lobbying or protest activity. For example, MSF did seek to influence policy through a coordinated lobbying campaign, but its credibility in policy circles emanated from its experience as a medical service provider in developing countries. MSF was one of the early adopters of ARVs and, like the physician Paul Farmer, played a key role in demonstrating the feasibility of extending treatment access in resource-poor settings. At the same time, MSF is a primary conduit for information on drug prices. Since 2001, its annual report, *Untangling the Web of Price Reductions*, served as a key guide to prices in an environment that had little information, until the creation of WHO's Global Price Reporting Mechanism in 2004. MSF also played an important role as an interlocutor with the Indian generic company Cipla as it made its foray into offering its products globally at reduced prices.

Other activists from civil society like ACT UP and Health GAP have played a more traditional role as strident activists, using dramatic protest activity, to target recalcitrant companies and politicians. Jamie Love of CPTech was a close ally, but he and his small organization relied more on their expertise in IP law both to shape the strategic direction of groups like Health GAP and also to advise governments like South Africa. Some organizations like the Global AIDS Alliance were similar in tone to Health GAP and ACT UP but focused their advocacy on more traditional lobbying in Washington DC. Although certainly insider strategies were part of ACT UP and Health GAP's repertoire of activities, more centrist advocacy organizations like DATA and the ONE Campaign focused on less confrontational insider tactics, using celebrity power and bipartisan allies to move the treatment agenda forward. Still other insider organizations, like church groups, relied on their connections to lawmakers and the testimony of the faith communities they worked with through overseas missionary activity.

Other advocates' groups played a central role in actual market organization. As described in Chapter 5, CHAI sought to organize both generic suppliers and buyers in the developing world. They drew their convening power from former President Clinton but helped provide a global public good through demand forecasts that allowed generic providers to envision forward pricing based on expanded volumes. Advocates on the inside of government and intergovernmental organizations like Peter Piot of UNAIDS, Richard Feachem of the Global Fund, and Mark Dybul of NIH and PEPFAR, proved to be key allies who helped steer their respective organizations to support the treatment agenda. Where Piot's role primarily involved coordinating information collection about the epidemic and using his "bully pulpit" to gain political and business support for an expanded treatment agenda, Feachem and Dybul were more operational, with Feachem guiding the policies of the new entity the Global Fund as a pass-through multilateral financing agency and Dybul as one of the lead actors in the bilateral US program.

As important as these diverse advocates were, their efforts would likely have remained stillborn were it not for the mobilization of communities of people living with AIDS in affected countries. While South Africa's TAC is perhaps the most well-known treatment advocacy organization, grass-roots groups of affected populations from a variety of other countries helped put AIDS treatment front and center on the agenda of the international community. TAC, like MSF, had a role in direct treatment provision, but it also had a strong advocacy role, first in challenging the legitimacy of the pharma company-led lawsuit against the South African government before turning its campaign skills to the South African government itself once AIDS denialism had taken root in the government of Nelson Mandela's successor, Thabo Mbeki. Part of TAC's role was to mobilize legal support for its cause, but where groups like Health GAP and ACT UP used dramatic, non-violent civil disobedience to attract media attention, TAC's strength often came from the large numbers of people that the campaign could mobilize through mass demonstrations.

Beyond South Africa's TAC, the ITPC's coalition of affected communities in different countries was important, particularly in the mid 2000s as the challenge moved to implementation of extended access at the national level. Focusing on the state level, Chorev described this process as the diffusion of strategies by governments seeking to take advantage of TRIPS flexibilities that permitted countries to override patent protections for health emergencies (Chorev 2012). The expansion of access was also championed by activists (for a deft exploration of these issues, particularly with respect to the supportive role played by activists in international negotiations, see Matthews 2011). Gonsalves, for his part, emphasized the role of local activists. He described the role of the ITPC as a "binding tie," with activists knitted together largely through email and listservs. If you had a map of the world, every continent has at least two or three very powerful voices. Around the world, you have a core of one or two dozen really intense AIDS activists, and as you go deeper, there are thousands of people involved (Gonsalves 2012b).

One of those was the Indian activist Loon Gangte, one of the founders of the Indian treatment advocacy group the Delhi Network of Positive

People (DNP+). Gangte was elected to be ITPC's South Asia representative in 2004. He described their work as efforts to defend the capacities of Indian generic companies to produce low-cost generics: "At DNP+ we have worked on IP/Patent issues since 2004. So far, we have filed approximately fifteen Pre-Grant Opposition [appeals to the Indian government opposing patents] on various ARV drugs and some other drugs, so each time we have a rally it is easy to relay and pass on the messages to our friends in different parts of the world seeking their support and solidarity" (Gangte 2012).

Similarly, in Thailand, a number of groups like the Thailand Network of People living with HIV/AIDS (TNP+) and the AIDS Access Foundation led the way in promoting access by challenging patents, leading a number of high-profile campaigns to steel the resolve of the Thai government with respect to access to ARVs. After campaigners challenged the government to issue a compulsory license for ddI from BMS, the Thai government took the issue to a national-level court and won in 2002, allowing local production of the drug (Kaplan 2002). The 2004 International AIDS Society meeting in Bangkok provided a focal point for continued mobilization. In 2006 and 2007, local activists and their international allies pressed the government to issue a compulsory license for Abbott's combination drug Kaletra and Merck's efavirenz (Fuller 2007). In the 2000s, the challenge increasingly became one of extending and overcoming barriers to access, with an emphasis on how communities affected by the virus could access treatment services and how, in turn, their governments could tap into the resources now made available for treatment from their own governments, the Global Fund, PEPFAR, and other donors. Here, newer groups like the Thai AIDS Treatment Action Group (TTAG) were instrumental in working with under-served and discriminated groups like intravenous drug users, prisoners, migrants, the transgendered population, and sex workers. Formed by Paisan Suwannawong, a founder of TNP+, TTAG focused its energies on preparing local leaders in the PWA community to have the knowledge and skills to secure access at the provincial level (Kaplan 2012).

As suggested above, transborder collaboration by activists in the ITPC network allowed local activists in developing countries to learn from each other, both in terms of effective advocacy but also programming, as resource-poor countries innovated by necessity. At the same time, Northern activists also sought to support their allies. Northern activists living in affected countries had long been some of the key interlocutors to local organizations and treatment access. For example, Richard Stern, through the Costa Rica-based Agua Buena Human Rights Association, has pressed for Central American treatment access since the late 1990s.[7] In the mid-to-late 2000s, some Western activists moved to work with affected communities. Gregg Gonsalves moved to South Africa for two years beginning in 2006, and Health GAP's Asia Russell and Paul Davis moved to Uganda and Kenya in 2010 and 2009, respectively. For her part, Karyn Kaplan, who had been active in Health GAP, moved back to Thailand in 2002 to launch TTAG with her partner, Paisan Suwannawong. She described the support role of Northern activists: "we should never be speaking for anybody. We should be standing alongside them. As a person from the global North working in the global South, we have very distinct value-added roles," allowing local actors to amplify their access to resources, information, and influence. For example, as an American citizen, she described how she was able to visit the USTR office in Washington and raise issues of concern to Thai activists. Together, they were able to communicate the concerns of the advocacy community (Kaplan 2012).

How the movement cohered

Greatly facilitated by the Internet, networks of like-minded individuals came to know each other through a variety of meetings, conferences, and personal connections. For example, leaders of TAC like Zackie Achmat had heard of the American advocacy movement ACT UP, and during a visit to New York in 2000, he came to know former ACT UP members Gregg Gonsalves and Mark Harrington through a mutual friend, Loring McAlpin. Gonsalves and other US activists assisted TAC later in the year in a series of treatment literacy workshops in South Africa (Grebe 2008, 25).

American activists also came to know each other through similar connections. In 1998, Gregg Pappas, acting head of international health in the Department of Health and Human Services, suggested to Jamie Love of CPTech that he meet with ACT UP Philadelphia, which is how Love came to speak at their January 1999 meeting where he got to know Paul Davis and Asia Russell (Sell 2001, 502).[8] Love's work and point of view were also given a platform in *AIDS Treatment News*, written by John S. James. Through contacts with Health GAP founding members Bob

---

[7] See www.aguabuena.org/ingles/index.php.
[8] Behrman's account has Love in New York attending the preliminary meeting of Health GAP in January 1999 along with Russell, Paul Davis, Bob Lederer, among others, fifteen or twenty activists all told (Behrman 2004, 137). Paul Davis is not listed on the official notes as an attendee (Health GAP Coalition 1999). Asia Russell suggested there may have been another late 1998 meeting between her, Davis, and Love (Russell 2012).

Lederer and John Riley, James came to know about Jamie Love (James 2012). Beginning in March 1999, James carried out a series of interviews with Love on compulsory licensing and other topics.[9]

Similarly, the story of Cipla's leadership in the production of ARVs also was one of serendipity and connections. In August 2000, David Langdon, a former Peace Corps volunteer, called on Bill Haddad, a former leading official in the early days of the Peace Corps who had gone on to become a leader in the generic drug business. Langdon asked Haddad to meet with Jamie Love from CPTech, Rob Weissman with Essential Action (which, like CPTech, was another Ralph Nader-founded organization), and Bill Richard. They discussed how to identify sources of raw materials for drugs that were not controlled by branded drug companies. Haddad called on a friend, Agnes Varis, who said in turn to contact Yusuf Hamied of Cipla (Haddad 2001). After talking with Hamied by phone, the group flew to London to meet with him in person, where Hamied suggested that his company's three ARV drug combination therapy cost $350 per patient per year at the factory door. They were able to help wangle a speaking slot for Dr. Hamied at a September 2000 European Commission meeting where Hamied made the offer to supply ARVs wholesale at $800 to $1,000 per patient. At that meeting, Hamied met Bernard Pécoul from MSF. Love then traveled to India in December 2000 to identify ways trade rules could be written to facilitate generic competition. There, he encouraged Cipla to draft letters to drug companies that held patents on AIDS drugs for a voluntary license to produce the drugs. A month later, Love was in Geneva for the World Health Assembly and attended a dinner party held by Pécoul, where he suggested that a $350 annual per patient ARV price might be possible. Love then encouraged Hamied to offer his triple cocktail at a dollar a day. In February 2001, Hamied offered to supply MSF clinics with the triple cocktail for $350 per patient per year. Soon thereafter, with Love's help, that offer was front page news around the world (McNeil Jr. 2001; Pearl and Freedman 2001).

International meetings also served as important occasions by which advocates came to know each other and develop deeper working relationships. For example, MSF on the heels of its Nobel Peace Prize, launched its Access Campaign in 1999. One of the first AIDS-related events was an important meeting on compulsory licensing in Geneva co-hosted by the Dutch-based Health Action International (HAI) and CPTech in March 1999.[10] Among the 120 meeting participants were Thai and American

---

[9] See http://ww1.aegis.org/pubs/atn/1999/.
[10] HAI and CPTech had collaborated on other endeavors for several years (Sell 2001).

activists, including Eric Sawyer and Asia Russell of ACT UP, as well as Bill Haddad, who would later go on to become a Cipla intermediary after helping activists make the initial connection (CPTech 1999a; HAI 1999a). In November 1999, the three organizations hosted a companion conference in Amsterdam in the lead-up to the disastrous WTO meeting that year in Seattle. Attended by 350 participants, the conference generated a statement on access to medicines at the meeting (CPTech 1999d). Among the presenters were Gro Harlem Brundtland and activists Asia Russell and Zackie Achmat, as well as Partners in Health co-founder Jim Kim (HAI 1999b). Similarly, Piot notes the importance of the World Economic Forum meetings in Davos, Switzerland, as providing a venue for meetings with pharmaceutical executives and activists (Piot 2012).

International AIDS conferences served as pivotal moments for advocates to get to know each other and coordinate strategy. For example, Piot met Eric Sawyer at the 1994 Paris Global AIDS Summit, a meeting organized by the French minister of health that brought together some members of civil society, researchers, and government officials. Sawyer was on the board of the Global Network for People Living with HIV (GNP+). Piot was seeking support from GNP+ and from Sawyer individually for his candidacy to become the first director of UNAIDS. Out of that meeting, Piot and Sawyer forged some common bonds, and while they would have differences of opinion on some issues, Sawyer describes the relationship that they sustained throughout Piot's tenure at UNAIDS. They had fairly frequent contact by phone and met in person if they were in the same city. They strategized about a number of things, and Piot would alert Sawyer about issues that were problematic, or new initiatives from UNAIDS. Sawyer attended a number of consultations associated with UNAIDS and the World Health Assembly. Coordination was especially vigorous around International AIDS conferences. Piot would solicit feedback and ask for ideas about how to distribute information, what would be the response of PWAs, and how it could be improved. Sawyer would also frequently reach out to him if problems on positions they were taking, or policies on WHO, UNAIDS, or other co-sponsors. In short, Sawyer said Piot was "always willing to listen" and that the two "agreed more often than disagreed" (Sawyer 2012).

Advocates also collaborated transnationally on joint actions at the International AIDS Society meetings, the 2000 meeting in Durban, South Africa, being particularly important, where the activists staged a joint march, and, at other gatherings like the UN General Assembly meeting that took place in June 2001. Some coalitions, like the Jubilee 2000 campaign for developing country debt relief, had a common platform that groups subscribed to when they joined the coalition, and different organizations also became shareholders in the central secretariat. The global AIDS treatment access movement was more fragmented, with no single organization at the center, but groups found other ways to coordinate their activities. As 't Hoen noted, there was some level of coordination at the very least not to "bite each other's tails." Both conference calls and international meetings served to help the different organizations coordinate ('t Hoen 2010). Pécoul also described the collaboration and coordination in similar terms, as "totally informal" and "very flexible." Although they were in permanent communication, there was "never signed any agreement with any of these groups" (however, advocates found other ways to generate periodic common platforms like the statement coming out of the 1999 Amsterdam meeting). The informal process, Pécoul suggested, facilitated swift action, as a more formal coalition would have meant that the activists spent all of their time trying to reach consensus (Pécoul 2012).

As is true for all contemporary late twentieth- and early twenty-first-century social movements, the internet has become a vital means to share information and coordinate actions, particularly internationally. Listservs including the IP-health listserv,[11] the Health GAP listserv,[12] and the Global Aids Alliance listserv[13] were among the more prominent examples. With many American treatment activists associated with Health GAP on the east coast of the United States, particularly in New York, Philadelphia and Washington DC, it was possible to have periodic in-person meetings. However, activists quickly found it easier to coordinate through conference calls. Health GAP, for example, would have a core conference call that preceded a larger conference call that included allies.

The most basic means of solidarity and support that groups used was the common sign-on letter. Gonsalves described the sign-on letter, where activists lend their name to an email letter or petition as the "default position" to get the message across. He suggested it was the easiest way to exert pressure to show support for some given issue. Such letters happen all the time, in the early days as often as once a month. In his view, it was rare to have people say no to such letters. They are generally items (like getting methadone on the essential medicines list) that activists have pretty broad consensus on and are not controversial within the movement (Gonsalves 2012b).

---

[11] http://lists.essential.org/pipermail/ip-health/.
[12] https://lists.critpath.org/pipermail/healthgap/. The list dates back further, to at least 2003.
[13] http://health.groups.yahoo.com/group/Global-AIDS-Alliance/.

These were quite frequent in this era, beginning with a sign-on letter associated with the first Health GAP action on African trade bills in 1999 (Love 1999a), followed by a letter to Vice President Gore on US pressure on South Africa's Medicines Act and another preceding the 1999 WTO meeting in Seattle (CPTech 1999b; c). In 2000, Health GAP actions focused on coordinated actions with TAC in the lead-up to the Durban AIDS conference in the summer. In 2001, international activists sent a letter to pharmaceutical companies urging them to desist in the lawsuit against the South African government (Health GAP Coalition 2001a). Later that year, they circulated a letter over the structure of the soon to be created Global Fund (Health GAP Coalition 2001b). In 2002, activists circulated letters to USTR Robert Zoellick and the TRIPS Council at the WTO about IPR rules for countries that lacked manufacturing capability to produce drugs (CPTech 2002a; b). The legal rights of these countries to import generic versions of drugs was left underspecified in the 2001 Doha Health exception. The following year, activists sent in separate but coordinated letters on the proposed Free Trade Act of the Americas (Health GAP Coalition 2003).

By 2004, actions focused on preserving the space opened up for generics. Advocates pressed Randall Tobias, the US global AIDS coordinator, to pursue the use of generic ARVs and other drugs through PEPFAR (Health GAP Coalition 2004a). Advocates also sent the Indian government a joint letter urging it to defend the rights of generic drug companies and the country's legal flexibilities as it became TRIPS compliant in 2005 (Health GAP Coalition 2004b). Additional letters were sent in subsequent years on G8 support for the MDGs (2005), Thailand's pursuit of a compulsory license (2006), Abbott's perceived retaliation in Thailand (2007), IMF gold sales and health funding (2008), and G7 countries and Global Fund financial support (2009) (Physicians for Human Rights 2005; CPTech 2006; Health GAP Coalition 2007, 2008, 2009).

Pre-convergence

Early on, even before more effective treatment options became available, American activists who were interested in the global dimensions of AIDS had difficulty finding support among their peers. Paul Boneberg was one such activist. In the 1980s, "Boneberg found himself alone" among American activists concerned about global issues (Behrman 2004, 120). During the transition to the Clinton administration, AIDS activists met to try to draft a position paper to influence the incoming administration. Boneberg pressed for global issues, and the response was: "[i]t's inappropriate for us to create something in the transition document that none of us have ever worked on or know about" (ibid., 124). Based on his earlier work organizing candlelight vigils around the world to remember those who had died from the disease, Boneberg founded the Global AIDS Action Network (GAAN) in 1994 to prod American AIDS organizations to take more seriously the global challenge.

Kate Krauss, an early ACT UP San Francisco activist who later relocated to Philadelphia after the 1996 AIDS meeting in Vancouver, also discussed the difficulty motivating her peers in the advocacy community to take on global issues. She said there was a lot of push back in the mid 1990s while she was still in California. At the time, a lot of people were dying. Her strategy was just to bring the issue up over and over again. She asked the group to sign on to a letter. She made the argument that you can't care about some of the people who are HIV+ positive unless you care about all of them (Krauss 2012).

Piot recounted that his early efforts to take on treatment in the developing world fell on deaf ears. At a 1996 meeting in Washington DC at the Red Cross, American activists told him "that they needed all their energy to ensure access to treatment in the United States and to support American AIDS patients who had lost jobs and home. They wished me good luck, but that was it" (Piot 2012, 252; for Paul Boneberg's similar account, see Behrman 2004, 126). Piot received the same reaction in response to his speech at the Vancouver International AIDS conference in the same year:

I remember very well when there was a conference in Vancouver in '96 when it became clear that there was effective treatment available – not a cure, but treatment. I gave a speech there also in the opening, and I immediately said, "Let's make sure that we do not exclude the majority of people living with HIV from that treatment." But nobody paid attention to that, because the agenda was "Let's get as many people as possible on treatment in the developed world." AIDS activists hadn't shown the slightest interest in AIDS in Africa, in the developing world. That was coming later, when treatment was accessible. (Frontline 2006)

Eric Sawyer, whom Piot described as a "rare, early convert to the global perspective," made a similar observation. At the 1996 summit, just as the evidence of PIs was giving people more hope of effective treatment therapies, Sawyer also gave a speech spurring conference-goers to think about the alarming number of people in developing countries that lacked access to even more basic medications to fight off opportunistic infections. He noted that he and Piot shared drafts of their speeches. In his speech, Sawyer called for tiered pricing by drug companies, and from donors a partnership to pay for it:

To the drug companies people with AIDS say it's time to drop your prices. Drug companies should consider developing a two tier pricing system that allows reasonable profits to be made from the rich. But, AIDS treatments must also be made available to the poor everywhere, at cost or at very minimal levels of profit. And if you drug companies don't make this shift voluntarily we will advocate for governmental regulations to mandate this and fight to have your patents taken away from you .... To the development agencies, UNAIDS and USAID PWAs say "we need a Global Initiative to get treatments to poor people, especially in developing countries." (Sawyer 1996)

Sawyer said the reaction among other treatment activists was swift and ferocious: "And that speech got a fair amount of press, and kind of jump-started the whole access to treatment for the developing world campaign. And not without huge negative reaction from the treatment activist community." Sawyer said even as he and Piot were thinking about strategy and next steps, the negative reaction from the treatment activists was striking:

And the treatment activist people were furious. They wouldn't even talk to me. Some of them were, "How fucking dare you. How dare you get up there and say that. Who do you think you are?" It was like, who the fuck do you think you are? Maybe you've got access to treatment, but what about the three million people that are going to die this year in the developing world, because they don't? I'm glad I was able to use my big mouth to bring voice to some of those issues. (Sawyer 2004)

Sawyer suggested that the response among senior activists was both to appeal to unmet needs in the United States and to the lack of capacity in the developing world:

Look, we can't meet the needs of clients in Manhattan, let alone Brooklyn or the Bronx. There is no way we are prepared to take on AIDS in the developing world or AIDS in Africa, especially since they don't have clean water or wood in Africa. Until we get everyone who needs treatment in the Bronx or until they get clean water in Africa, don't talk to us about AIDS in Africa. (quoted in Behrman 2004, 123)

Boneberg, in the inaugural Health GAP meeting in January 1999, was recorded as making a similar point:

What I don't know is if the AIDS group has the consensus and clout to mobilize the pharmaceutical companies quickly. I'm not sure if there is a consensus in the American AIDS community for global access issues .... The community is more ready than they were two years ago, but I think that AIDS activists in N.Y. could really start something. (Health GAP Coalition 1999)

Boneberg noted that once treatment became available in the United States, American AIDS groups understood the inequity: "As soon as they realized there was a discrepancy, they were there." However, even once they recognized the moral claims that others living with HIV around the world had, they still had a difficult decision about whether to prioritize resources and staff time to engage the issue directly. Some, like the San Francisco AIDS Foundation and the National Association for People With AIDS (NAPWA), did so wholeheartedly (Boneberg 2012).

Other activists, perhaps a little later to the scene than first-generation AIDS activists, experienced more favorable reactions to the push for treatment access. For her part, Asia Russell suggested that for the members of ACT UP Philadelphia, "as they learned about the issue, there was immediate resonance. There was no sentiment that this would be taking money from our backyard to people we don't know" (Russell 2012).

Convergence: drug access and prices

Even if the 1996 meeting in Vancouver did not generate immediate favorable reception for global treatment access, the possibility of effective treatment in Boneberg's view, changed everything (Behrman 2004, 135). As he noted, before HAART therapy became available in 1996, there was not the possibility of a divide between rich and poor countries (Boneberg 2012).[14] But the differences were not nearly as stark as when ARVs became available that transformed HIV into a chronic, manageable condition.

One can date the change and transformation in the aperture of American activists to consider the global implications of the problem when death rates from AIDS in the United States declined from a peak just above 40,000 in 1995. They fell to slightly more than 30,000 a year later, before declining to just above 16,000 in 1998, where it has hovered almost ever since (Behrman 2004, 134; see Slide 4 in CDC 2010).

While the turn to global treatment access did follow the decline in AIDS-related mortality in the United States, the change among American treatment activists was not immediate. Krauss talked about the transformation that gradually occurred. After she relocated to Philadelphia in 1996, there was still push back, but less. There was not a repudiation of focusing on local problems. She observed, "[a] moment of people opening their hearts" and suggested, "Once they did, [they] never had that problem again." In her view, this opening, which she saw simultaneously taking place in other AIDS treatment groups across the

---

[14] But, as Sawyer noted, there were huge inequalities in access to treatment to ward off opportunistic infections that some had been battling since the mid-to-late 1980s (Sawyer 2012).

United States, occurred about a year after she had been in Philadelphia, which would have been late 1997 or early 1998 (Krauss 2012).

Others see the general willingness to embrace global treatment access as occurring a bit later. Behrman notes that in 1998, when news of the tremendous decline in AIDS deaths in the United States became known, interest began to fade. In Sawyer's perspective, it still took several years for people to come around. "It really didn't change until probably in the 2000s. It was a kind of bit of holdover from resistance from the U.S.-based treatment activists." In part, he attributes the willingness of other American AIDS activists to join the global access movement as a product of the success of ACT UP and Health GAP, in partnership with CPTech and MSF, in putting the issues of compulsory licensing on the agenda. Initially, he said, activists like himself dealt with this opposition by "organizing around them" (Sawyer 2012).

For his part, Pécoul suggested that the first order of business was to build consensus within MSF itself before reaching out to other groups. The MSF Access Campaign began in 1998, supported by the prize money the group was awarded when it won the Nobel Prize in 1999. With MSF composed of 5 operational centers and 19 national sections, creating consensus within the organization was an initial challenge. Pécoul indicated there was initially a lot of disagreement and that the initial campaign was an internal one. Many MSF doctors in the field were finding large numbers of patients with HIV. Some registered concerns about cost-effectiveness and feasibility, particularly since ARVs have to be taken for the remainder of the person's life. He said that when there is disagreement within MSF, they generally start with a pilot project to test a new idea. In this case, pilot projects started in 1999 and 2000 in Thailand, Cameroon, South Africa, Cambodia, and Kenya in parallel with the campaign (Pécoul 2012).

How did activists converge on prices and access as the heart of their strategy? As the Health GAP coalition took shape, the branded pharmaceutical companies that produced ARVs seemed like "a logical target for the activists. The drug companies had by and large refused to entertain price adjustments for the developing world. Though price was only one impediment – though irrefutably a critical one – to ensuring global access, it was an obvious one" (Behrman 2004, 137). Mark Milano made a similar point about why activists focused on drug access. At the Durban conference, he made a speech noting that the problems of AIDS seemed overwhelming (given challenges of infrastructure, poverty, unemployment, oppression of women, stigma), but one thing, from his perspective, that could be fixed in the short-run, was that drugs could be put on the shelves of clinics. In Milano's view, if that happened, everything else would follow (Milano 2012). Piot made a similar point in his memoir, reflecting the convergence around drug access and pricing: "I thought, well, fixing the health systems across Africa is probably more than UNAIDS can handle right now. And promoting more testing, when the drugs weren't available, simply wouldn't work: there was no incentive. So my conclusion was that we needed to get the price of the drugs down before we worked on the rest" (Piot 2012, Kindle Location 5276).

By the early 2000s, as the activist Gregg Gonsalves noted, people rallied around treatment. He suggested that everybody in the AIDS advocacy community wanted money for treatment. Everybody involved knew they had to get prices down (Gonsalves 2012b). However, even if there was coherence about the need to get prices down, some members of the movement had slightly different strategies to approach the problem. Gonsalves identified a particular example around compulsory licensing:

[W]e do work with the Treatment Action Campaign in South Africa, and they had this competition case hearing against the drug companies in South Africa. And they just wanted to cut a deal for a low price for Glaxo, Bristol and Boehringer Ingelheim drugs. Jamie Love from Consumer [Project on] Technology in DC is like, "No, we have to get a compulsory license. We need to push this, and push this further." It's all about reforming intellectual property in the sphere of public health. And they're like, "No, it's really about us getting a cheaper price of the drug." (Gonsalves 2004)

The court case in South Africa levied by pharmaceutical companies in February 1998 against the country's Medicines Act also had a profound role in galvanizing the international AIDS community to focus on drug prices. It also helped spur TAC to be created. A February 1999 memo from the State Department was shared with activists and revealed that the Clinton administration was threatening South Africa with aggressive actions, including trade sanctions and cuts in foreign assistance (Sawyer 2002, 98). Once it became clear that the position of the branded pharmaceuticals industry was being supported by the Clinton administration, American AIDS activists began to identify a new target in the US government and sought to influence US trade policies that they deemed overly solicitous of restrictive IPR. More specifically, the Vice President, then an aspiring presidential candidate, was seen as an especially vulnerable target. Gore was serving as the co-chair of a binational commission with South Africa, a body established to deal with trade disputes (Behrman 2004, 144).

Milano captured the sentiment behind a series of campaign "zaps" where activists challenged Gore as he made his first few stops to announce his campaign: "When I was told that the U.S. government was actually trying to prevent South Africa from importing generic HIV meds, there was something specific we could do. I wasn't telling South Africa what their government should do. I was telling my government" (Milano 2012). Sawyer had a similar revelation. After meeting with Jamie Love, Sawyer realized that Gore would make a better target than companies or pending trade legislation with Africa, which had been Health GAP's previous focus. He said: "Forget this. We need to go after Al Gore for this bilateral stuff. He's about to announce that he's going to run for president. All of the attention will go after him. I don't want to do demonstrations about trade policies" (Sawyer 2012). Sawyer and other activists became convinced Gore was an important target after reading the State Department memo (Sawyer 2002, 98).

Interestingly, this episode reveals early tensions in the movement where Sawyer pressed to immediately shift the focus from pending African trade legislation to protests at the Vice President's house. Outvoted by his peers that such an action against the Vice President would divert attention from the already planned action, the plans to target Gore were deferred until later, when a dozen or so activists bused down to Carthage, Tennessee, and were able to infiltrate the Vice President's campaign announcement with audacious chants, signs, and t-shirts: "Gore's Greed Kills: AIDS Drugs for Africa." Campaigners were then able to "zap" Gore in seven of his first twelve campaign stops, including ones in New Hampshire, Boston, and New York, prompting Gore's people quickly to seek to resolve the issue (Sawyer 2002, 98–9, 2012; Milano 2007, 73). By year's end, the Clinton administration had reversed its aggressive position on supporting the pharmaceutical industry on IP and issued an executive order saying the United States would back-off from trade measures that might impinge on poor countries' access to medicines.

In this case, division over tactics resulted in a much more felicitous choice of timing when Sawyer's initial plans were outvoted. In other cases, prominent leaders pushed the envelope and defied the entreaties of coalition partners. For example, in 2000, South African activist Zackie Achmat rejected the demand by the South African trade union COSATU that he desist from illegally importing from Thailand generic fluconazole, a drug used to treat opportunistic fungal infections that often accompanied HIV (Grebe 2008). This effort, which garnered extensive media coverage, also helped enhance TAC's stature. However, despite these minor conflicts over specific tactical decisions, the broad contours of coordination and cooperation were relatively consensual. Sawyer noted that one way Western activists addressed potential transnational differences was to defer to advocates on the ground. He suggested that local organizations had veto power over things done in their country and priority over setting policies and priorities. For example, he noted that if US or Western activists had something in mind for Thailand's battle for compulsory licensing or internal drug registry rules, the local activists got control and final say (Sawyer 2012).

To a certain extent, this chapter has begged the question of where coherence comes from. The previous section, in sketching out the turn to global treatment access among American AIDS activists, provided a partial explanation, emphasizing the ripeness of the idea in 1997 and 1998 once domestic rollout of HAART had already successfully reduced AIDS-related mortality in the United States by more than 50 percent. That said, the emphasis in this chapter is structural: is the movement unified around a core objective or not?

In many ways, the AIDS treatment movement was aided in its search of coherence by dint of being relatively small, encompassing a handful of organizations and the individuals within them. Milano, reflecting on the success of a dozen or so activists who targeted the Gore campaign, and the small numbers who were involved in the November 1999 occupation of USTR Charlene Barshefsky's office, noted how small numbers of advocates were able to have immense influence:

So within three months, we changed trade policy. You did not need 400 people at ACT UP meetings to make major change. You could do things with a small, and what's the, Margaret Mead [quote], never doubt that a small group of committed individuals can change the world? That's what I was really going on [about]. I say, okay, everybody else has left. They're either bored with ACT UP; they're burned out; or they're being paid to do AIDS work, they're in organizations, so they can't do it, get arrested anymore; or they've got their triple-combination therapy, and they're not dying, and they're fine. Okay; we'll do it ourselves. We'll work with the people who want to stay here. And there were definitely people who wanted to do that. And we'll do these small, focused actions. (Milano 2007)

Sawyer made a similar point about how a May 1999 action against BMS, timed to correspond to its announcement of a $100 million Secure the Future initiative, was essentially planned and executed by himself and Jamie Love with the help of a few friends (Love 1999b; Sawyer 2012).

While the small size of the core group of individuals and organizations may have facilitated movement coherence, individual organizations faced significant internal stresses and coordination challenges, which are magnified when these groups attempt to "go global." Wong focuses on how such structural characteristics of individual organizations can impede collective action. She writes, "Before they can promote issues internationally, however, NGOs must be able to effectively set the internal agenda, and not all of them are equally capable of doing so because of their organizational structures" (Wong 2012a). She makes a nuanced argument about the degree of centralization that is required at the agenda-setting stage compared to the later implementation stage. From this perspective, MSF in general, given its decentralization and large number of national sections, is emblematic of the kinds of organizations that should have difficulty quickly taking on new initiatives (Wong 2012b, 78). However, as she notes, "MSF's Access campaign has a very particular, insulated structure that distinguishes it from much of the NGO's other témoignage [witnessing] work." She argues that the Access Campaign centralized both proposal and enforcement power, leaving implementation a bit more decentralized (ibid., 151). Governed by its own steering committee, Wong concludes that unlike the rest of the organization that operates by consensus, the Access Campaign relies on a "critical mass of support." Access statements do not have to be approved by all relevant actors in the organization and thus "decisions flow through with relative ease" (ibid., 176).

Pécoul, the first director of the MSF Access Campaign from 1998 to 2003, suggested that both the small size of the team and his own influence within the organization, having previously been the executive director of MSF-France, facilitated their decisiveness: "The campaign was a very small group of people. It started from my home with a computer and phone." The team for the first couple of years was three or four people, including Pécoul, 't Hoen, Daniel Berman, and Jacques Pinel. It was still composed of less than ten people after two years. He described the system as "light," with a small steering committee that delegated most of the work to a small executive committee (Pécoul 2012). Berman similarly noted that the standing of Pécoul within MSF provided him with unusual influence and stature (Berman 2012). Together, the small size of the initial coalition and the particular decision-making structure within one of the key coalition partners may help explain the degree of coherence the movement has experienced.

Conclusions

In this chapter, we explored the anatomy of AIDS treatment advocacy, from the NGO sector in the United States and Europe to the advocacy organizations on the ground in affected countries like South Africa, to their allies in governments and international organizations. We described the moments by which key individuals came to know each other, the venues that facilitated and focused collaboration, and the processes of coordination. After noting early divergence among advocates in the mid 1990s, we documented the growing unity among advocates that coalesced into a coherent global treatment advocacy movement in the late 1990s and early 2000s.

In terms of the questions and criteria to assess the coherence of the movement, while there was no single umbrella organization that coordinated activities, several nodes served as bridges/coalitional forces, including Health GAP, the Global Health Coalition, the International Treatment Preparedness Coalition, and UNAIDS itself. The coherence of the movement is more observable in the support for common platforms like the statements that were generated in 1999 conferences organized by MSF, CPTech, and HAI, and sign-on letters. While some of the nodes in the movement appeared to be relatively isolated from other pieces, namely, conservative activists in the United States, their goals on treatment access, including TRIPS flexibilities, price reductions, and generic competition, were not at odds with each other – very different from the prevention agenda. While new organizations like DATA and the ONE Campaign brought conservatives and celebrities to the cause in later years, their arrival, despite some potential friction, did not lead to open ruptures concerning treatment. Unlike the process of division that ACT UP experienced, groups tended to coordinate fairly effectively, and in the case of DATA and the ONE Campaign, the two organizations actually fused to become one in 2007 (ONE 2007).

With the success of the movement and the instantiation of many of its programmatic goals in governments and international organizations, the advocacy momentum started to wane, in keeping with the typical ebb of many movements. Indeed, some of the key organizations have subsequently shuttered their doors, including the Global AIDS Alliance, the Global Health Council (though it was being revived at the time of writing), and GAAN.

The Global Fund experienced something of a hostile takeover in 2011 as a result of perceived flaws in management and oversight. This action and the flatlining of AIDS funding in the face of the financial crisis prompted great concern by advocates that they were becoming something of a spent force. Gregg Gonsalves for his part wrote a spirited note in December 2011 on the Health GAP listserv bemoaning the inert state of the movement in response to the Global Fund cancelled funding round due to insufficient financial support: "More and more worried that civil society is locked into a let's-talk-more-about-it reaction to the failure of Round 11. I've heard no plans for any coordinated global strategy of lobbying, media work or demonstration in the past few weeks, though national level engagement is happening" (Gonsalves 2011b). In February 2012, he took the ONE Campaign to task on the Health GAP listserv, worried that its leadership had agreed that the US government can meet its commitments on HIV/AIDS even with budget cuts to PEPFAR, prompting Gonsalves to write: "I am tired of Bono presuming he can speak for people living with HIV/AIDS" (Gonsalves 2012a).

Moreover, a number of issues became increasingly contentious within the movement. In 2006, ACT UP Paris challenged some of the clinical trials that were being held in developing countries that were testing the effectiveness of pre-exposure prophylaxis (PreP), an intervention with ARVs for high-risk people that was later found to be highly effective in reducing the chance that someone not infected with the AIDS virus would later become infected. Gonsalves and Nathan Geffen wrote a spirited challenge of that activism in an essay entitled: "In defence of rational AIDS activism: How the irrationality of Act Up-Paris and others is risking the health of people with HIV or at risk of HIV infection" (Staley 2008).

In another example, the MPP also became a source of contention within the movement. The MPP was created in 2009, initially under the auspices of UNITAID, headed by former MSF activist Ellen 't Hoen. The pool sought to enlist branded pharmaceutical companies, among others, to provide their IP to the pool in exchange for modest compensation. Gilead was one such company that provided several ARVs to the pool with some restrictions for certain low- and middle-income countries, as well as which generic companies could produce their drugs (Baker 2011). A number of activists, including those associated with the New York-based I-MAK (Initiative For Medicines, Access & Knowledge), the ITPC, as well as other groups in the global South, raised concerns about the exclusivity of Gilead's agreement with the MPP. In October 2011, I-MAK circulated a petition asking for an overhaul of the MPP's agreement with Gilead. Knowledge Ecology International (KEI), the successor organization to CPTech run by Jamie Love, interestingly did not sign the petition, noting that it agreed with some parts and disagreed with others and that "[i]n our opinion, some parts of the petition repeat assertions that are not accurate, and do not provide a helpful or balanced view of what the Gilead licenses did and did not do" (Love 2011). In response, Jerome Martin of ACT UP Paris, posted the following: "So, James, what do you suggest now? To close the debate? And to the stupid activists to shut up because YOU only know better? Is it that what you call 'moving forward'?" (Martin 2011).

Gonsalves weighed in on this matter as well, and after issuing what he described as a "rant," suggested that what was happening within the movement was damaging: "I am very concerned about what is happening right now among us. What should be real substantive debates on technical and political matters have devolved into bitter recriminations, claims and counter-claims" (Gonsalves 2011a). It may be possible to unearth such heated exchanges from the entire tenure of the movement's history. As Milano noted, coordination in grassroots advocacy organizations at the best of times is a "pain in the ass" (Milano 2012). Nonetheless, while space forbids a more detailed discussion of this particular episode, the increasingly personalized tone of this debate, at a time of increasing scarcity of resources, is reminiscent of the tone, if not the substance, of the divisive battles that left the domestic AIDS advocacy movement in the United States in splinters in the early 1990s. Indeed, the sheer numbers of actors involved in the advocacy scene today may, as Hadden described for the climate arena, make coherence a much harder prospect going forward.

These internal challenges may be overcome in time. In 2012, new scientific developments, including the potential effectiveness of early treatment as a means of breaking the chain of transmission, emboldened activists. Coupled with news that more than 8 million people were on treatment in 2012, including 56 percent of those in need in Africa, advocates made a new push for an AIDS-free generation coinciding with the 2012 meeting of the International AIDS Society that was held in Washington DC (Busby 2012b). We will return to these themes about the future of global AIDS advocacy in the final chapter.

5   Advocacy strategies to address costs

> ... price is a man-made obstacle that we can change ...
> Alan Berkman, founder of Health GAP (cited in Smith
> and Siplon 2006, 56)

> So you have to develop a coherent critique of public policy ... If you
> can't persuade serious people you have a good idea, you are not going to
> go very far. You have to really have a persuasive argument why your
> policy will work, will get things done, will not destroy the incentive
> system, for example, for pharmaceuticals, or that it's a reasonable
> exception in the case of people with low incomes.
> Jamie Love, Director of the Consumer Project on Technology/Knowledge
> Ecology International, 2003

In the previous chapter we saw that the AIDS treatment movement was
able to cohere around universal access to treatment as its primary objective. But how could a universal access regime become (or at least
approach) reality? With ARV drugs costing thousands of dollars per
patient per year, there was no way that the international community
would mobilize around that objective. Yet by the late 1990s, drug prices
would begin to fall radically, with the expansion of "differential pricing"
by the branded pharmaceutical companies and, even more important,
the entry of generic manufacturers into the ARV market. These developments, however, were not simply a reflection of rational decision-making
by corporate executives who were seeking to maintain their share of the
AIDS marketplace. Instead, they were a product of advocates' strategies
that had as their explicit objective the reduction of ARV prices.

In this chapter, we explore those strategies to lower prices and extend
access. Lower prices, we argue, were crucial not just for AIDS patients but
to help advocates overcome decision-makers' concerns about the costliness
and feasibility of the treatment enterprise. As we hypothesized in Chapter 1,
"the higher the costs associated with achieving a market transformation,
the less likely it is that the transformation will be achieved." We also
hypothesized that the higher the opportunity costs of inaction for targets,
the more likely a market transformation will occur. As we discuss in what

follows, movement strategies to lower the costs and raise the opportunity costs were extremely relevant in this case.

With respect to AIDS treatment, there were two sets of costs that had to be faced in the first instance: the costs to pharmaceutical firms associated with lowering their prices while supplying the global market, and the costs to governments that had to pay for treatment in developing countries. "Big pharma" also faced the *potential* opportunity cost of threats to their IPR if they failed to be supportive of the universal access campaign. As we hypothesized in the introductory chapter, when costs for firms and governments remain high, the likelihood of a market transformation is diminished. Incumbent firms often have great political power and may oppose price reductions or policies like differential pricing if the costs are deemed too expensive. They may also challenge measures to reduce prices via generic entry or the introduction of IPR flexibilities. For potential new market entrants, the prospect of high costs, including those associated with battling the incumbents and government regulatory agencies, might dissuade them from moving ahead. And for governments that have to pay for AIDS treatment, higher costs could make universal access to ARVs seem unaffordable.

Advocates thus faced the challenge of devising strategies that addressed these costs, either through actions that accommodated the concerns of politically powerful incumbent firms, or by trying to change their cost–benefit calculus through "anti-corporate" campaigns aimed at damaging corporate reputations and challenging the IPR regime, or the so-called TRIPS Accord. For possible new entrants, advocates had to allay generic firms' fears that the developing world market for ARVs was too poor and disorganized to serve profitably, or that they would be subject to devastating reprisals by branded companies for IPR violations. To governments, advocates had to make the case that the costs were manageable both in terms of direct drug purchases, but also that the implementation costs and challenges were not so significant that service delivery in low-income countries would fail.

At the same time, advocates had to make a compelling argument that drug prices were the primary impediment to access rather than other dimensions of getting drugs into bodies, like the weak medical infrastructure found in many developing countries. In fact, when the idea of universal access to treatment was first floated during the late 1990s, there was hardly a consensus within the global health community that price was the sole, or even the major obstacle to rolling out ARVs across the developing world. Instead, poverty and inadequate health systems seemed to pose even greater problems. ARV treatment demanded sophisticated diagnostic equipment, careful monitoring by trained physicians and nurses, medical care for the ancillary diseases that often struck PWAs, and in many cases special diets and other lifestyle regimens. But as we noted in the previous chapter, prominent advocates like Peter Piot thought addressing price was more tractable than the much larger challenge of fixing health systems in Africa (Piot 2012, Kindle Location 5276).

Lowering the prices of AIDS drugs demanded taking steps beyond pleading with or cajoling the pharmaceutical sector. Again, so long as pharmaceutical executives could take cover behind the inadequacy of the AIDS infrastructure in the developing world, they could plausibly claim that lower prices would make no significant difference. Showing that rollout was possible in the setting of "resource constrained" economies was therefore critical to the process of getting these firms to the negotiating table, especially in the context of the existing institutional limitations.

In this chapter we therefore discuss the major steps that AIDS advocates took on the road toward universal treatment. We begin by examining how advocates addressed the concerns of governments that the drugs were so costly that extending treatment was simply unaffordable. We then show how the movement demonstrated "proof of concept" – that AIDS drugs could work effectively in the developing world.

Next, we turn our attention to firms' concerns about costs. Focusing on the fears of incumbent firms, we first look at the attacks made against the TRIPS regime by campaigners who wanted to punish big pharma through negative reputational sanctions and threats to the IPR regime, and we then show how other advocates encouraged differential pricing and generic entry as a more accommodating strategy. Turning to generic entrants, we discuss how efforts by CHAI helped organize demand and convince Indian and South African drug firms that the market would be there if they entered. Taken together, the advocates showed that an access to treatment regime could be developed at relatively low cost to governments that would pay for drug delivery and for incumbent firms and generics manufacturers that would produce the ARV medications.

Addressing the issue of costs to governments

Two sets of costs concerned governments, including both those states affected by the AIDS crisis and international donors who were called upon to assist in the response. First, given that prevailing ARV prices in the early 2000s were still about $10,000 per patient per year, governments could not imagine the possibility of treatment at anything like global scale. The price of drugs seemed simply out of reach to make a universal program feasible. Not only were the per individual costs daunting, but the aggregate costs of treatment *for life* would be immense, basically consuming entire health and foreign aid budgets.

Leaving aside the price of drugs, a second concern was the feasibility of extending access on the ground in resource-poor settings. There were many specialists in the AIDS community who saw this task as impossible, given the lack of infrastructure and existing behavioral patterns. Put a little differently, many skeptics of expanded treatment access simply thought that the implementation costs of treatment were too high, that the administrative burden, the infrastructure and supply chain needs, etc. were so onerous that the enterprise would fail. We address how advocates sought to address each of these concerns in turn.

Removing price as a barrier

Advocates sought to convince governments that price should not be a barrier to access by persuading and shaming branded firms to lower their prices and by enlisting generic drug companies to enter the market and lower their prices (more on both below). In the previous chapter, we described how advocates like Jamie Love enlisted Cipla to offer ARVs at more competitive prices, while challenging the TRIPS regime. While some advocates thought that these offers alone would lead governments to respond with large purchase orders, it took some time for this appreciation of the new possibilities and scope for expanded access to enter the political consciousness of leaders. Even at greatly reduced prices, the commitment to AIDS treatment still required an unprecedented expenditure of health and foreign aid dollars, and many other priorities – including in the health space – seemed equally deserving of scarce funds.

However, once it was understood that drugs no longer cost $10,000 a year, policy-makers had the same revelation ACT UP activists had in 1999 when Jamie Love pitched the idea of expanded access at the first Health GAP meeting. Indeed, in President George W. Bush's announcement of PEPFAR in his 2003 State of the Union address, he implicitly acknowledged the new generic offer: "And the cost of those drugs has dropped from $12,000 a year to under $300 a year, which places a tremendous possibility within our grasp" (Bush 2003). As Bush recalls in his memoir, once prices were that low, expanded access was possible: "For $25 a month, America could extend an AIDS patient's life for years" (Bush 2010, Kindle Location 6595). He told his team, "[W]e need to take advantage of the breakthrough."

Bush's speechwriter, Michael Gerson, made a similar point. He suggested that the decline in prices and the routinization of AIDS treatment regimens "allowed you to think bigger" and created more opportunity for scale than ever before (Gerson 2006). Jamie Love made a similar point in the documentary *Fire in the Blood*: "I talked to Mitch Daniels, the head of OMB, the people that do the purse strings for the federal government. When the price of AIDS drugs fell to a dollar a day, he felt they had an obligation to support treatment" (quoted in Gray 2012). Even as policymakers became more confident that treatment was affordable, advocates faced another challenge: convincing potential donors that it would also be effective.

Providing proof of concept

If ARVs were a complex and costly medication for the American medical system to handle, the situation was obviously much worse when it came to developing countries. Many, if not most, experts had little confidence that ARVs could effectively be deployed on a global basis, for reasons not only of cost, but also because of the severely limited medical infrastructure needed for AIDS diagnosis and testing. As a Harvard faculty group expressed it:

[O]bjections to AIDS treatment in poor countries fall into several categories. First, poor countries lack the adequate medical infrastructure to provide AIDS treatment safely and effectively. Second, difficulties with adherence to complicated medication regimens would promote and spread drug resistance. Third, antiretroviral drugs are expensive, and the treatment cost is too high for the United States and other wealthy countries to finance without siphoning resources away from HIV prevention programs and other worthy development goals. Finally, commitment from political leaders in Africa and other poor regions is not sufficient to underpin a major international effort towards providing AIDS treatment. (Individual Members of the Faculty of Harvard University 2001)

The near total absence of these drugs in the developing world, however, presented a disturbing contrast to at least some activists and policy entrepreneurs between the "haves and have-nots." A careful student of early AIDS policy, Greg Behrman, argues that "[m]ore than any other factor, the advent of effective drug therapy was the catalyst that helped galvanize the U.S. AIDS activist community to begin to fight the disease beyond America's borders" (Behrman 2004, 134). In fact, at the 1996 AIDS conference in Vancouver, American AIDS activist Eric Sawyer "demanded $3 billion from the United States to provide access to medicines in the developing world," while the charismatic Dr. Jonathan Mann, Director of WHO's AIDS program, called for a "new solidarity" (cited in Gartner 2009a, 35) with those who currently lacked access to

ARVs. For his part, UNAIDS Director Peter Piot asserted that "[i]t remains unacceptable that people living with AIDS, especially – but not only – in the developing world, should have to live without the essential drugs they need for their HIV-related illnesses" (cited in Knight 2008, 60). According to the official history of UNAIDS, Piot's speech "was the first time any of the UN organizations or any international development official had stated that pursuing treatment access in middle- and low-income countries would be a matter of policy" (Knight 2008, 60).

But at this time there was no plan or strategy for rolling out the drugs on a global basis. When journalist Laurie Garrett prodded Mann about what the "new solidarity" meant in practice for global ARV delivery, it soon became apparent to her "that he hadn't thought of it" (Garrett, quoted in Behrman 2004, 133). The costs of AIDS drugs were beyond the reach of developing countries, which in any case seemed to lack the medical infrastructure, much less the political leadership, to make AIDS a priority concern. As George W. Bush writes in his memoir, once he heard that ARV therapy was available and priced within reach, he echoed the concerns of many people by asking, "How will we get the drugs to the people?" (Bush 2010, Kindle Location 6596).

A number of ongoing programs in "resource constrained settings," however, were writing another story about the potential of ARV rollout. Most prominent of these were the scaling-up of ARVs in such countries as Brazil and Uganda, alongside pilot programs launched by Paul Farmer's Partners in Health in Haiti and by UNAIDS' Drug Access Initiative in four developing countries. These programs are reviewed briefly here to give a sense of how the demand side of the ARV market was constructed by treatment advocates during the late 1990s.

In 1996, Brazil became the first country to provide ARVs free to all AIDS patients. Accompanying this decision was a commitment to produce generic versions of ARV medications in Brazilian laboratories, both public and private (Coriat 2008). According to the US Institute of Medicine, "by 2001, public and private laboratories were manufacturing 63 percent of the ARVs available to Brazilians. Seven of the thirteen ARVs being used to treat Brazilians are domestically produced; others have been procured by the government on the international market through aggressive negotiation of prices" (Institute of Medicine 2005). In an important sense, this Brazilian approach to ARV treatment, which combined universal access on the one hand coupled with efforts at restructuring pharmaceutical markets on the other, became the "model" which the treatment advocacy movement sought to expand on a global basis.

The backbone of Brazil's ARV care is the national, or so-called "Unified Health System" (UHS), which was established in 1988. Similar to the British National Health Service, the UHS provides free health care to every Brazilian; indeed, the "right" to health care is enshrined in the Brazilian Constitution. AIDS activists in such countries as Venezuela and South Africa would also make use of such constitutional provisions in their pursuit of access to ARV medications (Torres 2002; Heywood 2009). In important respects, the spread of domestic demands for ARV treatment around the world in the 1990s, and particularly those movements based in developing countries, provided a political foundation for advocates who sought to extend the treatment regime globally (on this point, see Schwartländer, Grubb, and Perriëns 2006).

In 1997, the first year of the Brazilian program, about 36,000 AIDS patients received ARV medication. By 2003, Brazil provided 128,000 people with ARVs out of an estimated population of 600,000 with HIV infection and about half of that number with AIDS. As an important benefit of the ARV scale-up, more Brazilians voluntarily tested for HIV, and public information about the disease was widely disseminated. Brazilians credit this "holistic" program with a decline in HIV incidence as the country entered the new millennium (Institute of Medicine 2005). Accompanying the scale-up of the AIDS program was a dramatic increase in spending on HIV/AIDS care, which leaped from $34 million in 1996 to $232 million in 2001. While the cost-effectiveness of this and other AIDS programs has been the topic of sharp and continuing dispute (see Tren and Bate 2006), the Brazilian Ministry of Health itself – hardly an impartial source – reports cost savings of over $1 billion, due primarily to reduced hospital stays (Institute of Medicine 2005, 75).

A very different setting for the introduction of ARV treatment was found in Haiti, the poorest country in the Western hemisphere. There, Dr. Paul Farmer of Partners in Health had labored long and hard to provide the rural population with better health care, even arranging medical evacuation flights to Boston-area hospitals for some patients (Farmer was also a professor at Harvard Medical School) (Kidder 2003). It was in this setting that Farmer and Partners in Health developed an ARV regimen based primarily on directly observed therapy (DOT) versus expensive laboratory-based analysis of AIDS cases. The regimen was described by a group of medical faculty members as follows:

HAART is prescribed to patients based on easily observed clinical signs and symptoms, rather than advanced laboratory tests, such as CD4 cell counts and viral load, which are not currently available in this poor and rural setting . . . Each HIV-infected patient is assigned an *accompagnateur* (a "companion," most often a community health worker), who observes ingestion of the HAART medications daily and offers support to the patient and family. Directly observed therapy of HAART (or DOT-HAART) ensures that the HIV-infected patient is taking medications regularly, and this promotes the best clinical outcome for the patient and minimizes the opportunities for drug resistance to develop. (Individual Members of the Faculty of Harvard University 2001)

Alongside these programs in Brazil and Haiti, MSF also began a series of pilot programs in their clinics to establish the viability of expanded treatment in resource-poor settings. Pilot projects started in Thailand, Cameroon, South Africa, Cambodia, and Kenya in 1999 and 2000 in parallel with and, indeed, inspired by the Access Campaign. By 2003, MSF documented its experience with pilot projects in ten countries, serving more than 3,500 patients (Scouflaire, Macé, and Berman 2003).[1] According to Bernard Pécoul, who led MSF's Access Campaign, one important result of the pilot projects was documentation, not just on the effectiveness of ARVs in poor countries, but the specific effectiveness of triomune, Cipla's generic triple cocktail that, as we discussed previously, became available for a dollar a day in early 2001 (Laurent et al. 2004; Pécoul 2012).

In addition to these efforts by Brazil and pilot projects by prominent health NGOs, in 1996 UNAIDS began to formulate its "HIV Drug Access Initiative" (DAI). The purpose of this initiative was to determine whether ARV therapy would be effective in the developing world setting; it was basically another "proof of concept" operation. Peter Piot describes the rationale in his memoir. He told his governing board, "Let's go for a study. Just a pilot project – just to look at feasibility." He writes that at the time he thought, "If we could prove that the medication could be properly administered and utilized in developing countries, then, I felt, the moral case for action would be almost unassailable" (Piot 2012, Kindle Location 5296–314). Piot suggests that although money was a problem, the pilot was a success and "whisked away what had been the main argument of the pharmaceutical companies and donors: that there was no point in bringing down the price of treatment, because compliance was impossible. From that point on, their arguments were economic, thus exposing a certain amount of what was perceived by many people as greed" (ibid., Kindle Location 5349–66).

Even though there was already some experience with ARV rollout in countries like Brazil, Thailand, and Haiti, the pilot projects facilitated by UNAIDS and other UN agencies were important for at least three major reasons. First, as Badara Samb, who was among the leaders at UNAIDS of its DAI, noted, the Brazil experience at this time was not widely

---

[1] In mid 2003, MSF had enrolled 660 patients on ARVs in Cambodia, 260 in Cameroon, 436 in Guatemala, 65 in Honduras, 270 in Kenya, 607 in Malawi, 85 in Mozambique, 540 in South Africa, 615 in Thailand, and 18 in Ukraine.

known. UNAIDS was among the first agencies to document the Brazil case and see if its lessons were generalizable (Samb 2010). Second, as Perriëns has observed, the notion of getting five UN agencies to work with industry was unprecedented and had "unique visibility" in the global health community (Perriëns 2010). Third, it was not clear that the experience of the pilot projects in countries like Brazil, Thailand, and Haiti would generalize to Africa and other parts of Asia. Ian Grubb, who served as a policy adviser at WHO and later at the Global Fund, provided additional support for why additional approaches to the rollout of treatment were thought necessary. Because Brazil was perceived as a relatively well-off, middle-income country with its own drug production capabilities, it was not clear that its experience could generalize. As for Haiti's special system of *accompagnateurs*, it was feared the Haitian model might not be replicable in larger countries like Zambia (Grubb 2010).

Unlike other proof of concept trials, the DAI was grounded on a basic bargain between the UN and the pharmaceutical industry: that if DAI demonstrated that ARV rollout in the developing world were effective, and if the pharmas provided the ARVs at lower prices to these countries, UNAIDS (and its partner organization in this endeavor, the WHO), would stand firmly behind pharmaceutical patent protection and would urge their developing world member governments to do so as well. In the following section, when we discuss the advocates' attack on the TRIPS regime, we will more fully understand the appeal of this bargain.

On 16 June 1997 UNAIDS met with representatives of the pharmaceutical industry to discuss "the feasibility and implications of the initiative." According to Dr. Joseph Saba, who was then a senior official at UNAIDS, "the companies regarded the protection of intellectual property rights as a critical issue." UNAIDS accepted that protection as a condition for their participation in the DAI; "governments of the pilot countries agree to provide protection of intellectual property on drugs purchased through the initiative" (Saba 1998). The initiative was officially launched later that year, with four pilot countries, including Côte d'Ivoire, Vietnam, Chile, and Uganda.

Over the period 1998–2000, DAI successfully enrolled just a small number of people on treatment – about 4,000 in all (Schwartländer, Grubb, and Perriëns 2006, 542). Some of the efforts worked better than others. The Vietnam initiative never really got off the ground, as they could never agree on terms that price reduction would be made available to clients (Perriëns 2010). In Côte d'Ivoire, the program suffered from frequent stockouts due to funding issues and logistics (Piot 2012, Kindle Location 5351–68). But, on the whole, the results of independent evaluations by the CDC and the French National Agency for AIDS research were encouraging. As Piot notes: "[T]he conclusion was that compliance in the developing world could in many cases actually be *better* than in Europe and North America. People ... could very clearly see that the drugs were keeping them alive, so they were strongly motivated to adhere to the protocols" (Piot 2012, Kindle Location 5351–68, emphasis in original).

On the basis of these various programs, initiatives, and calls to action, opinion leaders in the world of public health came to view treatment as a promising option for the developing world. In 2001, for example, a group of Harvard professors signed a "consensus statement" on ARV therapy that read:

We believe that the objections to HIV treatment in low-income countries are not persuasive and that there are compelling arguments in favor of a widespread treatment effort . . . . [O]bstacles to treatment such as poor infrastructure can be overcome through well-designed and well-financed international efforts ... A considerable body of evidence suggests that effective AIDS treatment is now possible in low-income countries. (Individual Members of the Faculty of Harvard University 2001)

Ian Grubb said these demonstration projects ultimately were "incredibly important politically to show you could do it" (Grubb 2010). But, as we suggest in the next section, firms had their own concerns about costs that had to be allayed.

Addressing the issue of costs to firms

Firms, both branded and generic pharmaceutical companies, had their own concerns about the costs of lowering prices and extending access to ARVs to people in poor countries. Branded drug companies worried that accepting flexibilities on IPR rules would undermine their business model, setting a precedent for demands to make a range of other "essential" drugs available at low prices. With emerging markets in India, China, and Brazil set to become growth centers for firms, the long-run costs of accepting low prices for one disease for a small market, largely in Africa, were still seen as too high. Moreover, branded drug companies worried that consumers and, in turn, government agencies in Western markets, would also come to see the price differential between products in industrialized and developing countries and either illicitly try to re-import drugs from poor countries or, at the very least, demand that drug prices come down. In short, they were worried about what the industry called "reference pricing," where industrialized world governments would ultimately use developing world prices as reflective of the appropriate cost of drugs (Piot 2012, Kindle Location 5349–66).

For generic companies, the costs were somewhat different. For them, first they had to worry that there would be no market for their drugs if they entered the market on a larger scale. Some had dabbled in the ARV market in developing countries, but some firms had soured on the experience as orders were small, contracts were not always paid on time, and there was a greater risk of corruption. Indeed, the registration process for trying to sell one's products in many different small markets was seen as so onerous that few firms regarded them as an important market. At the same time, generic companies also had to worry that changing IPR rules would make it harder for them to develop and sell their products in poor countries. While Indian firms were assured that they could produce generic drugs for their home market given India's patent laws (at least, until India phased in TRIPS rules), it was unclear whether exports would be subject to such freedom.

Advocates therefore had a number of strategies meant to convince firms that the costs of supporting expanded treatment access were worthwhile. For some campaigners, particularly the likes of Jamie Love, Health GAP, and South Africa's TAC, the choice was to change the relative cost–benefit calculation of firms by raising the reputational costs of inaction. Other prominent advocates, more of them on the inside of international organizations like Peter Piot, sought a different bargain, as already noted: convince the firms to lower their prices in exchange for protection of IP in other domains. With respect to the fears of generic companies, advocates, acting through CHAI, sought to persuade them that the market for their products would exist through credible purchase orders. At the same time, campaigners also challenged global IPR rules, first in court cases, foremost by countering the case the big pharmaceutical companies had brought against the South African government and then through the WTO. We start with these cases, as the outcomes both raised the reputational costs of obstruction by branded companies and paved the way for generic firms to enter the market.

Suing Mandela and attacking TRIPS

As noted in Chapter 2, given the fluidity of rules regarding how the global IP or TRIPS regime would be applied in important respects, perhaps most prominently in the area of public health policy, it was only a matter of time before it would be tested by WTO member governments. Encouraged by AIDS advocates, the most prominent early cases occurred over access to ARV medications, first in South Africa and later in Brazil. In both cases the interests of developing countries were pitted against those of "big pharma," and, thanks to effective framing of the issue by the advocacy movement, public sympathy was decisively on the side of the "South." These cases would play a major role in subsequent pharma actions and policies with respect to ARV access (the best review of the relationship between TRIPS and public health remains Devereaux, Lawrence, and Watkins 2006).

In 1997, just two years after TRIPS was adopted as part of the Uruguay Round of trade negotiations, South African president Nelson Mandela signed into law the South African Medicines and Medical Devices Regulatory Act (hereinafter the Medicines Act). The Medicines Act had as its main purpose the granting of power to the minister of health to authorize compulsory licenses to South African companies to produce drugs or import generic versions of medications needed to face public health emergencies. It also contained language that seemed to suggest that the minister of health could overturn the patents on "any medicine" at any time. While the law was general in its application, it was specifically prompted by the high cost of patented ARV drugs. In fact, in 1996 South Africa had "requested that the United States provide access to drugs at a reduced cost to tackle AIDS," and when no positive response was forthcoming, the government passed the Act enabling it to obtain generic substitutes from overseas suppliers, chiefly based in India (Ragavan 2004).

In 1998, over forty pharmaceutical companies operating in South Africa filed a legal challenge to the Medicines Act before the country's Constitutional Court. The companies, along with the South African Pharmaceutical Manufacturers Association (SA-PMA), contended that the Act violated both South African law and the country's obligations under TRIPS. These actions were supported by the US government, which threatened South Africa with various trade sanctions if it did not rescind the Act (Thomas 2001).

Whatever the legal merits of the suit, it provoked an international firestorm of controversy; in essence, it became a "focal point" for the ills of the TRIPS system and placed the blame for public health disasters at the feet of big pharma. As the suit dragged on, it ran up against the American presidential campaign of 2004, and AIDS activists used the occasion to disrupt Vice President Al Gore's speeches and events (it was widely noted by the activists that, while serving as Clinton's Vice President, Gore had co-chaired a US–South Africa commission on bilateral ties). NGOs like Oxfam and MSF entered the fray with an intensive advocacy campaign that pitted patents and profits against human lives. As Stanford's Barton writes, "The suit became a public relations debacle for the (pharmaceutical) industry, and ... the industry settled in April 2001" (Barton 2004). The ability of advocates to impose costs on target actors is a frequent theme in the international relations literature on shaming (Keck and Sikkink 1998; Greenhill and Busby 2008; Busby 2010a; Demeritt 2012; Hendrix and Wong 2012) as well as the social movements literature (Luders 2006 offers a nuanced account distinguishing between the disruptive costs of protests compared to the costs of acquiescing to movement demands). Whether a confrontational strategy can succeed over the longer term is another question, one we address at the end of this chapter and in the book's conclusion in Chapter 8.

South Africa was not the only developing nation putting the heat on the pharmaceutical companies over pricing and patent rights. Brazil also joined the fray a few years later by demanding that Merck lower the price of two locally marketed ARVs or face the prospect of compulsory licensing. In January 2001, after months of unsuccessful negotiations, the US government asked the WTO to assemble a dispute panel focused on Brazil's application of patent laws (Thomas 2001). In June 2001, the United States unexpectedly withdrew its complaint, a move that received widespread applause from the activist community (Crossette 2001).

The South African lawsuit had a catalytic effect on the global AIDS movement. Shortly after the case was brought to court, a group of AIDS activists met in 1998 to form the Health GAP Coalition, "an association of . . . organizations united to fight global AIDS, with a particular focus on making drugs accessible around the globe" (Behrman 2004, 136). They had an informal discussion centered on how to advance global access to ARVs, and they soon turned their attention to the issue of drug pricing. Price was but one problem facing advocates, but as we noted in the previous chapter, it was "an obvious one" (Behrman 2004, 137; on the origins of Health GAP, see also Smith and Siplon 2006).

As discussed in the previous chapter, Jamie Love joined Health GAP's deliberations in January 1999 and played a critical role in forging its strategy. Love worked with Ralph Nader on health issues, focusing on the question of how IPR and patent laws impeded patient access to low-cost treatments for diseases such as cancer. While Love had initially concentrated on the situation in the United States, testifying before Congress regarding how pharmaceutical companies took advantage of IP developed with US government support, he soon became so well known in the health policy arena that some developing countries began demanding his advice on how to acquire AIDS drugs at lower costs. A former business reporter said that Love started out with a fundamental premise: "If the taxpayers paid for the development of the intellectual property, then they ought to get some kind of return on their investment" (cited in Lindsey 2001).

After having five minutes to present views on compulsory licensing at Health GAP's January 1999 meeting, two-and-a-half hours of the February meeting was dedicated to the topic. For AIDS activists, Love suggested that this perspective on the mutability of patents was new information (Love 2003). At Health GAP's second meeting, Love explained how patents provided drug companies with monopoly power and how the US government worked hand in glove with the firms to ensure that these drugs were not pirated or produced illicitly, even at the expense of access to medicines by the poor. However, Love believed that the government's position could be changed if it faced the wrath of the activist community; he asserted that no politician wanted to be "accused of preventing tens of millions of poverty-stricken people in the developing world from getting access to lifesaving drugs. *Politicians would be vulnerable in a way that executives were not*" (cited in Behrman 2004, 140, emphasis added).

Love therefore outlined a two-pronged strategy that included putting pressure on American politicians who appeared to be in big pharma's pocket on the one hand, while working directly with developing countries and generic manufacturers on the other to promote the development and use of low-cost generic ARVs. Activist Eric Sawyer, who attended the meeting, found Love's presentation persuasive: "I immediately realized that Jamie Love had given us the key to unlock the door" (cited in ibid.).

Love's political strategy was predicated on the foundational view that price stood as the major impediment to ARV rollout in the developing world and could be lowered by attacking pharmaceutical patent rights. For its part, the industry increasingly realized that it would not succeed in fighting developing countries based on TRIPS infringements and that a new strategy had to be devised for ensuring that property rights would be respected. During the late 1990s, therefore, in consultations with UNAIDS and the WHO, the drug companies began to raise the possibility of "differential pricing" for the developing world. The idea was that drug prices should remain high in industrialized countries, compensating for R&D costs, while they could be reduced in the developing world to something nearer the marginal costs of production. However, any such agreement had to be based on the international community's acceptance of the drug companies' property rights, and on the industrialized world's commitment not to use developing world prices as "reference prices" for their own consumers (Schwartländer, Grubb, and Perriëns 2006; Knight 2008; Piot 2012). The development and impact of differential pricing are the topic of the following section.

Differential pricing: theory and practice

In an earlier section we have seen that one of the early efforts at "proof of concept" regarding ARV rollout in the developing world was the DAI sponsored by UNAIDS. Unlike other proof of concept projects, DAI was based on a fundamental bargain between the UN and the pharmaceutical industry, namely, lower prices in exchange for support regarding corporate property rights. Specifically, the pharmaceutical industry agreed to provide ARV medications based on the principle of "differential pricing." But what did differential pricing mean, both in theory and practice? What were the consequences of the differential pricing regime for ARV access? And does differential pricing provide a "model" for the pharmaceutical industry for how *all* drugs should be priced?

Briefly, differential pricing, at least in theory, offered a promising method for reconciling the interests of R&D-intensive pharmaceutical firms with those of ARV consumers who had differing abilities to pay for these drugs. The fundamental idea is that the costs of pharmaceutical R&D could be spread across consumers according to their ability (and willingness) to pay. In short, differential or "Ramsey" pricing "implies prices that vary across markets inversely with each market's price sensitivity or demand elasticity" (Danzon and Towse 2003). To use a simple example, imagine a water utility in a resort town that, like many tourist traps, has tourists with high incomes on the one hand and service workers – who live in the town year-around – with relatively low incomes on the other. The water utility will charge the local hotels high prices for water, which are then paid for by affluent consumers as part of their bill, and lower prices for local consumers, who are also, of course, voters. In essence, the hotels and their tourist occupants will subsidize the water consumption of the poorer local population.

As health economist Danzon emphasizes, "a necessary condition for maintaining appropriate price differentials is that markets are separable, such that if manufacturers charge low prices (in LDCs), these low prices do not spill over" to the Organisation for Economic Cooperation and Development (OECD) economies. Danzon continues:

In practice, markets are not separate because governments in many countries regulate their domestic prices based on lower prices in other countries ("external referencing") and intermediaries can import products from low to high price countries ("parallel trade"). Given these linkages across markets, basic economics predicts that manufacturers will rationally seek to maintain much higher prices in LDCs than they would require if markets were separate and price linkages do not occur ... *except when forced by political or other pressure.* (Danzon 2001, emphasis added)

What Danzon emphasized, and in this she was joined by several other economists, including F.M. Scherer at Harvard (Scherer 1993; Scherer and Watal 2002) and Jean Lanjouw at Berkeley (Lanjouw 2003; Jack and Lanjouw 2005), was that differential pricing could only be achieved if the international community built an institutional framework – a set of stable agreements – in support of this practice. Indeed, this is precisely what the DAI and the AAI tried to accomplish. As Piot writes in his memoir:

> What I proposed to industry was a new social contract: in return for reasonable profits in high-income markets and a monopoly on new products (in other words, functioning patents), the pharmaceutical industry would invest in R&D for much-needed new medication, and provide new essential drugs immediately at cost (plus a small margin) to developing countries, instead of waiting for their patents to expire. (Piot 2012, Kindle Location 5399)

In return for differential pricing, it called upon the UN to support the IP of the firms and the OECD nations to refrain from parallel importing and reference pricing. And while hardly a firm commitment, the pharmas accepted this bargain because they were, in fact, under intense political pressure. Simply stated, for the firms, an informal agreement with UNAIDS was better than some formal "code of conduct" that the WHO might enact, as it had done against Nestlé and other baby food manufacturers with its code on the marketing of breast-milk substitutes (Sikkink 1986).

A successor to the DAI, the AAI, was launched in May 2000 by UNAIDS and the WHO and sought to expand the use of differential pricing by research-based pharmaceutical companies. Participating companies included Abbott Laboratories; Boehringer Ingelheim GmbH; BMS; GSK; F. Hoffmann-La Roche Ltd; and Merck & Co., Inc. Price reductions were concluded with 39 countries. Prices were expected to be about 80 percent below US prices (Behrman 2004, 134). By June 2003, three years after the start of the program, industry estimated that 76,300 people were on ARVs in Africa as a result of the program, up from 9,300 in the third quarter of 2000 (Sturchio 2003). Six months later, in December 2003, the number of people on ARVs through the AAI reached 150,000 (Sturchio 2004). But agreements with participating countries had to be negotiated individually, which slowed down rollout of the program (as a point of comparison, the Global Fund was able to enlist 770,000 in its first three years of operation (Global Fund 2011a).

Despite the limitations of the AAI, Schwärtlander, Grubb, and Perriëns, and Sturchio (all of whom were involved in creating the program) credit the scheme in helping drive down prices of ARVs (Schwartländer, Grubb, and Perriëns 2006; Sturchio 2004). Perhaps even more important was the early demonstration effect of the DAI and AAI, along with programs in Haiti, Brazil, and elsewhere, which showed that access could be extended to people in poor countries. According to Joseph Perriëns, the UNAIDS official who had been in charge of the DAI and played a key role in AAI, both programs were "very important to alter the perception that ARV therapy was impossible in developing countries. Donors could not agree [to pay for ARVs] if they had not seen demonstration of feasibility" (Perriëns 2010).

Why did insider advocates like Peter Piot embrace differential pricing rather than some wholesale challenge to IPR rules favored by campaigners like Jamie Love, Health GAP, and MSF? MSF's Bernard Pécoul said dismissively of the initiative, "it's like an elephant giving birth to a mouse" (MSF 2000b). Piot acknowledges that although the entry of generic companies was a "game-changer" for widespread HIV treatment, "I also learned that simplistic views about the 'good' generics producers and the 'bad' propriety-based companies were wrong. The companies just employed different business models, and by definition generics would not exist without the originals" (Piot 2012, Kindle Location 5366). He sought to take advantage of the pressure on drug companies to have "serious negotiations" and also use study tours with drug executives like Ken Weg of BMS and Ray Gilmartin of Merck to see the problem first-hand. As Piot writes, "I could feel that they were both struggling with the ethics of the situation, though some of the other pharma men were entirely impervious to any argument outside profit and shareholders" (Piot 2012, Kindle Location 5366). With Gro Harlem Brundtland's support (what Piot calls a "welcome shift"), a "proactive" Piot pursued an agreement with the branded drug companies.

Piot explains that UNAIDS was heavily criticized for these efforts by campaigners who thought generic firms should have been enlisted at the outset. He suggests at the time he was worried that drug quality was "not always up to international standards." Given the contested nature of IPR rules, generics might also have fallen foul of international trade rules. He writes that "the legal framework for using them was still shaky at best" (Piot 2012, Kindle Location 5382). Moreover, Piot rejects the absolutism of some activist groups:

Groups like Médecins sans Frontières, Health GAP, and Jamie Love's Knowledge Ecology International – which argued that patent rights make medicines more expensive, are therefore evil, and should be eliminated – had some valid points in an ideal world, but they were not dealing with the urgency of reality, nor with the fact that we would need new HIV drugs when the older ones lost their effectiveness, which was more or less unavoidable. (Piot 2012, Kindle Location 5382–99)

He suggests he would continue to meet with pharma companies even if others would not: "So if ActUp didn't want to sit down with Evil Big Pharma, so be it, but Big Pharma was still invited, and we would continue to also deal with ActUp" (ibid., Kindle Location 5382).

Piot describes some of the efforts to persuade branded companies to lower their prices. At Davos in January 2000, Piot and Brundtland appealed to Merck Chief Executive Officer (CEO) Gilmartin to continue the tradition they established with Mectizan on river blindness by making a similar humanitarian gesture on HIV/AIDS. Gilmartin's initial reply was dismissive, saying "his shareholders would never accept an agreement to give the company's expensive new medication away at cost." Piot admits that he and Brundtland left the meeting thinking "another waste of time" (Piot 2012, Kindle Location 5400–16). Merck's Jeff Sturchio, however, recalled the meeting actually took place a year later in 2001. He said that, even though Merck had already announced tiered pricing a year earlier as part of the AAI, that on the plane ride home from the 2001 meeting where Piot and Brundtland pressed for greater reductions and more transparent pricing Gilmartin started to come around, saying: "Maybe we should do more" (Sturchio 2009, 2013). A few weeks later, both Gilmartin and Weg from BMS were ready to make a deal in exchange for assurances on re-importation of drugs (Piot 2012, Kindle Location 5426–33).

What made the branded companies reconsider? For the companies, the initiative was potentially attractive, given the negative fallout from the South African court case that was still pending and would only be resolved the following year. As Joseph Perriëns argued, business could have acted unilaterally and not had the endorsement of the UN, but the program made it much easier to motivate countries to take the risk of introducing drugs that were still very expensive in their programs. For the companies, association with a UN-supported initiative also offered "goodwill" benefits (Perriëns 2010).

As Sturchio noted, the branded companies were under intense pressure to re-think their strategy. However, they tended to be conservative, and no single firm wanted to be the first to drop their prices. A common initiative made it possible for all the firms to take action. He suggested the impetus was provided by the ARV pioneer GlaxoWellcome, per the initiative of its CEO Richard Sykes. By the end of 1999, a series of structured discussions were launched using shuttle diplomacy that involved industry, UNAIDS, WHO, and some other UN agencies (Sturchio 2009).

Even in the context of adopting "differential pricing," each company adopted its own approach. Merck, for example, offered tiered pricing, one for low-income countries, another for low middle-income countries, and a third for market prices. Other companies offered two tiers, one for LDCs and another for all others. Some companies decided not to pursue differential pricing and instead donated drugs in certain cases, with Pfizer offering access to fluconazole (a drug used to treat fungal infections seen frequently in people with AIDS) being the most prominent case in point (Perriëns 2010). Sturchio suggested each company established final decisions on how to price rather than having a coordinated pricing arrangement because of concerns about antitrust (Sturchio 2009).

Ben Plumley, who represented GlaxoWellcome at AAI negotiations and then moved to UNAIDS to staff the initiative, described some of the impetus for industry. They were worried about a public relations disaster at the biannual international AIDS meeting in Durban, not just that their exhibition booths might be attacked by AIDS activists, but that they could be subject to intense criticism by the international community. There was an increasing sense that if industry did not change its business model for HIV medicines in developing countries, its entire business model could be under threat. He suggested that people should not underestimate the power of the advocacy community. Plumley confirmed that Glaxo's Sykes was among those most enthusiastic on the industry side, with both GlaxoWellcome and Merck in competition over which company was the most philanthropic. For industry, the rationale of bringing in the UN was, as Plumley described it, "political cover" for coordinated activities, including mobilization of Indian generics manufacturers. Peter Piot's leadership was critical in this regard, because both UNAIDS and the WHO were extremely hostile to the private sector at the time (Plumley 2010).

But in practice, how much difference did differential pricing schemes really make? In the case of the DAI pilot countries, big pharma reduced its prices from somewhere in the area of $12,000 per year for ARV treatment to about $7,200 per year (Knight 2008), a figure that was still quite elevated by developing world standards and, of course, well beyond the reach of all but the wealthiest consumers. In fact, the DAI pilot programs only provided drug access to a relatively small number of people living with AIDS; AAI, for its part, helped drive prices lower. Perriëns suggested that the average branded price per patient per year dropped to about $1,200 (Perriëns 2010; this is also confirmed in Schwartländer, Grubb, and Perriëns 2006, 542; Piot 2012, Kindle Location 5414). From Sturchio's point of view, the big price declines in ARVs were a function of the AAI initiative, which brought prices down below $2,000 before the end of 2000 (Sturchio 2004, 121). Although the timing makes it appear industry was responding to generic competition, the decision to lower prices had been made long before Cipla went forward with its offer to the European Union (EU) Commission in September 2000 (Sturchio 2009). Sturchio attested: "the tiered prices had been made available in May 2000, four months before Hamied's dramatic announcement, and 10 months before Cipla began to supply at lower prices in March 2001" (Sturchio 2013). Perriëns speculated that branded companies may well have heard that the UN was considering going to generic companies (Perriëns 2010). Sturchio, for his part, defends the effort:

> While everybody on the outside was jeering that this was too little, too late and the prices were still too high, the reality of the AAI was different. It wasn't until some of the senior people at our companies could see that it was possible to work with UNAIDS and WHO and other agencies, that the pharmaceutical industry could make progress on actually implementing programs that would help people who needed the medicines. (quoted in Knight 2008, 123–4)

Ellen 't Hoen, who led MSF's advocacy efforts, disputed the AAI's contribution to big price declines. She suggested it was not useful and that it put a huge damper on the political movement for generic competition (which, of course, may have been one of big pharma's objectives). She said that it did help to create a culture in companies that they should produce ARVs for others besides people in advanced industrialized countries. History has shown, she said, the AAI deals were not all that good, as later steep declines through robust generic competition showed ('t Hoen 2010). Interestingly, where Sturchio's chart of price declines credits AAI for the major price movements of the early 2000s, MSF's annual series, *Untangling the Web*, emphasizes the price movements wrought by generics, starting with Brazil's prices in 2000. The UNAIDS ten-year history also notes that whether the AAI or generic competition led to price reductions remains disputed (Knight 2008). Given that generics have become the dominant providers, it is fair to say that they were willing to offer lower prices than the branded companies, even if both sides take credit for the initial downward movement in prices.

For his part, Piot suggests that the outcome of the AAI was a bit disappointing for different reasons. "Our big gap," he writes "remained the absence of a funding mechanism: even with the price discounted, someone still had to pay. My bet was that with drastically reduced prices, we could now convince donors to pay for treatment." However, both African governments and activists poured cold water on the idea. Without international funding, "uptake was poor" (Piot 2012, Kindle Location 5433). Nonetheless, even if the scale of those receiving treatment remained low given the scale of the need, the DAI and AAI provided big pharma with a framework for addressing developing world AIDS issues, offering differential prices in those regions while preserving their property rights and higher prices in the industrialized countries. One issue that we will take up in the final chapters of this book is whether the differential pricing model could be extended to other diseases and what its implications might be.

While the AAI sought to accelerate access, the model was a difficult one from the start, as the participating firms were reluctant to share information with each other and the public. In part because of antitrust reasons, each firm set the terms for what prices it would charge for its drugs, with rules for differential pricing varying between companies. As Piot later admits, "We had made a mistake in accepting that the final price negotiations had to happen country by country, as industry wanted to keep control over the sensitive cost structure of their drugs" (Piot 2012, Kindle Location 5433–49).[2] The purchasing arrangements through the AAI remained tightly controlled by individual firms. As Schwartländer et al. note, "the roll-out was slow and hindered by individual countries having to negotiate price and conditions" (Schwartländer, Grubb, and Perriëns 2006, 542). Although the initiative reported the collective number of people on treatment and some of the details about individual firms' deals, little information about these purchasing arrangements was publicly available.

At the same time, there were ongoing rivalries between the WHO and UNAIDS. Staff members at the WHO were especially skeptical of the private sector. Branded companies embraced the initiative with different motivations between and within them. Some companies and some individuals within companies were convinced that access had to be extended to more people, in part given the need, and in part because the industry's position on IPR access and AIDS drugs was endangering their entire business model. Other companies and individuals were more convinced that the optics of the AAI, given its public relations role, were more important than scaling-up the number of recipients. For those actors, accelerating access meant a slow, gradual rollout, not an ambitious timetable that would rapidly close the gap between current supply and total need.

Major pricing reductions on ARV drugs would not be achieved until generic competition came on the ARV scene after 2000, a few years after the DAI scheme was launched. And it was the promise of cheap generics, rather than the differential prices of branded products, that really made the

---

[2] As noted above, the poorest countries were eligible for one price while middle-income countries potentially faced a different, higher price (WHO and UNAIDS 2002; Waning et al. 2009).

idea of "universal access to treatment" more than a pipedream. With drastically lower prices for ARVs, the concept of a treatment-driven approach to AIDS would become overwhelmingly compelling to a broad coalition of movement stakeholders. Still, the DAI and AAI, along with the other "proof of concept" initiatives we have mentioned, gave further evidence that widespread ARV rollout was feasible in resource-constrained settings.

By 2003, the AAI had largely run its course, according to Plumley. It was a bit of an anachronism to have a program made up of only the branded companies now that generics were entering the market. At first, however, branded companies had trouble interacting with generic firms. That tension began to ease by 2003–4, as individual branded firms like BMS and Gilead signed licensing groups and forged strategic partnerships with generic manufacturers (Plumley 2010). Initially, branded companies sought to keep generic companies out of the AAI. They did not see them as legitimate partners. That began to change as the WHO's Prequalification Program, discussed in the next chapter, demonstrated that the drug quality of generic companies would not bring the industry into disrepute (Perriëns 2010).

Branded companies ultimately were not willing to go as far as their generic competitors on price. Although the AAI embraced differential pricing and significantly lowered the prices of ARVs for developing countries, generic firms had been willing to offer lower prices for their ARVs than branded companies (GAO 2006; Waning, Kaplan *et al.* 2010). Those prices were not a natural evolution of the market, but were also politically constructed by bundling demand, a theme to which we now turn.

Bringing in the generics

Efforts like the DAI and the AAI were intended to allay the fears of big pharma that extending ARV access could be achieved without fundamentally undermining their business model, which was based on patent protection and high prices in the industrialized world. Where these programs somewhat neutralized the political objections by branded firms to the idea of extending access, the results were disappointing from the perspective of advocates, given the scale of the need.

Campaigners from civil society, and increasingly, international organizations, thus pinned their hopes on generic companies in India and South Africa. But there, too, despite an initial offer from Cipla's Yusuf Hamied in September 2000 at the European Commission to provide a triple cocktail for as little as $600–$800 a year (described in more detail in the previous chapter), that offer did not translate into orders overnight. As Singhal and Rogers write: "Dr. Hamied left the Brussels meeting expecting a bombshell of rapid reaction. Several ministers of health and heads of state of African countries were present at the Brussels meeting. But to Dr. Hamied's surprise, nothing happened" (Singhal and Rogers 2003, 152). This shows that lower prices, on their own, did not immediately translate into greater demand. In Hamied's view, things changed dramatically after he made his February 2001 announcement to provide the triple cocktail at a "humanitarian price" of $350 per patient per year to groups like MSF. He suggested that with the media coverage that accompanied his announcement, especially after Donald McNeil's story in *The New York Times*, the "floodgates opened." Thereafter, many of his competitors in the Indian generic pharmaceuticals industry "joined the bandwagon" (Hamied 2012). But increased media attention also provides only part of the generics story.

By the end of 2002, the number of people on ARVs was still paltry, hovering well below 500,000. By 2010, in contrast, in excess of 6 million people were estimated to be on treatment (UNAIDS 2011b). What changed? As the next chapter details, the Global Fund and PEPFAR, which ultimately became the two largest procurers of ARVs, were created in 2002 and 2003, respectively. However, the role of CHAI,[3] a project of President Bill Clinton's foundation, looms large, as it not only further secured price reductions, but more importantly, it fundamentally helped to organize and pool demand into larger volumes, beginning with its first agreement announced in October 2003. David Ripin of CHAI described it as "organizing the market on two sides" (Ripin 2012). This organization of the developing world market for ARVs, coupled with foreign aid funding to buy the drugs, was crucial to generic entry.

Ira Magaziner, the architect of the Clinton initiative, described why the offers of price reductions from companies like Cipla had difficulty scaling-up demand. Before CHAI, you had a "scattered market" and nobody was aggregating volume. Companies were selling some ARVs, but it was not a large amount by volume. The ARV market in most poor countries was not a priority, given other health challenges and extremely limited funding and infrastructure. Companies looked at all the different countries with separate registrations, potential corruption in bids, and delayed payment, and concluded that the ARV market in developing countries "wasn't something worth pursuing very hard or likely to yield much success" (Magaziner 2012). Kate Condliffe, who joined CHAI in 2003 to lead its Access Program, suggested that the generic companies shared a number of fears that first had to be overcome. They had a

---

[3] CHAI was renamed the Clinton Health Access Initiative in January 2010 and spun off as an independent organization.

healthy and fair skepticism about volumes. They had been getting a lot of pressure from many different groups for a long time to lower prices in expectation of large volumes that had not really come to fruition. This was, she noted, before PEPFAR had announced their willingness to buy generic drugs and before there had been significant growth in the number of people on treatment, and there was a lot of uncertainty in the marketplace (Condliffe 2012).

Magaziner described how the Clinton Foundation arrived at its approach. President Clinton wanted a new agenda for his foundation, focusing on economic development, but the AIDS crisis kept cropping up in his conversations with developing world leaders, because, due to AIDS deaths, two people had to be hired for every one position. Even though ARV prices had already come down thanks to differential pricing, they were still too expensive and the systems were not in place to deliver the drugs effectively, so not enough people were on treatment; indeed, even generics prices were too high for most governments. At the same time, efforts to provide treatment by MSF and Partners in Health operated on a very small scale. Magaziner urged Clinton that someone needed to step in to provide leadership in this space by assisting governments to scale-up treatment. As CHAI helped governments to develop scale-up plans and tried to raise money from potential donors, in late 2002 and early 2003 Magaziner went to US and European drug companies to see if they were interested in lowering prices for higher volumes. Unfortunately, given concerns that low-priced drugs from the developing world would find their way to developed country markets, and concerns about prices more generally, they felt they had done enough through their previous initiatives, so Magaziner and CHAI turned to generic companies in India and South Africa (Magaziner 2012).

In October 2003, CHAI announced the first deal with four generics companies: three Indian firms (Cipla, Ranbaxy, and Matrix), and the South African firm, Aspen. The first agreement lowered the prices for the commonly used generic triple cocktail (of nevirapine, 3TC, and either AZT or d4T) by about one-third, from 0.55 cents to 0.38 cents a day, or $140 dollars a year (Schoofs 2003). The first agreement provided cheaper prices for a "consortium" of four countries in Africa (Mozambique, Rwanda, South Africa, and Tanzania) and twelve different countries/territories in the Caribbean[4] (Altman 2003). For members of the

---

[4] Bahamas, Dominican Republic, Haiti, and members of the Organization of Eastern Caribbean States (which includes Antigua and Barbuda, Dominica, Grenada, Saint Kitts and Nevis, St. Lucia, Saint Vincent and the Grenadines, and three territories, Montserrat, Anguilla, and the British Virgin Islands).

consortium, the prices that were quoted were equally available to all (Waning *et al.* 2009). Twenty-two consortium members are also partner countries where CHAI helps with capacity-building by creating large-scale, integrated HIV/AIDS treatment and prevention programs.

Since the initial agreement, CHAI has concluded a number of other agreements aimed at reducing prices of ARVs and HIV diagnostic tests. They range from one in July 2005 with producers of the ARVs' active pharmaceutical ingredients,[5] to another in January 2006 with manufacturers of diagnostic tests, to a focus in November 2006 on lowering the price of pediatric AIDS drugs,[6] to a May 2007 effort aimed at second-line ARV therapies, to the present, as therapies lose patents and new approaches to treatment come on-line.[7] By September 2008, the number of members of the Clinton consortium had increased to 71 countries, including 36 African countries, 11 Asian countries, 2 Eastern European countries, and 22 Latin American and Caribbean members (counting the members of the Organization of Eastern Caribbean States as a single unit), giving the organization as a whole much greater market power than any one country would have on its own (CHAI 2008a).

In November 2006, CHAI and UNITAID (a new UN agency whose budget for purchasing AIDS drugs comes from taxes on airline tickets) announced their partnership. In January 2010, the HIV/AIDS initiative became a separate non-profit organization and was renamed the Clinton Health Access Initiative. CHAI estimates 2 million people as beneficiaries of drugs purchased through its pricing agreements. Together, CHAI has concluded ARV price reductions with eight different suppliers and 40 different drug formulations, and another 16 price reductions on HIV/AIDS diagnostic tests from 12 suppliers.[8] In all, CHAI estimates its price

---

[5] http://foundationcenter.org/pnd/news/story.jhtml?id=112700008.

[6] http://foundationcenter.org/pnd/news/story.jhtml?id=163600004.

[7] CHAI has concluded a number of agreements to reduce prices of ARVs and HIV diagnostic tests. The complete list includes the following: July 2005 (active pharmaceutical ingredients), January 2006 (diagnostics and ARVs), July 2006 (diagnostic tests), November 2006 (pediatric AIDS drugs), May 2007 (second-line ARV therapies), April 2008 (second-line and children's ARVs), April 2009 (second-line and heat stable Kaletra), August 2009 (second-line and TB drugs), and May 2011 (tenofovir and second-line).

[8] CHAI concluded agreements with eight manufacturers of ARV formulations, active pharmaceutical ingredients and/or pharmaceutical intermediates including: Aurobindo Pharma, Cipla Ltd., Emcure Pharmaceuticals, Hetero Drugs, Matrix Laboratories, Micro Labs Ltd., Ranbaxy Laboratories and Strides Arcolabs. The ARVs in CHAI's pricing agreements include: abacavir (ABC), atazanavir (ATV), efavirenz (EFV), emtricitabine (FTC), lamivudine (3TC), lopinavir/ritonavir (LPV/r), nevirapine (NVP), ritonavir (RTV), stavudine (d4T), tenofovir (TDF), and zidovudine (AZT) (CHAI 2011).

reductions have reduced the cost of first-line drugs by 50 percent, pediatric drugs by 90 percent, and second-line drugs by about 30 percent. More recently, it has expanded its work to malarial medications, among other areas (CHAI undated).

In essence, CHAI negotiations helped transform the business model for the ARV industry. After rounding up putative purchase orders from governments, CHAI negotiators approached Indian generic firms and asked them to lower their prices. Former President Clinton describes the rationale, noting that governments had previously overpaid for ARVs, as they faced steep price mark-ups by middlemen. He says, "It got me to thinking about how once more we had a public-goods market that was not only underfinanced; it was disorganized." Clinton elaborates, "What we tried to do was to get them to go from what I call a 'jewelry-store model' to a 'grocery-store model' – from a high-profit, low-volume, uncertain-payment business to a low-margin, high-volume, certain-payment business" (see Rauch 2007). As Waning *et al.* argue, the Clinton Foundation's early efforts did not try to bring procurement under a single roof like the pooled procurement programs of PEPFAR, UNITAID, and the Voluntary Procurement Pool. Rather, CHAI relied on making "ARVs more affordable by negotiating price ceilings that reflect suppliers' costs plus reasonable and sustainable profit margins" (Waning *et al.* 2009, 520).

For governments, the new prices meant that "[a]ll of a sudden, they could treat six times as many people for the same amount of money" (Dugger 2006). *The Wall Street Journal* concluded that "[e]ssentially, the Clinton Foundation is becoming a market maker" (Schoofs 2003). For generic firms, this was critical, as Yusuf Hamied of Cipla noted, "This is the first time a group has come forward with predictable volumes" (Schoofs 2003). CHAI's influence went beyond bargaining and securing bulk prices. It helped generic firms realize savings through application of business consulting skills. Magaziner "called in a network of volunteers, some of them donated by McKinsey, and had them dissect the supply chain for ARVs" (McLean 2006). The companies, according to *The Wall Street Journal*, "opened their books and manufacturing processes to a group of Clinton business advisers. Then the [CHAI] advisers and the companies hunted for ways to cut costs, starting with raw-material suppliers in China and ending with the products' packaging" (Schoofs 2003). Magaziner described the process as follows:

We worked for several months with the companies trying to analyze their costs of production. We went all the way back and talked to the raw material suppliers, the people who produce the active pharmaceutical ingredients, and then the final formulations, analyzed the production costs and projected ahead with them with their engineers that if we scaled-up productions and could provide them with predictable large volumes, what could happen to the cost of production, how much they could come down, and therefore how we could lower prices. (Magaziner 2004)

The specific contribution of CHAI to help firms lower their prices is potentially a sensitive topic for generic firms, proud of their achievements and their technical abilities. Cipla's CEO, Yusuf Hamied, was known to have an encyclopedic knowledge of active pharmaceutical ingredient (API) prices (Love 2009). As Bill Haddad argued:

Suffice it to say that when the Clinton team visited Cipla, they were novices about producing either AIDS drugs or other medicines generically. But the doors of knowledge were willingly opened to them. Dr. Hamied opened up his books for their review ... which you never do ... and took them on a tour of how the raw and finished product were developed and manufactured. I do not know of one generic AIDS manufacturer that was lectured or influenced by any of the Clinton consultants on how to manufacture their products. ... There is no need for any of the sidekicks to blow a horn to enhance President Clinton's influence or recognition of the urgent need for AIDS medicines and financing. Early on, after he left office he added his influential voice and concern to let the world realize that affordable medicines were available and he actually offered Cipla as an example of what was possible. He helped in creating a universal understanding of the needs of the poor nations and he sought through the Foundation and personally, needed financing. (Haddad 2011)

Hamied echoed these views, "When the Clinton people came to see us, they knew nothing about HIV." He said that he got on well with Ira Magaziner and told the Clinton folks that the backbone of supplying anti-AIDS drugs were the people who made raw materials and gave them their names. He elaborated, "The people who came were very good managers, they were not accountants, they were not god almighty .... They were the buying group. We sat with them and educated them. We didn't hide anything." While worried that Cipla never seemed to get sufficient credit for its efforts, Hamied acknowledged, "I'm not saying the Clinton Foundation didn't help, didn't assist, it was a team effort. You can't clap with one hand only" (Hamied 2012).

Certainly, CHAI representatives took pains to portray their efforts with Indian firms to identify opportunities for realizing economies of scale as collaborative. Condliffe described the process. Around April or May 2003, Condliffe and four or five volunteers spent several weeks at manufacturing sites in India to build an analytical model that formed the basis of negotiations. She described it as "getting to know the companies" through a series of introductory visits and meetings at the senior level with the CEOs. The aim was to put together something similar to a "buying club," an informal consortium of countries expecting significant growth in treatment that would therefore generate an expected volume of demand for the companies. CHAI consultants sat down with the R&D teams to understand their business and what they were thinking about ARVs. They then worked remotely to build up cost models and spent time on where efficiencies might come from.

Given the importance of API in the overall cost of final drugs, Condliffe and the team took a trip to China in summer 2003 to visit intermediate suppliers. She gave the suppliers a sense of the volume forecast to see what impact it might have on their willingness to bring prices down for API. As the team worked with the companies on the final text of the agreement in advance of the October 2003 announcement, CHAI folks worked in parallel to support a series of national governments to develop country scale-up plans and raising money from donors to pay for the initiative (Condliffe 2012).

While acknowledging that the generic companies could have carried out this exercise on their own, Condliffe suggested that their meetings helped accelerate the process by which the companies considered the implications of expanded purchase orders. They discussed running longer and continuous batches, reducing down time, the possibilities of moving to larger vessels as volumes grew, when that might be possible, and where the most cost-effective intermediate suppliers might be (ibid.). Magaziner expressed a similar view, saying "if you know anything about drug production, it's like cooking. If you can do it in larger vats, you get economies of scale. If you can run a long production run, you reduce your costs because every time you change over, you have to wash the vat and are down a day" (Magaziner 2012).

Magaziner described these efforts to identify potential cost savings with expanded purchase orders as "dynamic costing," which allowed for "forward pricing." CHAI used the negotiations to set a ceiling price on the drugs, focusing initially on five drugs. What made the commitments credible, Magaziner said, along with the country plans for particular countries like Mozambique, Tanzania, Rwanda, and countries in the Caribbean, were commitments from Canada, Sweden, Ireland, and Norway to support those procurement plans of particular countries (Magaziner 2012).

By allying with the access advocates on ARVs, Indian generic companies could help secure some of their industry's own goals with respect to IP. As Roemer-Mahler argued: "The access to medicines campaign presented a context in which Indian companies could undertake a new attempt to influence global IP regulation to include more flexible standards" (Roemer-Mahler 2010a). For his part, what Hamied found attractive about the offer was the direct face-to-face discussion and transparency. He described it as different from a tender process. Rather, the Clinton folks said, "[W]e have so many dollars to spend," and they agreed on price and volume. Hamied contrasted that process with the current tender system for some contracts as "he who offers the lowest tender takes it all." He suggested that some of the generic firms put up huge factories, lost out on tenders to South Africa, and could not supply for two years (Hamied 2012).

Sandeep Juneja, formerly head of the HIV project at Ranbaxy from 2001 to 2007, echoed this perspective. Juneja, who had been working in southern Africa and looking for new business opportunities, initially prompted Ranbaxy's entry into the ARV market. During 2001 and 2002, he was in South Africa and observed the court case with branded companies. He noted that Ranbaxy's costs, which had already gotten into the ARV market in India, were much cheaper than branded companies. He suggested that, given the scale of the need in Africa, Ranbaxy enter the ARV market in Africa. The head of the pharma business offered Juneja a new job in running the effort out of New Delhi. At the time, Juneja said he was only vaguely aware of what other competitors like Cipla were doing. In June 2001, once he assumed his new position, Juneja began surveying what the market looked like, what products Ranbaxy would develop, the sources of API, and so forth. With the backing of the head of the pharma business, Juneja was able to get management to fast-track a few products.

This initial mission was motivated in large part by Corporate Social Responsibility (CSR) rather than as a source of profits. Still, it had to be "self-sustainable." Part of what made this mission a bit more attractive was that the funding stream would likely be donor driven where funding sources were secure, and money would come in on time. Given good credit deals with API suppliers, this new effort would not affect the working capital of the company. As another point in their favor, none of the ARVs, Juneja noted, required special manufacturing capabilities. The ARVs could be made alongside drugs for diabetes and painkillers, and did not require separate isolation.

Ranbaxy also saw this mission as a way to build its reputation in emerging markets, particularly the public sector, where the company was not as strong. What Ranbaxy did not anticipate is that its market entry would have a positive impact on its reputation in North America and Europe, which helped deepen the company's commitment to the initiative. However, he described its first couple of years as "pretty bare" in the order books. The company thought Cipla's offer would help elicit a larger market. Juneja personally did a lot of promotional work with African ambassadors in India in the lead-up to the 2001 winter holidays. They identified health ministers and had local Ranbaxy staff follow up, but despite offering a price of less than $300 per year, they did not get that many responses (Juneja 2012).

When CHAI approached Ranbaxy in 2002, Juneja said demand was picking up, though "still weak." Since the intentions were very good in the company, they decided to hold on and continue to work on an incremental cost basis. Any additional demand would be welcome and help Ranbaxy ramp up economies of scale and lower cost. CHAI suggested that they could put the developing countries together in a kind of pooled procurement. Their idea was to put the people together to form a sort of "buying club." CHAI, Juneja argued, "brought us into their vision of having a very low mark-up." He said CHAI asked us to "take a leap of faith that this will happen. And we did" (Juneja 2012).

Other generic firms described what made the CHAI process attractive to them in similar terms. Stavros Nicolaou, senior executive at South Africa's Aspen Pharmacare, described his firm's entry into the ARV market and its subsequent collaboration with CHAI. In late 2000 and early 2001, South Africa was coming to terms with the magnitude of its HIV pandemic. Faced with an unprecedented pandemic, Aspen decided that as the largest pharma in South Africa, it had to play a role in meeting the crisis. But prices had to come down, and in South Africa, patents were a barrier. Aspen was not a proponent of lobbying for compulsory licenses or more flexibility in TRIPS, as executives there believed that such moves would scare off potential foreign direct investors and have other consequences for the country. Aspen needed to maintain a dialogue with R&D companies to win potential licensing arrangements with them. With a video of a clinic near his ancestral home that Nelson Mandela had asked Aspen to sponsor, a group of Aspen executives went hat in hand to Paris to talk to BMS about a voluntary license for the production of some AIDS drugs. As confidence built around this license, later voluntary licenses shared R&D, then intellectual data, and finally full technology transfer. This model of voluntary licensing was then extended gradually to agreements with other companies. By introducing generics licenses in 2001 and 2002 and its first generic ARV in 2003, Aspen was able to bring prices down in the South African market. At around the same time, CHAI started to increase its image and efforts around HIV and was instrumental in negotiating lower API prices. This helped Aspen reduce prices and made treatment affordable to millions (Nicolaou 2012).

When the Clinton team approached Aspen, Nicolaou suggested that his firm's participation with CHAI initially "had to be a leap of faith" because the communal procurement process was "unprecedented." Nicolaou suggested that someone needed to coordinate volumes in the highly fragmented market, because by coordinating volumes, economies of scale and forward discounted prices of API could be realized. It took a lot of risk, and not everything CHAI tried succeeded, but a lot did (ibid.).

Another Indian generic company executive suggested that the initial CHAI model was very attractive, although it became somewhat problematic later on. He suggested that CHAI's model is different from what it subsequently became, which he described as a "facilitating agency." In the beginning, CHAI had a broader role. In his words, "[CHAI] gave us a proposal with an average price of $200 per patient per year." The company thought it could get some "good mileage out of" participating in CHAI's effort. The company initially waited for orders directly from CHAI, "but nothing materialized." Countries then ultimately began to approach the firm directly after two to three years. When the company offered those countries prices on their individual orders, CHAI might reappear and remind it of the CHAI price, which in some cases was lower (Indian Generics Firm Representative 2012).

The CHAI story raises the question of whether generic entry would have happened "on its own" without intervention by the Clinton Foundation or other advocates aimed at organizing the market. To this Magaziner responded that it may have happened eventually, but it "sure would have taken a lot longer," with many thousands of lives lost in the process. He pointed out that "[a] fair number of people are alive because we were able to get it done." He noted that the WHO had earlier debated internally the idea of organizing demand for a year and a half and did not pursue it in the end. He also emphasized that despite discussions in 2002 and 2003, neither the Global Fund nor WHO had moved forward with pooled procurement.

Further, at the time CHAI began its operations, the Global Fund was new and PEPFAR was not yet launched, so there was no major funding source for ARV purchases in the international community, providing a major inducement to generic entry. If CHAI had not brought buyers and sellers together, the market would have stayed fragmented, and it "would have been years and years" for the same results to be achieved by PEPFAR or the Global Fund (Magaziner 2012). Kate Condliffe, who joined CHAI in 2003 to launch its Drug Access Program, made a similar point, suggesting that by negotiating forward pricing based on future expected volumes, CHAI accelerated the development of the generics market and the price reductions that come with scale. In her view, these changes would not otherwise have happened for several years (Condliffe 2012). David Ripin, who joined CHAI in 2007 as part of its pharmaceuticals team, suggested that a "local equilibrium" can be reached with a stable situation that may not be optimal. Outside actors are needed to catalyze and disrupt the market to get over the barrier. He summed up the organization's perspective: "Some of what we and others have done in the market may very well have happened in the absence of intervention, but how much longer would it have taken and how many patients would not have had access to treatment as a result?" (Ripin 2012).

Leaving aside the technical role played by CHAI representatives, the initiative has been an important agent in driving down drug prices. One study looking at transactions conducted between July 2002 and October 2007 found that for 9 of 13 dosage forms, CHAI-negotiated prices were statistically significantly lower than non-CHAI purchases. Prices for CHAI drugs were lower by 6 to 36 percent below non-CHAI purchases (Waning et al. 2009, 525).[9] Indeed, CHAI's efforts may have been so successful that there are increasing concerns by producers that the prices have been driven so low as to discourage firms from staying in or entering the market, a theme to which we return in the final chapter.

As this market has matured, CHAI's role has transformed and expanded. No longer is it possible simply to use expanded volume as a way to drive prices down. CHAI has sought other avenues, including process improvements, to understand where there are technological and market bottlenecks in different areas from ARVs, to malaria, to vaccines (Magaziner 2012; Ripin 2012). For example, working with its own in-house technical capacity and collaboration with university scientists, CHAI was able to support the development of a new process to produce tenofovir, which reduced costs by 20 percent (Schoofs 2011). Thus, CHAI has continued to find ways to intervene in drug markets to bring more drugs to patients in the developing world.

Conclusions

The economist's view of the ARV market is that prices would have come down "naturally" once generic manufacturers entered the scene. As we have shown in this chapter, however, the ARV market had to be created, given disorganized demand among poor, developing countries and patent protection on several ARV medications that helped keep prices high. By attacking the TRIPS regime on the one hand and by pooling demand on the other, AIDS advocates advanced the cause of universal access to treatment regime. However, these changes ultimately had to be accompanied by purchase commitments from donor governments to make the generic ARV market a reality.

---

[9] The study also looked at products eligible for differential prices and compared the price of branded products to non-CHAI generics. Here, 15 of the 18 branded drug dosage forms were statistically more expensive than non-CHAI generics (which themselves were more expensive than CHAI generics), with margins ranging from 23 to 498. Only two branded drugs were cheaper than non-CHAI generics (Waning et al. 2009).

In pursuing their strategy, the advocates were attentive to the costs associated with a global treatment regime. They saw no path toward universal access if prices remained at or near industrialized world levels of around $10,000 per patient per year. At the same time, although this view was not universally shared by all advocates, price reductions had to be carried out in a way that did not impose inordinately high costs on the major players in the market, including incumbent firms, generics manufacturers, and governments in the developing and industrialized worlds.

In that respect, patent rights challenged the advocacy community as a potential dividing line. On one side were activists like Jamie Love, who believed that the patent regime was fundamentally illegitimate. On the other were UNAIDS officials like Peter Piot, who believed that industry was necessary to any long-term solution to the AIDS pandemic, as it held the keys to R&D and future AIDS therapies and cures. These perspectives did not ultimately stand in the way of expanded access. India's freedom to make and export many first-line generics until it fully had to adopt TRIPS rules bought the world time and removed some of the exigency of finding an immediate accommodation between health needs and industry concerns.

However, these contesting visions raise questions about the efficacy of different strategies of contestation and, in particular, whether oppositional tactics in the face of persistent industry power can succeed over the long term. While social movements often have a life cycle of movement mobilization and decline, large multinational enterprises, despite the vicissitudes of industrial change, may endure and live to fight another battle. Although advocates of the confrontational stripe may have won a few skirmishes like the South Africa court case and even, as we discuss in the next chapter, the 2001 Doha health exception, incumbent firms are resilient and can enlist the help of powerful allies at a later date to secure bilateral agreements between governments. Indeed, the pursuit of so-called TRIPS-plus programs has allowed firms to ring-fence ARVs as special and defend their interests in other domains, leading some analysts, like Drahos and Drezner, to question the lasting influence of advocates (Drahos 2007; Drezner 2007). As we discuss in the final chapter, these initiatives continue to proliferate, including the proposed India–EU bilateral agreement and the Trans-Pacific Partnership that the United States and a number of countries in Asia were negotiating in 2012.

For generics manufacturers, the patent issue was also explosive. Again, on the one hand they could enter markets that refused to uphold TRIPS disciplines for reasons of public health emergencies. On the other, to the extent that they wanted to engage in licensing agreements or to move toward innovative R&D themselves, then they also had an interest in supporting the patent regime. With patent issues looming large now that India is fully integrated into the TRIPS regime, these issues remain live areas of contention. Indeed, although voluntary licenses between branded and generics firms exist for a range of ARVs, generics companies have found themselves in conflict with branded firms. We return to these themes in the concluding chapter.

The strategy adopted for advancing universal access to treatment tried to reconcile some of these potentially divisive positions. By promoting the AAI, for example, pieces of the advocacy movement accepted the patent rights of big pharma in return for lower, differential prices, which at the time seemed like a major advance in the global rollout of AIDS drugs. At the same time, by pooling demand, advocates convinced generics manufacturers that a viable market for these drugs existed, even in the developing world.

Further, as we argued in this chapter and discuss in more detail in the next, the price reductions brought about through differential pricing and generic competition meant that the industrialized nations no longer had an excuse to stand by and donate only paltry sums to the fight against global AIDS. Advocates could lobby government agencies to increase their budgets for ARV drug procurement, and politicians who wanted to join this fight no longer had the high price of drugs standing in their way. In essence, lower prices gave those politicians who wanted to make global AIDS an issue some political cover.

In order to endure, however, an advocacy strategy for advancing market transformation, no matter how effective at a given moment in time, needs to be institutionalized: the operations of the transformed market, including its funding, its rules, and its market structures, need to be stabilized to set expectations for participating agents about the new rules of the game (Fligstein 2002). It is to these institutional issues that we turn in the following chapter.

6   Institutions to stabilize the market

> The emergence of a market for generic ARVs was shaped by public policies, notably the provision of donor funding for treatment and the creation of an international regulatory structure for drug quality approval.
>
> Anne Roemer-Mahler, 2010.

Until the Global Fund for AIDS, TB, and Malaria was created in 2002, if you were diagnosed with HIV, your fortunes were largely dependent upon where you were born. If you were born poor in Africa, you almost certainly were going to die. Access to ARV drugs was determined by market prices and your ability to pay. By contrast, if you were HIV+ in an advanced industrialized country, chances are that, by the late 1990s, you could get access to ARVs through national health systems or private insurance. Even the United States, which lacked a national insurance health scheme, provided poor Americans access to ARVs through programs like the AIDS Drug Assistance Programs, which came into being when the Ryan White CARE Act was passed in 1990.

Of course, rich and middle-income countries did not develop these programs overnight in pragmatic response to the AIDS pandemic. With AIDS initially viewed by the "mainstream" as a disease of the deviant, the community most immediately threatened by it had to mobilize to help create the political momentum for extending access to AIDS drugs to all who needed them. However, in most of the leading countries, the market and medical institutions required to diagnose, counsel, procure, dispense, treat, and pay for this access were already present and extensive. While many programs to test and treat the disease were new or even experimental, the broader edifice of health systems was in place.

At the beginning of the 2000s, the global response to AIDS experienced what analysts describe as a "revolution" (Fidler 2008). An enormous shift of resources, organization building, and effort took place in a short period of time, transforming the nature and form of global public health with extensive implications for other domains, including foreign assistance. In the process, global health policy became part and parcel of regular meetings of leaders of advanced industrialized countries, elevating these problems from low politics to higher, if not high, politics.

For AIDS, this "revolution" resulted in tremendous changes. In less than a decade, the number of people with access to treatment in low- and middle-income countries went up from about 200,000 in 2002 (three-quarters of whom were in Brazil) to 5.2 million by the end of 2009 (CFR 2010; WHO 2010a). This amount only covered about a third of the people sick enough to need treatment, but it was still regarded as an incredible triumph by advocates, largely unthinkable a decade earlier (although analysts have raised questions about the long-run sustainability of this policy (Over 2008)).

What changes made it possible to extend AIDS treatment to that number of people? As we have argued throughout this book, the institutions and rules changed such that the market allocation of drugs based on ability to pay (either directly or via national health insurance coverage) was replaced by the notion that all people, regardless of station, should ultimately have access to these drugs. While the transformation of ARVs from private into merit goods remains an aspirational goal to a large extent, given that many who are infected with HIV still do not receive treatment, international institutions now promote delivery of AIDS drugs to poor countries, and they have become a high-volume, low-margin good.

For that market transformation to happen, a number of changes in the international organizational landscape were needed. Namely, the creation of the Global Fund, PEPFAR, and UNITAID (described in more detail in this chapter) made it possible to correct for the demand-side failures of low-income countries and gave suppliers – increasingly generic producers – the incentive to enter the market and provide drugs to people in poor countries. These bilateral and multilateral funding mechanisms came into being once ARV prices began to fall and the "proof of concept" that they could be effective in resource-constrained settings had been demonstrated.

That said, we recognize that the delivery of AIDS treatment and the story of how those changes happened involves a host of other actors and organizations as well, both within and outside the global health arena. Unlike most health challenges, AIDS has become part of a broader complex of institutions; while the disease is nested mainly in the issue of global public health, aspects of the problem overlap with other domains such as trade and national security as well (Alter and Meunier 2009; Fidler 2010). For that reason, organizations like the WTO and such UN bodies as the General Assembly and Security Council, have taken an interest in various aspects of the AIDS pandemic. Indeed, the pervasive nature of AIDS and its actual or potential influence on the security environment (particularly in Africa), as well as on global health, helped create a large coalition of interests behind a treatment regime.

This chapter seeks to explain how increasing access to ARVs was shaped by the rule-making processes of organizations involved in the global AIDS arena. Our starting assumption is that markets require institutions that provide certain "stabilizing" services in order to function (Fligstein 2002). For pharmaceutical companies, for example, these institutions include property rights regimes and health care systems that provide incentives for medical innovation on the one hand and an outlet for new technologies and treatments on the other. The same market for drugs, however, can create undesirable allocations from the perspective of at least some social groups. Changing the principle of access to ARVs was a key objective of treatment activists, but that required both challenging and altering (or building from scratch) the institutional structure for global AIDS policy.

As we have maintained throughout the book, this new market did not emerge spontaneously owing to the "natural" forces of supply and demand but was politically constructed. Universal access to treatment would have been stunted at birth without political intervention to stabilize the market around this new principle of drug allocation. That political intervention primarily involved standard-setting policies over drugs and procurement policies that enabled developing countries to acquire medications and diagnostic tests and equipment. How these new institutions and rules were built is the main topic of this chapter.

The chapter is divided into six sections. The first reviews the market-stabilizing functions of international institutions in general, and the rules that stabilized the ARV drug access regime in particular. The second section explores the most important institutional innovations that have stabilized the market in support of access, namely, the Global Fund and PEPFAR, with some discussion of UNITAID as well. The remaining sections elaborate on five elements of standard-setting – the decisions in 2001 and 2003 over IPR and drug patents; the WHO's treatment guidelines that were created in 2002 and amended in 2003, 2006, and 2010; the WHO's pre-certification policies for drugs which were created in 2001; and the US FDA parallel certification standard, which was created in 2004.

Explaining AIDS governance, rule changes, and ARV access

International rule-making can lead to changes in the behavior of both states and private sector actors. New trade rules, for example, may limit the ability of states to impose restrictive tariffs, while providing incentives for firms to import and export a range of goods and services. On balance, the expectation is that these rules ought to be to the advantage of all states that participate in the international institutions, if states freely enter into the agreements. Kapstein, for example, argues that international institutions must be inclusive, participatory, and welfare-enhancing (Kapstein 2006a). As such, international rules should be self-reinforcing (North 1990).

However, as the Nobel Prize-winning economic historian, Douglass North, has shown, economically inefficient rules can persist over time, advantaging some interests over others (North 1990). Building on this argument, Fligstein contends that most rules work on behalf of incumbent firms and that politics is about creating and sustaining institutions that privilege their interests. Even if international institutions are "freely" created by states and supposed to serve their interests, unequal power relations can influence negotiations and enforcement dynamics such that it is unclear if the content of international rule-making is in fact consistent with the long-run interests of all states (Barnett and Duvall 2005; Fligstein 2008).

Institutions perform a number of functions that enable markets to clear. These include ensuring that contracts are honored, that disputes can be resolved peacefully, and that property rights are respected. Information asymmetries must also be contained so that buyers and sellers can reach agreements over prices and quantities. If the rules of the game for market transactions are constantly being rewritten, a firm cannot reliably depend on a particular income stream. For firms that have major multi-million or billion dollar investments in infrastructure and research that take many years to amortize, the uncertainty wrought by unstable institutional bargains will diminish their willingness to invest. States can impose different burdens on firms in terms of what costs they have to incur to do business in their territory, but everywhere firms seek policy stability.[1]

As Robert Keohane wrote in the 1980s, international institutions are ostensibly useful to states for similar reasons. They provide a set of functions to states and private sector actors that make them attractive, including reducing transactions costs, providing information, and improving monitoring and enforcement to detect and deter cheating.

---

[1] As the varieties of capitalism literature has suggested, firms can flourish under different systems of rules that impose more or less costs (Hall and Soskice 2001). The overall level of costs is important but as, if not more, important is the certainty of the rules that actors can take as given when they plan their activities. Instability and volatility of rules, practices, and behavior may be the enemy of market activity more so than the high costs of doing business. In an increasingly globalized world, even if there is some variation in rule-making between countries, firms have sought both more uniformity of treatment (at least by kind of country) and more secure rules to stabilize their expectations.

Because of their usefulness to states, the scope for cooperation in the absence of hierarchy (i.e. there is no world government) in the international system may be extensive (Keohane 1982; see also Abbott and Snidal 1998). As Robert Axelrod pointed out, institutions may allow states to extend their time horizons to look beyond the current period and recognize the cooperative opportunities wrought by repeated interactions with others (Axelrod 1984).

To understand the landscape of institutions and organizations involved in reinforcing the principle of access to AIDS treatment, it can be helpful to ask the question, "What tasks or functions does the regime complex need to perform?"[2] Many of these functions are universal to other substantive arenas, but here we focus on the core market-stabilizing functions essential for treatment access. Beyond proper diagnosis of the disease, getting large numbers of people on ARV therapy requires a continuous and credible source of funding for needed medications, along with distribution mechanisms that are cost-effective in getting drugs into bodies. Property rights rules must balance concerns about future innovation against present-day access, while quality assurance mechanisms and treatment guidelines must ensure that the right drugs, appropriately vetted, get to the people who need them.

In this chapter, we focus primarily on institutions that mobilize finance and provide standard-setting related to patent rights, drug guidelines, and quality assurance mechanisms. Given that many patients lacked purchasing power to buy drugs on their own, credible commitments of money to purchase ARVs were essential for the universal access market to function. At the same time, decisions about patent rights, what medications should be taken, and whether or not drugs met certain quality standards ultimately determined which ARVs could be bought and sold in the newly created global market.

Together, these effects reflect *market stabilization* around a new principle of universal access. Whereas before, the principle of access was based on

---

[2] (Keohane and Victor 2010; Busby 2010b). One study suggested the tasks of global health included seven core functions: (1) convening, (2) defining shared values, (3) ensuring coherence, (4) establishing standards and regulatory frameworks, (5) providing direction (establishing priorities), (6) mobilizing and aligning resources, and (7) promoting research (Sridhar, Khagram, and Pang 2010, 2). For a similar list of global health functions, see Ruger and Yach 2008. Their list includes norms and standards, global action, professional management, financial resource transfer, scientific research capacity, and leadership. Will, quoting David Kay, identifies a comparable list that included: (1) problem identification, agenda setting, consciousness raising, (2) monitoring and evaluation, (3) data gathering and information collection, (4) risk evaluation/impact assessment, (5) information exchange and dissemination, (6) facilitation of coordination, (7) normative pronouncements, (8) standard setting and rule-making, (9) supervision of norms, and (10) operational activity (Will 1991).

ability to pay, the new principle of access, though aspirational, was based on need. Adoption of this new principle implied a change in the market structure for ARVs, from low volumes/high margins to high volumes/low margins. In the transition period leading to market stabilization around the new principle of access, institutions – that is, the rules that shape market incentives – had to coalesce around the objective of putting larger numbers of people on treatment at the least possible cost.

Market stability does not mean that markets no longer evolve and change. Indeed, given the size of the unmet need for ARV medications, market stability around the new access principle was contingent upon it being scalable. Simply put, this meant that either additional funds had to be made available to buy more drugs from pharmaceutical manufacturers or drug prices had to continue to decline to meet greater needs at given levels of funding, say, due to innovation in the ARV space. In other words, if the new principle of access was to endure over time, the following had to happen: (1) expanding volumes of products being made available, (2) falling prices, and (3) credible commitments of finance for drug purchases. To the extent that market stability around the new principle of access invites entry by low-cost producers, we would also expect (4) to see firm entry into the ARV market-place. In the medium- to longer-run, however, as Waning and her co-authors warn, competition (combined with government pressure) could drive prices for ARVs too far down, meaning that profit margins are inadequate to spur innovation, or even to keep existing firms in the game (Waning, Kyle *et al.* 2010, 17). This may ultimately mean that governments will somehow subsidize the production of these medications.

Other observable indications of a transformed market include greater use of generic ARVs by developing countries (especially in light of the 2001 WTO declaration on TRIPS and public health); the use of compulsory licensing and TRIPS flexibilities; and, finally, exploitation of the 2003 "August 30th" WTO provision to allow exports of drugs made under compulsory license to third countries without production capabilities. The remaining sections of this chapter examine how institutional creation and rule changes shaped and sought to stabilize a new market structure based on expanded access to treatment.

Mobilizing finance: the Global Fund, PEPFAR, and UNITAID

Arguably, the two most important institutional innovations that have facilitated access to treatment are the Global Fund to Fight AIDS, Tuberculosis, and Malaria and PEPFAR, the US bilateral AIDS response. A third program, UNITAID, has also become an important source of finance for ARV procurement, based largely on a tax on airline tickets that some countries have put into force.

The Global Fund, with a small secretariat located in Geneva, was created in 2002 as an independent pass-through financing entity and has largely, though not exclusively, been funded through financing rounds from supporting member governments. Interestingly, the Global Fund is not in the UN family of organizations, and as a consequence, possesses interesting design features, with civil society formally represented on its board, a feature not possible in member state-governed UN organizations. PEPFAR, created under the aegis of President George W. Bush in 2003, is a bilateral program funded through US Congressional appropriations. Its proponents also promised that it would serve as a radical departure from existing US foreign aid ventures with its swift disbursement of funds mainly to fifteen focus countries, most of them in Africa and the Caribbean.

Given their scale, the Global Fund and PEPFAR are the most significant of the programs that have financed large-scale purchases of ARVs. Since 2002, the Fund has had ten funding rounds, with an eleventh that was set to open in August 2011 cancelled due to deterioration in the Fund's financial status and contestation over its management. As of December 31, 2010, the Fund had mobilized $21.7 billion for more than 600 programs in 150 countries. Given its wider mandate, of course, not all of these funds were dedicated to addressing the HIV/AIDS crisis (Global Fund 2010a). The Fund, as of January 1, 2010, had allocated about 57 percent of its grant resources to HIV/AIDS (Global Fund 2010b). A significant portion of Global Fund expenditure supports drug procurement. Eighteen percent of the Fund's portfolio has supported the purchase of medicines and pharmaceutical products; another 17 percent has supported health products and health equipment (Global Fund undated). The Global Fund estimates that it was supporting nearly 3 million people on ARV therapy as of December 2010 (potentially co-financed by other partners), up from 130,000 people in 2004 (Global Fund 2011a).

For its part, PEPFAR mobilized $38.923 billion (in nominal dollars) between fiscal years (FY) 2004 and 2011 (see Table 6.1). This total includes a significant amount of money for the Global Fund, to which the United States is also the largest donor. Through FY 2010, US contributions to the Global Fund totaled $5.7bn. Like the Global Fund, a significant share of PEPFAR's bilateral resources is dedicated to treatment. In the early years of the program, this share was set by Congress at 55 percent. When PEPFAR was re-authorized in 2008, these directives were relaxed, with at least half the money to be spent on treatment and care. In FY 2009, 35 percent of PEPFAR's $4.2 billion in bilateral funding was directed towards treatment (Kaiser Family Foundation 2011a). PEPFAR reported

Table 6.1: *PEPFAR appropriations by FY 2004–12*

Fiscal year (FY)	Appropriations (in $ billions)
2004	2.311
2005	2.719
2006	3.29
2007	4.518
2008	6.031
2009	6.68
2010	6.687
2011	6.687
2012*	7.154

Source: Kaiser Family Foundation 2011a.
* FY 2012 figure is US President Barack Obama's budget request only.

that its programs supported 3.2 million people on ARVs as of September 30, 2010 (Office of the US Global AIDS Coordinator 2010).[3]

The volume of donor funds disbursed for global health, led primarily by investments in the Global Fund and PEPFAR, increased dramatically in the 2000s, from $4.5 billion in 2002 to $17.2 billion in 2009 (Kaiser Family Foundation 2011b). Both the Global Fund and PEPFAR represented significant departures from past practice in terms of the volume of funds that were leveraged and, as suggested above, also in terms of institutional design. The Global Fund was an independent financing agency outside the UN family, whereas PEPFAR was created as a program outside the traditional bilateral foreign assistance program USAID. In this context, it is interesting to understand how both came about and took the form they did, not least because other movements have been inspired by the process of their founding and their unique design. In both cases, the role of civil society in their creation remains contested, but the important point for our purposes is that these institutions exist to support and sustain the new principle of universal access to treatment.[4]

[3] It should be noted that PEPFAR does not support the full costs of treatment, but shares the costs with other donors. A 2012 PEPFAR study estimated that for first-line therapies, the estimated average PEPFAR contribution was $305 of the $708 in annual treatment costs (Office of the US Global AIDS Coordinator 2012).
[4] A variety of actors can take some credit for contributing to the founding of the Global Fund. Jeff Sachs called for such a fund at the 2000 Durban meeting. Peter Piot suggested that the ideas for the Fund's size came out of a study led by UNAIDS' Bernhard Schwartländer (Piot 2012, Kindle Location 5062–79) and identifies a number of different proponents, including US Representatives Barbara Lee and Jim Leach, as well as Dave Nabarro of the UK DFID (ibid., Kindle Location 5551–69). US Senate

Given that UN Secretary General (at the time) Kofi Annan is often cited as the lead advocate for the Global Fund, the question may be asked, why did it not end up becoming part of the UN family? Richard Feachem, the Global Fund's first executive director, put the decision in context in an interview with the authors. Although there had been some successful efforts at AIDS containment in a few places like Brazil, basically the "HIV pandemic was raging completely out of control and ... collective efforts to attenuate it up until the 2000s had achieved nothing." Establishing the first global financing mechanism since Bretton Woods, rather than creating a new International Development Association (IDA) replenishment window at the World Bank or a financing arm of WHO, was therefore a major decision. However, given that the existing institutions had clearly failed, including the UN and the World Bank, activists, NGOs, and officials in the US government all recognized that whatever entity was created had to be "new and different" in order to justify substantial new funding (Feachem 2012).

In Feachem's view, though a number of wealthy governments were indifferent about potentially locating the Global Fund in the UN family, there were enough voices opposed, including the US and Japanese governments, that the Fund ultimately became an independent entity. Feachem recalls a meeting in 2006 when Annan visited the Fund. Asked about the initial decision, Annan said, "At the time, 2001, I wanted it to be part of the UN and now in 2006, I'm glad that I lost the argument. Had you been part of the UN, you would not have achieved what you have." Although there have been some enclaves of success in the UN system, including the smallpox eradication initiative that was based at the WHO, Feachem suggested that the "dead hand of bureaucracy," particularly in hiring and firing, would have prohibited the kinds of innovation and success the Global Fund was able to achieve as an independent agency (Feachem 2012).

Christoph Benn, director of external relations for the Global Fund, suggested that it was "most remarkable" that an independent fund was strongly supported by Annan and WHO's Director, Gro Harlem Brundtland. In Benn's view, Brundtland strongly promoted the creation of such a

---

Majority Leader Bill Frist and other US lawmakers were working on legislation that was the predecessor to the Global Fund (Russell 2012). The Japanese credit the idea to the January 2000 G8 summit in Okinawa, where the hosts proposed an initiative on infectious disease (Ministry of Foreign Affairs of Japan 2000). For his part, Kofi Annan is often identified as the main champion for Global Fund. Building on the 2000 UN Security Council meeting, Annan set in motion the international process that culminated in the Fund in January 2002. His April 2001 speech in Abuja, Nigeria, calling for the Fund, and the subsequent UN General Assembly meeting in June 2011, are often identified as two key meetings that led to the Fund (Schocken undated).

Fund and never insisted that it should be part of the UN. It was important that the Fund be independent and flexible, with governance decided by all parties, including civil society and the private sector (Benn 2010). As both Benn and Feachem noted, no UN entity can include NGO representatives as full members, since that status is limited to member states. Both regarded the Fund's formal incorporation of NGO representatives on the board as a critical attribute of the new organization (Benn 2010; Feachem 2012). Similar issues apply to the Global Fund's relation to the private sector and the private sector board seat.

Piot noted that the suggestion from David Nabarro of the UK's Department for International Development (DFID) was to have the Fund associated with UNAIDS. In Piot's view, "we would not be *able* to operate transfers of huge amounts of money with any degree of efficiency," being so dependent on WHO and the United Nations Development Programme (UNDP)'s administrative systems that he regarded as "slow, bound up in red tape." While other co-sponsoring agencies were "keen on a UN fund" (except for UNDP's Mark Malloch Brown), Piot recognized that the United States would not accept a new UN agency in control of this program. Piot's view was shared by both Kofi Annan and his deputy, Louis Frechette: "Louis had an even darker view of UN efficiency than I did, and Annan felt that no US Congress would vote for billions of dollars in new funding for anything to do with the UN" (Piot 2012, Kindle Location 5551–69). With a variety of proposals circulating in early 2001 for special multilateral AIDS funds, UN agencies and donors started coalescing around the idea of a single fund, though WHO remained a holdout until the April 2001 meeting in Abuja, where Annan and Brundtland ironed out remaining differences (ibid., Kindle Location 5569–86).

The negotiations over the course of 2001 leading up to the Fund's creation were contentious. Piot notes that the working group faced greatly divergent views: "But the major donor countries and the European Commission agreed on one thing: they were on a war path against the UN." France suggested replacing UNAIDS on the working group with a pharmaceutical company representative, while the UK regretted that UNAIDS did not "voluntarily" withdraw from the group, as it was becoming too large. Bill Steiger, who led the Bush administration's negotiations, "tried to remove UNAIDS and WHO from the working group completely" and though socially likable, "he was ferocious in his never-ending attacks on the UN and WHO" (Piot 2012, Kindle Location 5586–603).

Piot suggests that the outside pressure from AIDS activists was "intense" and that the major points of contention were whether the Fund "should be independent or hosted by the World Bank, where it should be based, who should head it up, which health problems it would finance in addition to AIDS, which countries could benefit, whether it would only pay for commodities such as drugs and condoms or also for actual programs, who would decide where the money would go, and much, much more" (ibid., Kindle Location 5603–20). By January 2002, these differences had been ironed out in time for the fund's creation, head-quartered in Geneva, with three NGO representatives formally on the board. Of this story, which we can only begin to capture here, Piot said, "I'm sure a few Ph.D. theses will come out of it" (ibid., Kindle Location 5604–20).

While the process leading up to the creation of the Global Fund had some space for advocacy groups to contribute to its founding, PEPFAR, as suggested in Chapter 3 on movement coherence, was created by a handful of people inside the US government, outside of normal channels of inter-agency deliberation. Mark Dybul suggested why this was necessary: "If it went through the normal interagency process, we would still be talking about it" (Dybul 2009). The narrative of the internal deliberations has been told both by journalists and scholars, as well as in a number of different memoirs by former President George W. Bush, Secretary of State Condoleezza Rice, speechwriter Michael Gerson, domestic policy adviser Jay Lefkowitz, and Senate majority leader Bill Frist (Behrman 2004; Gerson 2007; Messac 2008; Frist 2009; Lefkowitz 2009; Gartner 2009a; Bush 2010; Busby 2010c; Rice 2011; Donnelly 2012).

Most accounts focus on the moral convictions of the president, and the advice he received from Rice and Gerson, among others, in the lead-up to the formal announcement to move forward with the plan. Bush himself is credited with giving Anthony Fauci (of the National Institute of Allergy and Infectious Diseases) the instruction to "Think big!" and envision a program with a much larger budget than had been developed as part of an earlier $200 million program to prevent the transmission from mothers to their children. Both Bush and a number of his advisers pushed Fauci and Dybul to demonstrate the feasibility of treatment. In previous work, one of us assessed other explanations for the program's announcement in early 2003, including the imminent war in Iraq and the role of pharmaceutical companies, neither of which were regarded as especially relevant. As Dybul confirmed to us again, the notion that Iraq had something to do with this process was unfounded: "As one of the people engaged from day one, that is just nonsense." The subject never came up. Moreover, pharma companies had "zero [role]. No involvement whatsoever" (Dybul 2009).

While the various histories of PEPFAR provide some flavor of the process that led to the announcement in President Bush's 2003 State of the Union address, a 2012 article by John Donnelly provides some interesting detail that suggests the importance of pilot or proof of concept projects, both in justification for PEPFAR overall as well as for its specific design. Donnelly describes the process in the following terms: "In 2001 Fauci and Dybul helped start a series of clinical trials in Africa to test various approaches in antiretroviral treatment. The idea was to find a way to lessen the cost of treatment so as to put more people on medication, while still making sure people didn't develop resistance to the drugs." In Uganda, Dybul observed the efforts in Kampala by Dr. Peter Mugyenyi, who would later be President Bush's guest of honor at his 2003 speech. Those treatment programs were largely successful, but Dybul pressed further to see if programs in rural areas might also be a success. In the town of Tororo near the Kenyan border, Dybul, along with colleagues from the CDC, found pilot projects run by TASO, a Ugandan NGO. With health care workers on scooters visiting patients in distant locations to ensure that they were taking their medications, eating well, and in good health, Dybul concluded: "Here was an opportunity to really get access to people. It showed me that it was possible to treat AIDS both in clinic and through rural outreach" (quoted in Donnelly 2012, 1391).

Even as these visits were persuasive, a few of the experts consulted in the lead-up to the announcement understood that scaling-up treatment would be a tremendous challenge. Paul Farmer was one of those invited for a November 2002 meeting at the White House. As Donnelly writes:

Farmer also was secretly worried. When he looked at himself and the three others, he realized that altogether they had treated only a few hundred patients. He was the only one of the four treating AIDS patients in a rural setting, and he had just 100 people under his care. And now they were talking not thousands or hundreds of thousands of patients, but millions. (Donnelly 2012, 1395)

Despite his reservations, he remained hopeful: "[W]e had faith in this, almost unwavering faith, about the slender amount of data on which to base a major health initiative. There was no reason to believe that the treatment of Africans would be any different than the treatment of Americans" (ibid.). In the end, President Bush decided to support the effort and administration members threw their weight behind it with an announcement of $15 billion. As Dybul attested, the reason was simple: "President Bush cared about it deep in his heart." He had a personal interest and directed his staff to do it and do it well. It was not because anyone whispered in his ear. He had a deep religious belief. There was this overwhelming catastrophe killing the most productive members of society, and something had to be done (Dybul 2009).

As largely taxpayer-funded programs, both the Global Fund and PEP-FAR might suffer from a problem of credible commitments as consistent and reliable sources of long-term finance. Donors may cut back, or at least curtail the expansion of funding sources in difficult economic times. That reduction has happened with respect to AIDS funding since the financial crisis of 2008, although the flat-lining and slight decline in commitments and disbursements are not as great as some have feared. However, in the early years of both programs, appropriations of money did materialize in large amounts, providing at least a credible present opportunity for service and drug providers. That said, recognizing the potential cyclical volatility of funding sources based on foreign assistance, supporters of the Global Fund and global health sought more broadly to develop alternative financing schemes that were counter-cyclical, or at the very least provided an alternative funding stream to government appropriations. For example, celebrities like Bono created Product RED in 2006, a line of consumer products from retailers like Gap, Armani, and Apple, with a portion of proceeds of t-shirt sales, sunglasses, and other items destined for the Global Fund.[5]

More significantly, with funding from the world's first global tax, levied on airline travel, UNITAID was created in September 2006, with proceeds aimed to help partners like the Global Fund and the United Nations (International) Children's (Emergency) Fund (UNICEF) procure drugs and supplies for AIDS, TB, and malaria at low cost (generating more than $1 billion in its first three years of operation).[6] UNITAID is considerably smaller than the Global Fund and PEPFAR. By 2011, it had mobilized almost $2 billion for a variety of activities, including drug procurement for ARVs (Douste-Blazy 2011). Since 2006, UNITAID has leveraged more than $790 million for HIV-related products, including drugs and diagnostics, helping treat nearly a million people. UNITAID, through partnering with CHAI (discussed in the last chapter) has focused on pediatric AIDS, becoming the largest funder of pediatric AIDS drugs in low-income countries (UNITAID 2011).

Where the Global Fund had its origins in Kofi Annan's vigorous advocacy, and PEPFAR is a US government-directed initiative that President George W. Bush set in motion, UNITAID is a multilateral initiative with bilateral roots. Housed under the auspices of the WHO,

---

[5] Product RED raised more than $160 million for the Global Fund between 2006 and 2010. See also www.joinred.com/red/; www.theglobalfund.org/en/resources/?lang=en.

[6] See www.unitaid.eu/. Parallel efforts to support long-term finance include the International Financing Facility for Immunisation (IFFIm), which seeks to issue bonds in capital markets from rich countries to support GAVI's activities. See www.iff-immunisation.org/. Another new initiative, Debt2Health, was created in 2007 and allows countries to swap foreign debt in exchange for freeing up additional resources for Global Fund-supported programs. See www.theglobalfund.org/en/innovativefinancing/debt2health/. Through mid 2012, four agreements have been reached leveraging more than $100m for the Global Fund.

UNITAID has its own governance structure with a 12-person executive board that includes representatives of the WHO, founding countries, regional representatives of affected countries, civil society, and foundations. UNITAID was strongly influenced by the French under the leadership of its then-President Jacques Chirac. The idiosyncrasies of its formation are described in the memoir by the French politician Philippe Douste-Blazy. He describes the process that led to UNITAID's creation: "As Jacques Chirac settled into his second term as president, he undoubtedly realized that he would be seventy-four at its conclusion. He had already begun to think about ways to cement his status as a great leader .... [H]e chose the Millennium Development Goals as his challenge" (Douste-Blazy and Altman 2010, 15). Chirac sought a way to connect a desire to do something meaningful on international development that would be supported by a tax on financial transactions or airlines. With a tax on financial transactions running into opposition, Chirac settled on an airline tax.

In his efforts to identify a suitable target, Douste-Blazy, after becoming foreign minister, stumbled on one after meeting with Bill Clinton in 2005. Clinton told him he should work on HIV/AIDS and said, "You have to say to the drug companies, I'm giving you money, not for one year but for several years, for example, three hundred million dollars per year for five years. How much do you agree to decrease the price?" (Douste-Blazy and Altman 2010, 22). Upon his return, during a visit with Brazil's President Lula, Chirac asked Douste-Blazy: "You've both spoken about an airline ticket tax, but what is it for?" (ibid., 23). Lula said hunger, Chirac said AIDS, and Douste-Blazy was allowed to break the tie and supported AIDS and a financing initiative for drug purchases.

After successfully broaching the idea in September 2005 with Lee Jong-Wook of the WHO, Peter Piot of UNAIDS, Richard Feachem of the Global Fund, and Ira Magaziner of CHAI, they wrote a communiqué outlining what the fund would do. In December 2005, Douste-Blazy was able to relay the memo to Chirac, who blessed it: "It's a good idea. Perfect, Philippe. Move forward" (Douste-Blazy and Altman 2010, 26). In 2006, Douste-Blazy then worked out the logistics to enlist other countries, including a number of developing countries, to bless the airline tax or find other ways to support the initiative. The early champions of the fund also included Brazil, Chile, the UK, and Norway. At the time, the effort was going to be called FIAM (Facilité Internationale d'Achats de Médicaments). After meeting with a young radio personality who thought the name sounded too inaccessible, a new name was suggested: *Tous Unis pour Aider* (Everyone United to Help) which, contracted, became UNITAID (Douste-Blazy and Altman 2010, 30). In September 2006, UNITAID was born.

How have these three programs leveraged ARV drug procurement? Once the Fund was created in January and Feachem was appointed as its first Executive Director in April 2002, a whole host of operating procedures had to be established, and staff had to be hired. As Feachem noted, even though the interim leadership had approved some initial funding decisions, there was no proper office, no bank account, and no employees, just a name on a door in a suburb in Geneva. Procurement rules were among the key issues in those early months. Everything was put in place with the team that they built. According to Feachem, the procurement rules were always buy branded or generic, Indian or otherwise, provided that the purchase was legal in national and international law. They wanted quality assurance, either through the WHO prequalification scheme (discussed below) or, preferably, a "stringent regulatory authority," of which there are about half a dozen in the world. In short, they wanted legality, assured quality, and best prices from day one. Interestingly, with respect to generics, Feachem said "board delegations that might have objected, didn't." He suggested that the board "behaved extremely well on that issue" and that powerful board members, like the United States, did not object (Feachem 2012). Thus, generic drug purchases became part and parcel of the Global Fund's procurement system from the outset.

The same was not true of PEPFAR, whose procurement practices were, as Feachem noted, initially "strikingly different." As discussed later in the chapter, PEPFAR's supporters always envisioned a role for generics, but initially it only purchased branded ARVs and did not accept the WHO quality assurance prequalified list of medicines. What this meant is that clinics that received funding from both the Global Fund and PEPFAR had to keep careful records on the different drugs that could be bought under each program, naturally adding to their administrative and reporting costs. It also meant that treatment costs per patient were much higher for PEP-FAR than for the Global Fund (Feachem 2012). As we discuss in the section on the FDA fast-track approval process, once approved in mid 2004, both programs could increasingly procure the same drugs.

Until 2007, the Global Fund's ARV procurement policy was disaggregated, with countries purchasing ARVs individually, informed by the WHO treatment guidelines and the list of prequalified medicines. In April 2007, the Global Fund board decided to create the Voluntary Pooled Procurement (VPP) program that became operational in 2009. With over 40 percent of its funds dedicated to procurement of drugs and other medical supplies, the VPP was intended to drive the prices down further and ensure faster delivery as well as higher quality products. In the 18 months of operation between June 2009 and December 2010, $70.9m worth of ARVs were purchased through the VPP.

Table 6.2: *Percentage global market share by volume of new first-line ARVs by PEPFAR, UNITAID, and Global Fund, 2008*

Drug	PEPFAR	UNITAID	Global Fund	Total market share
ABC	11	42	30	83
FTC	39	45	6	90
TDF	28	49	12	89

Source: Waning, Kyle *et al.* 2010.

Feachem suggested resistance from donor countries in Europe, who were trying to build local capacity in procurement, delayed deployment of pooled procurement. Feachem argued that he pushed for pooled procurement from "day minus 1." He wanted a procurement scheme with teeth modeled on GAVI (formerly the Global Alliance for Vaccines and Immunisation) that negotiated a common price for recipient countries. Recipients were free to negotiate their own individual deals on vaccines, but they would only be reimbursed for the price that GAVI had negotiated, a move that could obviate the potential for misappropriation of funds, low-quality products, or sweetheart deals between the supplier and the individual agent in the recipient country. Some board members, particularly European donors whose bilateral programs supported technical capacity, saw this pooled procurement as top-down imposition and undermining of local procurement skills. Despite support from the United States and Japan, pooled procurement languished, and ultimately only a "watered down" version was implemented (Feachem 2012).

Both PEPFAR and UNITAID have had pooled procurement schemes for longer than the Global Fund (Global Fund 2011b). PEPFAR's pooled procurement has been handled by the Supply Chain Management System (SCMS), a consortium of NGOs and private sector providers that was created in late 2005. CHAI has been responsible for pooled procurement for UNITAID since it was created in 2006, although its history of brokering price reductions for ARVs dates back to October 2003 when it announced its first agreement with generic pharmaceutical companies.

Together, these three programs account for most of the market share of drug procurement. For example, for older first-line ARVs such as EFV, 3TC, NVP, d4T, and ZDV, Waning *et al.* estimated that in 2008 PEPFAR accounted for 27–34 percent of market by volume, with the Global Fund accounting for 47–57 percent. Table 6.2 provides more detail on drug purchases of newer first-line ARVs (Waning, Kyle *et al.* 2010, 8, 13).

Similar results can be observed when looking at purchases of triple-cocktail FDCs. The FDC 3TC/NVP/d4T cocktail was only approved by the FDA fast-track process in November 2006, making it eligible for use through PEPFAR in 2007. Until then, the Global Fund was the main purchaser. By 2008, PEPFAR represented 40 percent of the market for this FDC, split between two companies, Strides and Cipla. Similarly, in 2008, PEPFAR accounted for 28 percent of the purchases of the 3TC/NVP/ZDV combination. Purchases were split among three companies, of which more than 90 percent came from a single firm, Aurobindo. Meanwhile, the Global Fund's purchases, which reflected its then still-disaggregated procurement process, were spread more evenly across four-to-five manufacturers (Waning, Kyle *et al.* 2010, 8). For small firms like Aurobindo, PEPFAR purchase orders consti-tuted a significant part of their business, nearly 9 percent of their total revenues in 2007. For larger firms like Cipla and Ranbaxy, PEPFAR was an important, though less significant share of their revenue, more on the order of 1-to-2 percent of total annual revenues (Roemer-Mahler 2010b, 47).

What the various procurement programs under the Global Fund, PEPFAR, and UNITAID have in common is that they have delivered affordable medicines to patients at scale. With the Global Fund and PEPFAR each taking credit for 3 million-plus patients on ARVs, and UNITAID providing ARV services to almost a million people, that was demonstrated. While branded pharmaceuticals have been crucial sources of ARV supply, particularly for PEPFAR before the FDA expedited approval for generics, low-cost generic ARVs, aside from procurement and distribution systems, have enabled these programs to ramp up to wider numbers of people.

What enabled PEPFAR, the Global Fund, and UNITAID to scale more broadly and quickly compared to the industry-led DAI and AAI efforts discussed in the last chapter? Whereas PEPFAR relied more on bilateral, embassy-based procedures to swiftly roll out programs, the Global Fund sought broader country ownership through locally con-trolled coordinating mechanisms. All three – PEPFAR, the Global Fund, and UNITAID – were underpinned by standard operating procedures that sought to regularize the procedures for access and to translate the process of drug procurement into an efficient delivery mechanism from application to service provision. Because the spon-soring agencies were firmly committed to swift rollout of access, they subsidized the cost and provided technical assistance to recipient countries to enable them to get the paperwork right in applying for funds and services.

Mobilization of finance to procure ARVs is only part of the institutional story. In order to purchase drugs, particularly low-cost generic versions of ARVs, they had to be available in the first place. A host of other decisions, on IPRs, drug regimen guidelines, and quality assurance, had to come together to make it possible for generic firms to make the drugs and for procurement agencies to buy them.

WTO rule-making

The January 1995 agreement that brought into existence the WTO included language on TRIPS. By creating minimum standards for IP, TRIPS sought to narrow the flexibility countries previously had in administering their national IP regimes. TRIPS mandated that countries had to offer twenty years of patent exclusivity from the filing date of a patent application, although it extended the implementation period for LDCs until the end of 2005.

Despite these limitations, TRIPS allowed countries in principle to retain the possibility of issuing compulsory licenses for drugs to generics manufacturers, requiring that they do so (1) with specific review and authorization, (2) that rights holders be compensated, and (3) that a reasonable attempt to obtain a voluntary license had to be made. In instances of national emergencies, countries did not even have to seek a voluntary license from manufacturers (Fink 2008). However, the United States and other advanced countries sought to protect IP and limit the use of compulsory licensing through pressure and bilateral trade agreements (so-called TRIPS-plus measures), which left developing countries less secure about what rights they effectively possessed under TRIPS. This lack of clarity would give rise to the 2001 Doha Declaration on TRIPS and public health, which specified what rights developing countries had with respect to pharmaceutical drugs and health emergencies.

In November 2001, in Doha the WTO elaborated the rights of poor countries to override pharmaceutical patents and issue compulsory licenses for public health emergencies, and it extended the transition period from 2006 to 2016 within which LDCs had to offer patent protection to the pharmaceutical industry under the provisions of the TRIPS regime. In these negotiations, developing countries were advised by such organizations as Oxfam and CPTech (Fleet and N'Daw 2008). The 2001 exception specified the rights of producing countries to grant compulsory licenses. However, for countries that lacked manufacturing capacity, the 2003 "August 30th" decision (also known as the "paragraph 6 solution") created a process to allow countries with ARV production capacity to export to them (Fink 2005; Elliott and Fink 2008; Fink and Elliott 2008).

Has either of these decisions affected access? The 2001 declaration has been more consequential than the 2003 decision, as few countries without production capacity of their own have availed themselves of the elaborate rules associated with the more recent initiative. In part, they have not had to. Under pressure from activists, some branded companies have issued voluntary licenses for their ARVs. Moreover, as 't Hoen argues, for countries that lack production capacity, there have been other options, as many first-line drugs lack patents in India and therefore could be produced by generic companies:

The lack of use of the mechanism can partly be explained by the fact that many of the 1st line AIDS drugs needed today are "pre-TRIPS" – that is, they are not patented in India and are still available as generics. A single compulsory license, government use order or non-enforcement statement suffices to allow for the import of these products when a valid patent exists in the importing country. ('t Hoen 2009, 37)

More than 60 developing countries have made use of TRIPS flexibilities to procure lower-cost medicines. Seventeen low- and middle-income countries – including Cameroon, Ghana, Guinea, Mozambique, Eritrea, Swaziland, and Zambia – have issued compulsory licenses or government use licenses for AIDS drugs since the 2003 WTO decision.[7] Twenty-six of 32 countries that are "least-developed" and members of the WTO explicitly referenced the Doha Declaration in their decision to allow imports of generic ARVs ('t Hoen et al. 2011).

Thus, the salience of making use of the 2003 mechanism may have been deferred for several years until second-line therapies – many of which are under patent in India – are needed (as a developing country, India had until 2005 to institute TRIPS provisions). By 2010, advocates increasingly warned that those patent restrictions were increasingly constrictive, particularly for PIs.

That said, several other developments continued to facilitate access to newer therapies. India's patent office vigorously defended access to AIDS treatment by rejecting patent applications in September 2009 for ARVs by some firms, including Gilead's tenofovir, and darunavir from an Irish firm, Tibotec Pharmaceuticals (Majumdar 2009). In January 2011, the Indian government also rejected Abbott's patent application for Kaletra, a combination of lopinavir/ritonavir, which is a preferred second-line therapy for

---

[7] Middle-income countries like Thailand and Brazil have also issued compulsory licenses for drugs (Love 2007). For an updated assessment of the challenges of using these flexibilities, see UNAIDS and WHO 2011.

drug-resistant HIV (Kaiser Family Foundation 2011c). Gilead's patent on another important drug, tenofovir, marketed as Viread, has also been quite shaky.[8] Gilead did provide a voluntary license to a number of Indian firms which limited where they could sell generic versions of the drug worldwide, particularly to middle-income countries. However, Cipla rejected such an agreement, since the drug was not yet patented in India. As a result, Cipla was free to market generic versions of the drug around the world. In 2010, the FDA approved a generic version of the drug through its quality assurance process, described later in this chapter (Dance with Shadows/Pillscribe 2010).

Beyond the lack of immediate need to take advantage of the 2003 provision, Drahos argues that the complexity of implementing the 2003 agreement made it more difficult for countries to take advantage of (Drahos 2007). Countries making use of the mechanism had to adapt local legislation to permit the process. The mechanism requires that the exporting country as well as the importing country (if the drug is patented in the importing country) grant a compulsory license. For each instance, countries had to specify how much of the drug would be exported. For the next shipment, countries would have to go through the same process all over again.[9] However, the specific provision of the 2003 WTO decision has only been applied once. Rwanda, as importing country, and Canada, as exporting country, used the mechanism in 2007 (UNAIDS and WHO 2011, 6). Although Rwanda had other options, this mechanism was used to demonstrate its complexity and limited utility (Perez-Casas 2011).

The WTO rule changes on their own did not create market demand for ARV products, as many poor people in developing countries lacked purchasing power at almost any price. Thus, the procurement decisions by donors, including the Global Fund, and later PEPFAR, as well as decisions by other donors and affected country governments, were important in compensating for poor people's and poor countries' lack of demand. The rule changes did, however, create a permissive environment for more generic ARV products to enter the market.

Perhaps more importantly, branded pharmaceutical companies had suffered a public relations debacle in the wake of their lawsuit against the South African government, which was dropped in April 2001. The WTO rule changes continued to put pressure on branded pharmaceutical companies to offer their own products at differential prices to poor countries, to refrain from enforcing patent rights in the developing world, and, as

---

[8] The US Patent Office also invalidated four patents related to the drug in 2008 (Basheer 2008).

[9] See www.wto.org/english/tratop_e/trips_e/implem_para6_e.htm.

mentioned above, to agree to voluntary transfer of licenses to producers in developing countries. In March 2001, BMS announced that it would not object to South Africa licensing or producing generic versions of d4T (originally produced by Yale University and licensed to BMS) and ddI (Suleman 2001). In June 2001, BMS granted South African-based Aspen Pharmacare a voluntary license to make d4t (Yale AIDS Network 2003). In October 2001, Glaxo, for example, granted a voluntary license to allow generic production of AZT and 3TC (essentialdrugs.org 2001).

As previously discussed, Attaran and Gillespie-White, in an October 2001 article, had questioned whether patents were the main barrier to access in developing countries, noting that of the 15 ARV drugs used in 53 countries, very few countries had patents on those drugs, and of the countries that did, only a few drugs were under patent (Attaran and Gillespie-White 2001). However, Love in his response that same year, noted that patents did exist for some of the most important drug combinations in particularly important developing world markets with large HIV+ populations, such as South Africa. Several three-drug combinations were under patent, as were a number of two-drug combinations: "All of the least expensive generic cocktails – those that can be currently manufactured for less than $500 per year – are blocked by patents on 3TC, AZT, AZT+3TC or Nevirapine" (Love 2001a).

No matter which side of the patent debate one falls on, most observers would agree that the WTO decision of 2001 helped solidify the confidence of developing countries to pursue strategies that defended public health without great risk of falling foul of the international patent regime. Beginning in 2002, with a large swath of resources for HIV directed through the Global Fund, which approved of generic drug purchases by recipient countries, generics began to have a larger and larger market share.

Until that time, there were more limited purchases of drugs, including generic drugs, particularly by African countries. The Global Fund's reporting mechanism was launched when it was created in 2002. Prior to that time, there are only patchy records of ARV procurement. Lucchini *et al.* obtained pricing data for 13 African countries and Brazil for the years 1997–2002.[10] Brazil's observations dominate the dataset, constituting more than 90 percent of the purchases, mostly generics.[11] In the African sample, most of them occurred in 2001 and 2002,[12] and Nigerian drug

---

[10] African countries covered include Benin, Botswana, Burkina Faso, Burundi, Cameroon, Côte d'Ivoire, Gabon, Kenya, Malawi, Mali, Nigeria, Republic of Congo, and Togo.

[11] By quantity, Brazil's purchases amount to 94.3% of the NRTIs, 91.0% of the NNRTIs, 98.6% for PIs, and 95.6% for multi-combination drugs (Lucchini *et al.* 2003, 187).

[12] More than 90% of African purchases of the sample occurred in 2001 and 2002.

purchases, most of them generics, dominate for many classes of drugs.[13] However, the majority of African countries in the sample purchased few generics.[14] As important as the percentage of generics are the actual volumes; Nigeria, for example, which purchased the largest total volume of AIDS drugs in Africa in the sample, only purchased 6 million daily dosages of NRTIs between 2001 and 2002. Maximally, this could provide for about 8,100 people taking a daily dosage a day for two years.

By the end of 2009, more than 5.2 million people in low- and middle-income countries were on ARVs, including 3.91 million people in sub-Saharan Africa, up from negligible numbers in 2002 (UNAIDS 2010). By the end of 2010, the estimated number of people receiving treatment in low- and middle-income countries had increased sharply to 6.6 million (UNAIDS 2011a). Since 2006, Indian-produced generic ARVs have accounted for more than 80 percent of the donor-funded developing country market, and comprised 87 percent of ARV purchase volumes in 2008 (Waning, Diedrichsen, and Moon 2010). Between 2002 and 2008, generic ARVs comprised 63 percent of the WHO's procurements reported on its Global Price Reporting Mechanism database (Waning, Kaplan et al. 2010, 164) (see Table 6.3).[15]

While the percentage of generic drugs did not increase unambiguously over time as a percentage of the total, generics, with an anomalous year from mid 2004 to mid 2005, provided the lion's share of ARV drugs over time as the number of people on treatment dramatically increased. One reason the percentage of generic drugs probably has not grown even higher is due to the fact that a small but increasing percentage of people on ARVs need second-line drug therapies, products that have largely been produced by branded companies.

The conclusion we can draw from these figures is that as the WTO began to support greater flexibility for developing countries to produce and later to import "cheap" generic ARVs, international donors began to scale-up their commitments to finance treatment in the developing world. The

---

[13] By dosage numbers, Nigeria's ARV purchases constituted nearly 60% of NRTIs and nearly 75% of NNRTIs, all of which were generics. Of these purchases, including Brazil's, more than 90% of NRTIs were generics, 39.3% of NNRTIs were generics, 21.6% were of PIs, and 74.6% were of multi-combination drugs.

[14] Five of the African countries – Benin, Botswana, Burkina Faso, Gabon, and Republic of Congo, purchased no generic drugs for any of the four classes. Côte d'Ivoire purchased branded drugs exclusively, except for 10.2% of its NRTIs; likewise, Togo purchased all branded drugs, save for 21.7% of its multi-drug combination purchases (Lucchini et al. 2003, 188–9).

[15] This mirrors the findings from Chien over the period 2004–6 which found the same percentage of generic use (63%) using the WHO's GPRM data (Chien 2007).

Table 6.3: *Percentage of generic ARV purchases, WHO Global Reporting Mechanism*

All ARV purchases in GPRM	**Subset of 32 oral solid ARV dosage forms**						
July 2002–June 2008	*July 2002–June 2003*	*July 2003–June 2004*	*July 2004–June 2005*	*July 2005–June 2006*	*July 2006–June 2007*	*July 2007–June 2008*	*TOTAL*
63	92	69	48	64	74	69	66

Source: (Waning, Kaplan *et al.* 2010, 164).

subsequent sections document the other rule changes that facilitated this transformation, beginning with the WHO treatment guidelines.

WHO treatment guidelines

We can observe the importance of rule changes by identifying the emergence of and changes in the WHO treatment guidelines for scaling-up ARV therapy in low-income countries. In April 2002, 10 ARVs were added to the WHO list of essential medicines, and the WHO released its first treatment guidelines for scaling-up ARV therapy in "resource-limited settings" (WHO 2002). The guidelines were subsequently revised in 2003, 2006, and 2010, with additional guidance released in 2012 for "sero-discordant" couples, where one partner has HIV and the other does not (WHO 2010b). WHO ARV treatment guidelines are not legally binding, but do serve as an important signal for a variety of users (including public health practitioners, donors, and drug companies) about what drugs should be taken, at what stage of the illness, in what combination, by whom, and so on. "WHO treatment guidelines," as Quick and Moore note, "have no inherent authority over diagnosis, treatment, clinical monitoring, or patient care" (Quick and Moore 2010, 423).

The 2002 guidelines included seven regimens with combinations of 10 different ARVs, including PIs, which were relatively expensive (WHO 2002). The 2003 revision, launched to accompany the WHO's "3 by 5 campaign" (3 million people on ARVs by 2005), identified four regimens with combinations of five ARVs including EFV, 3TC, NVP, d4T, and ZDV, and no PIs (WHO 2003). The 2006 revision provided more flexibility for providers with 24 first-line regimens ("standard") and eight "alternative" regimens. Three additional ARVs were added, in addition to the other five: ABC, TDF, and FTC. The 2006 revision also encouraged practitioners to begin planning on phasing-out stavudine (d4T) because of its side-effects and toxicity to patients (WHO 2006). The 2010 revision includes six key first-line regimens comprised of six ARVs for those who have never taken them before, simplifying and focusing the 2006 regimen (Waning, Kyle *et al.* 2010, 5).[16]

The 2010 revision, announced in November 2009 (WHO 2009b), but officially launched at the International AIDS Society meeting in July 2010 (*Lilongwe Times* 2010), recommended starting ARV therapy earlier, when CD4 counts dropped below 350 cells/mm^3 or less.[17] The 2006 guidelines had recommended starting treatment later, after a patient CD4 count had already dropped to 200 cells/mm^3 or less. The 2010 revision also recommended phasing-out first-line drug stavudine (d4T) in favor of less-toxic ARVs.

[16] WHO Recommended Treatment Regimens 2002–10.

2002 (7)	2003 (4)	2006 (24)	2010 (6)
EFV+3TC+ZDV	3TC+NVP+d4T	**Standard**	EFV+3TC+ZDV
3TC+NVP+ZDV	EFV+3TC+d4T	3TC+NVP+ZDV	3TC+NVP+ZDV
ABC+3TC+ZDV	3TC+NVP+ZDV	EFV+3TC+ZDV	EFV+3TC+TDF
IDV/	EFV+3TC+ZDV	3TC+NVP+d4T	EFV+FTC+TDF
r+3TC+ZDV		EFV+3TC+d4T	3TC+NVP+TDF
3TC+LPV/		FTC + NVP + ZDV	FTC+NVP+TDF
r+ZDV		EFV+FTC+ZDV	
3TC+SQV/		FTC+NVP+d4T	
r+ZDV		EFV+FTC+d4T	
3TC+NFV+ZDV		3TC+NVP+TDF	
		EFV+3TC+TDF	
		FTC+NVP+TDF	
		EFV+FTC+TDF	
		ABC+3TC+NVP	
		ABC+EFV+3TC	
		ABC+FTC+NVP	
		ABC+EFV+FTC	
		Alternatives	
		3TC+TDF+ZDV	
		ABC+3TC+ZDV	
		FTC+TDF+ZDV	
		ABC+FTC+ZDV	
		3TC+d4T+TDF	
		ABC+3TC+d4T	
		FTC+d4T+TDF	
		ABC+FTC+d4T	

[17] These are the number of cells per cubic millimeter.

The guidelines emphasized that ART should include an NNRTI, either nevirapine (NVP) or efavirenz (EFV), and two NRTIs. Among the NRTIs, the guidelines said that one should be zidovudine (AZT, also known as ZDV) or tenofovir (TDF), and the other should be lamivudine (3TC) or FTC (emtricitabine). d4T is an NRTI that had been used extensively; AZT and TDF are alternatives, but they are more expensive (WHO 2010a).

Thus, if these guidelines are meaningful, we should observe a shift away from the procurement of d4T, beginning with the 2006 revision. Waning et al. document procurement trends in their assessment of the Global Price Reporting Mechanism and the Global Fund's Price Quality Report between 2002 and 2008, which encompass a majority of total ARV purchases by low- and middle-income countries during this time period.[18] From 2006 to 2008, even as treatment greatly expanded, Waning et al. document only a modest increase in d4T purchases, from 515,000 person-years to 895,000. Given the greater than five-times increase in its main competitor, ZDV, from 139,000 person-years to more than 733,000 person-years over that time period, they attribute this small increase to the guidelines. From 2009 on, we should observe a more marked shift away from d4T (Waning, Kyle et al. 2010, 5). In response to the change in guidelines, a number of countries, including Kenya, India, and Zimbabwe, announced in late 2010 and early 2011 that they would eventually phase out d4T (Zimbabwe Broadcasting Corporation 2011; Indian Express 2011; IRIN News 2010a). In addition to the impact of the changed guidelines on phasing out d4T, Waning et al. document a more than fifteen-fold increase in purchases of the newly recommended emtricitabine and tenofovir from 2006 to 2008 (Waning, Kyle et al. 2010).

With respect to d4T, it may take some time to see the phase-out in procurement patterns. When we look at the procurement of d4T, procurement peaked in 2007 after the WHO's initial 2006 recommendation that d4t be considered for phase-out. After rebounding a bit in 2010, orders were down in 2011 and provisional numbers through March 2012 suggest quite low orders (see Figure 6.1).

Similarly, with respect to the triple cocktail of 3TC + NVP + d4T (which includes six formulations), the peak occurs in 2010, with

---

[18] Their data captures procurements reported to the Global Fund and WHO, mostly funded by the Global Fund, PEPFAR, and UNITAID. It does not include national purchases by larger, middle-income countries. They estimate that their data captures about 27% of purchases by Brazil, South Africa, and Thailand and thus captures most purchases by developing countries (Waning, Kyle et al. 2010).

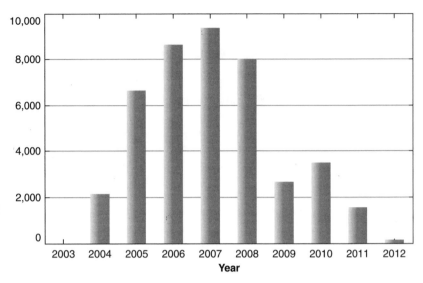

Figure 6.1: Procurement patterns of d4T (1mg) – number of treatment years
Source: Global Price Reporting Mechanism.

a marked decline in 2011 and the first three months of 2012 (see Figure 6.2).

As the news stories about the decisions by Kenya, Zimbabwe, and India suggested, phasing out of d4T, which is considerably cheaper than alternative therapies, may take some time. As a result, we may not yet observe the full force of implementation of the WHO guidelines. These observations notwithstanding, coupled with the WHO prequalification standards for medicines, the treatment guidelines have had an important effect on procurement patterns of particular drugs and combinations of ARVs. The next section elaborates the effects of the prequalification standards.

WHO prequalification standards

In March 2001, the WHO appointed its first manager and initiated its Prequalification of Medicines program, along with UN partners UNICEF, UNAIDS, and the United Nations Population Fund (UNFPA). It was not until March 2002 that the first list of WHO prequalified medicines was announced to help guide procurement by UN agencies such as UNICEF. As Roemer-Mahler argues, public policies helped create this market by linking procurement and regulation:

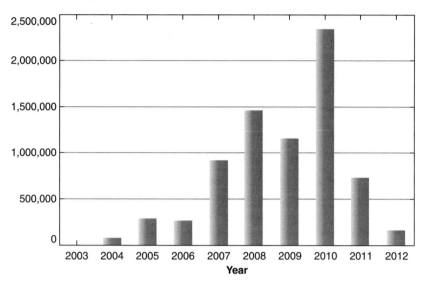

Figure 6.2: Procurement patterns of 3TC + NVP + d4T – number of treatment years
Source: Global Price Reporting Mechanism.
Note: Includes all formulations: 60 mg + 100 mg + 12 mg, 40 mg + 70 mg + 10 mg, 30 mg + 50 mg + 6 mg, 20 mg + 35 mg + 5 mg, 150 mg + 200 mg + 40 mg, 150 mg + 200 mg + 30 mg

Governments and international organizations shaped the market for low cost generic ARVs by taking on the task of buying drugs for people living with HIV in developing countries. Furthermore, they influenced the market by creating a regulatory environment that determined which companies can participate in this market. (Roemer-Mahler 2010a, 9)

The prequalification program was essential in this regard, as it directly informs the procurement strategies of most major funders of ARV purchasers, including the Global Fund, various UN agencies, as well as the World Bank and UNITAID. For the vast majority of developing countries lacking the capacity to verify the quality of drugs, particularly those produced overseas, the WHO's prequalification process provides a useful service.

Activists also regarded the prequalification scheme as absolutely essential for generic competition. Donors would not procure generic drugs if they could not be assured of their quality (Perez-Casas 2011). Coming on the heels of Cipla CEO Yusuf Hamied's announcement in February 2001 that he would provide a triple cocktail of ARVs for less than a dollar a day, activists pressed for a quality assurance scheme in

Geneva. Generic industry veteran Bill Haddad described efforts to enlist the WHO to create a universal drug qualification scheme in mid 2001:

> Within the week, Dr. Hamied, the leader of Doctors without Borders and I went to the World Health Organization and laid out our case. If WHO did not create a one-stop approval process, the multinationals would drag us from one courtroom in one country to another courtroom elsewhere, trying to wear us out. WHO agreed and Canada, the EU, Scandinavia and South Africa created an airtight regulatory pathway that was as stringent as any in the world including FDA – they and we could not afford a mistake. (Haddad 2007)

Despite the creation of the prequalification scheme, the WHO is not a supranational regulatory body and has no national legal authority with the prequalification of drugs (WHO 2004a). In practice, for countries that lack national regulatory capacity, the WHO has become a *de facto*, if not *de jure* regulator, despite a small staff and limited funding.[19] Many countries take their purchasing cues from the WHO, although, as noted in the subsequent section on the FDA fast-track drug approval process, certain countries like the United States have privileged their own national drug certification process over the international one.

The aim of the effort was to establish "unified standards of quality, safety and efficacy for HIV/AIDS, malaria and tuberculosis" medications (WHO 2011a). Initially supported by UNAIDS, UNICEF, UNFPA, and the World Bank, the prequalification program enables companies that would like their products to be prequalified to apply. Both the drugs and the manufacturers that produce them have to be prequalified (*The Lancet* 2004). Manufacturers have to provide extensive documentation prior to a visit from an inspection team, including basic description of the drugs, clinical data, and inspection information (Zimmerman 2002).

For generics producers, the WHO requires companies to present proof of "bioequivalence" – that the drugs in question "satisfy the same standards as those applicable to the originator's product." Bioequivalence also means that "reasonable assurance must be provided that they are, as intended, clinically interchangeable with nominally equivalent market products" (Welink 2010). Put a little differently, bioequivalence "means that the active ingredient in a generic medicine is absorbed into the body

---

[19] In its first two years, the program was initially staffed by one manager and one assistant. An inspector was added by the French government in 2003. By 2011, the program had grown to an overall program manager, a chief inspector and five inspectors, a head of assessments and seven assessors, eight support staff, and one person for each of the following areas – liaison, capacity building and training, and sampling and monitoring. In 2006, the Gates Foundation funded expansion of the program, with most of the program's resources now provided by UNITAID (Van Zyl 2011a)

at the same rate and amount as in the brand-name product" (Generic Pharmaceutical Association undated). Since performing new clinical trials for the drugs would be prohibitively expensive, generics firms typically contract with a so-called Contract Research Organization (CRO) to perform the bioequivalence check. Bioequivalence can be established in multiple ways, but typically it includes comparing the branded product with the comparable generic product using volunteer test subjects. Officials from different national drug regulatory authorities review these dossiers.

The first inspection team visit from the WHO and UNICEF lasted up to two weeks at each factory; later, the visits came to last at least three consecutive days at a minimum. The inspection teams regularly include both WHO officials and national regulatory authorities deputized by the WHO to carry out the inspections (WHO undated). The inspection team assesses the extent to which the manufacturer complies with WHO Good Manufacturing Practices (GMP) standards. Alternatively, inspections can be carried out by so-called "stringent regulatory authorities" that are recognized by the WHO. A stringent regulatory authority includes those that are (1) members of the International Conference of Harmonisation (ICH) like the United States and member states of the EU, (2) ICH observers, or (3) a regulatory authority associated with an ICH member via a mutual recognition agreement.[20]

After the inspections are concluded, the WHO completes its Public Inspection Report and decides on the prequalification listing. Provided there are no problems, the review can take anywhere from two-to-four months; longer if documentation is not in order or there are problems with the inspections, which may trigger a Notice of Concern (NOC). In 2010, the median time to prequalify a branded product was 4.3 months, while generic products took significantly longer, a median of 31.6 months (WHO 2010c). Once a drug and its manufacturer are prequalified, the drug is listed on the prequalified list of medicines for treating priority diseases, and UN agencies are permitted to procure the drug. Drugs and facilities periodically (normally every three years) have to be re-qualified.

The WHO's first list was released in March 2002 and comprised 41 drug formulations, including 11 ARVs and 5 drugs for infections that

---

[20] ICH members include member states of the EU, the United States, and Japan. ICH observers include the European Free Trade Association (EFTA) as represented by SwissMedic, Health Canada, and the WHO. Regulatory authority that has mutual recognition agreements with ICH members include Australia, Norway, Iceland, and Liechtenstein (WHO 2011b).

often accompany HIV. Four branded producers, including GSK, BMS, Roche Holding, and Abbott Laboratories, provided 26 of the drugs. Ten were from the Indian generics firm Cipla, including nevirapine, zidovudine (AZT), and lamivudine (3TC), which made up its triple-cocktail formula. Other Cipla products prequalified included acyclovir for shingles, ciprofloxacin for bacterial infections, and vinblastine and vincristine sulfate for Kaposi's sarcoma. In addition to Cipla, three small European generics producers also had drugs prequalified in the first approval process. To encourage competition, the WHO approved several producers of AZT, including the original patent holder, GSK, as well as Cipla and Combino Pharma, a Spanish generics firm that produced the drug for MSF to supply clinics in Gabon, Tunisia, and Côte d'Ivoire. The WHO initially solicited applications for 16 ARVs and 24 drugs for other conditions that affected the immune system of HIV+ individuals. The WHO was open to both branded pharmaceuticals and generics, so long as the company was legally registered in its country of origin (McNeil Jr. 2002).

The WHO has conducted periodic reviews of bioequivalence studies to ensure they meet standards for quality and accuracy. In some cases, this has meant that drugs that were previously prequalified had to be de-listed because of failure to meet certain quality control standards for clinical and laboratory practice. For example, in May 2004, Cipla temporarily had to pull two ARVs, 3TC and AZT, from the pre-approved drug list after the WHO found fault with the paperwork produced by the CRO contracted to perform the bioequivalence tests (both returned to the list in November 2004) (Altman and McNeil Jr. 2004; WHO 2004a; b). The Indian generic firm Ranbaxy had three of its ARV drugs de-listed for similar reasons in August 2004. In the wake of those CRO inspections, both Ranbaxy and another Indian firm, Hetero, voluntarily withdrew 7 and 6 ARVs, respectively, from the list in November 2004 (WHO 2004c; d). Although most of these de-listings occurred early in the years of the prequalification program, de-listings periodically continue in the event of some concerns about product quality.

In October 2010, the WHO announced that it would also begin prequalifying APIs, the precursor ingredients to finished pharmaceutical products. The aim was to reduce the time to prequalify finished products, if they were made from APIs already prequalified. The WHO also prequalifies quality control laboratories (QCL). At the end of 2010, the WHO list of prequalified medicines totaled 252 products manufactured in 20 countries. In 2009, 44 medicinal products were prequalified, of which 39 were generics. In 2010, the WHO

Table 6.4: *Number of products prequalified accepted*

	2001	2002	2003	2004	2005	2006	2007	2008	2009	2010
No. of HIV/ AIDS products prequalified	0	61	13	13	17	33	13	29	24	24

Source: Van Zyl 2011a.

prequalified 36 products, thirty of them generics (WHO 2011c). As of March 31, 2011, there were 187 HIV-related products prequalified by the WHO, more than 60 percent of which were generics (WHO 2012b). By another estimate, there were more than 225 different HIV/AIDS products that had been prequalified since 2001 (see Table 6.4).

In terms of our expectations, we should see increases in procurements in the Global Price Reporting Mechanism (GPRM) dataset following prequalification, particularly by UN agencies. Where delisting lasts long enough, we should also observe declines in procurement. Detecting procurement declines for particular drugs may be difficult to observe, as procurement for ARVs increased dramatically during this time period. Moreover, the GPRM dataset also includes purchases brokered by CHAI and those procured through PEPFAR, which have somewhat distinct quality control mechanisms from the WHO prequalification scheme.[21]

In addition, the Global Fund and the World Bank endorsed the WHO prequalification program but did not preclude purchases of drugs that were not WHO prequalified (World Bank 2003).[22] For this reason, it may be difficult to discern the precise impact of the WHO prequalification program on drug procurement, since the dataset encompasses purchases

---

[21] PEPFAR purchases those drugs that have been approved by the FDA. CHAI's quality assurance criteria include: (1) drugs approved through the WHO prequalification process, (2) those approved by the FDA or another stringent regulatory authority (SRA), (3) those submitted to the WHO, FDA, or another SRA, and (4) those imminently expecting to submit to the WHO or FDA and from a facility already compliant with GMP (CHAI 2008b; 2010).

[22] For example, the Global Fund allowed countries to purchase ARVs that were prequalified through the WHO (option A), authorized by an SRA (option B), or authorized by the National Drug Regulatory Authorities (NDRA) in recipient countries (option C). Option C was to be phased out by December 31, 2004, but it was initially extended to April 30, 2005. Various exceptions continue as part of Global Fund procurement strategies such that countries, if they cannot identify qualifying drugs under options A and B, can still access needed drugs, subject to certain constraints (Global Fund 2004; 2006; 2009; 2010c).

by non-UN actors, some of which were responsive to other drug quality standard-setting bodies (PEPFAR) or were encouraged but not mandated to follow WHO prequalification (Global Fund, World Bank).

Andre van Zyl, the former manager of the Prequalification Program, explained why procurement trends do not necessarily adjust in a short period of time:

> One may not see a difference [in procurement] in a short while. Once a product is prequalified, the company still has to register the product in each country where they want to sell it (like the FDA process). This itself can take months to years in many countries. Thereafter, the company (in most cases) has to offer the product on a tender (competing with other companies). Countries can buy non prequalified products with their own funding (and it happens in cases) – as these are often cheaper than prequalified products meeting international standards (e.g. purity of the API used). (Van Zyl 2011b)

When one looks at procurement trends in the GPRM dataset, the patterns of purchases are consistent, but not conclusive with respect to WHO prequalification. For example, Cipla's lamivudine (150mg) and its lamivudine/ziduvodine combination (3TC [150mg] + AZT [300mg]) were de-listed in April 2004 following problems with the CRO bioequivalence report. Following the de-listing, procurements of both declined, or languished at low levels. Cipla's version of the drugs returned to the list in November 2004, after which time significant but fluctuating levels of both dosage levels can be observed (see Figures 6.3 and 6.4).

Observing procurement trends for one generic company's drugs early on in the prequalification scheme history, of course, is not fully dispositive. We can also observe the effects of WHO listing by looking at procurement trends for other drugs, including branded ones, later on in the history of the WHO prequalification program. For example, Gilead's tenofovir was prequalified in March 2006 (see Figure 6.5). Like the purchases of Cipla's drugs, tenofovir was purchased in increasing quantities after being prequalified, with considerable monthly variation.

As we suggested earlier, not all states have accepted the WHO prequalification standards as a guide to procurement. In the US context, the Bush administration backed a rival process through the US FDA. Like PEPFAR's relationship to the Global Fund, over time the two schemes have become more integrated, with drugs approved by the US FDA also reflected on the WHO prequalification lists (as well as drugs approved by Health Canada). This practice began in December 2005. For example, Matrix's generic version of tenofovir, which was approved by the FDA, was added to the WHO list in December 2007. Like other listings, procurement of Matrix's tenofovir increased after listing, with substantial variation between months (see Figure 6.6).

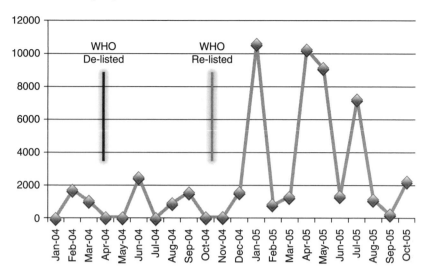

Figure 6.3: Cipla Lamivudine (3TC) 150mg procurement – number of treatment years
Source: Global Price Reporting Mechanism.

The results reported here are suggestive of the influence of WHO prequalification on subsequent procurement. Coupled with official policy, it is clear that UN agencies privilege procurement of drugs that are prequalified through the WHO and that drugs approved through other regulatory agencies are regarded as a second-best solution.[23] Despite the preference for WHO prequalified products in the procurement decisions by most international organizations and national governments, a notable exception is the separate procedure the United States initially had through the FDA. The origins and effects of the FDA process and its impact on PEPFAR procurement are discussed in the next section.

[23] For example, UNICEF encourages purchase of WHO prequalified medicines, but in the event of their unavailability will allow drugs approved by the US FDA, the EMA, or drugs approved through independent quality evaluations (UNICEF 2007). Similarly, most non-UN agencies also privilege WHO prequalification. The Global Fund's updated December 2010 policy on procurement of medicines only allows its funds to be used on drugs that are prequalified by the WHO, a stringent regulatory authority, or, in the event of necessity, on the recommendation of an expert review panel (ERP). The ERP process is an elaborate review process that seeks to limit and make exceptional the use of what the Global Fund earlier called option C, the procurement of drugs not prequalified through normal WHO or SRA channels (Global Fund 2010c).

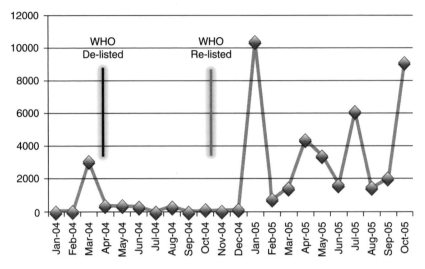

Figure 6.4: Cipla Lamivudine (3TC 150mg) + Zidovudine (AZT 300mg) procurement – number of treatment years
Source: Global Price Reporting Mechanism.

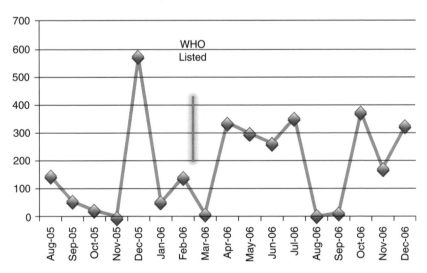

Figure 6.5: Gilead Tenofovir (300mg) procurement – number of treatment years
Source: Global Price Reporting Mechanism.

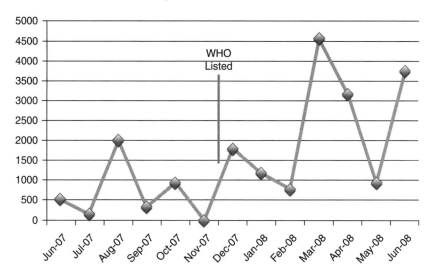

Figure 6.6: Matrix Tenofovir (300mg) procurement – number of
treatment years
Source: Global Price Reporting Mechanism.

The FDA fast-track procedure

In his January 2003 State of the Union address, President Bush committed $15bn over five years in support of PEPFAR. In his remarks,
Bush acknowledged that drug prices had fallen from $12,000 to less
than $300 a year, implicitly accepting the important role played by
generics. The original US legislation authorizing PEPFAR specified that
55 percent of the funds be allocated to treatment, with 20 percent for
prevention, 15 percent for palliative care, and 10 percent for orphans
and vulnerable children.[24] With a significant share of PEPFAR
funds committed to treatment, regulation of drug quality became a
significant issue.

Despite the WHO prequalification procedure for ARVs, the Bush
administration balked at adoption of the WHO standards, raising suspi-
cions by the advocacy community that PEPFAR would merely serve as a
vehicle to enrich branded pharmaceutical companies. While advocates
lobbied the administration explicitly to embrace generics in the legislation authorizing appropriations, generic drugs were not specifically

[24] These were recommendations for the first two years of PEPFAR; beginning in FY 2006,
they were mandated by law (Kaiser Family Foundation 2006).

mentioned in H.R. 1298, which was signed by the president in May 2003.[25] In June 2003, Congressional allies of the NGO community – specifically Senators Daschle, McCain, and Kennedy – requested a study by the GAO to assess the costs of ARVs and how best the United States could meet its ambitious treatment goals at lowest costs (Daschle, McCain, and Kennedy 2003).

Advocates' concerns that the Bush administration would favor branded pharmaceuticals over generic ARVs were bolstered when Randall Tobias, a former Eli Lilly pharmaceutical executive, was appointed to be the first Global AIDS Coordinator in July 2003. While Bush administration officials said that they were open to generic drug purchases as part of PEPFAR, they rejected the WHO as the appropriate organization to assess drug quality. At a July 2003 international AIDS conference in Paris, Anthony Fauci, the director of the US National Institute of Allergy and Infectious Diseases, explained the US strategy:

We certainly want to get the highest quality at the lowest price …. That may mean getting it from the [brand-name] companies who bring their price low enough so it is feasible to be part of the programme. It does not exclude generic drugs. (quoted in Hirschler 2003)

Bill Haddad, the American generics drug manufacturer who, along with Jamie Love, initially enlisted Cipla's Hamied to produce low-cost generics in 2001, charged that underlings in the Bush administration were responsible for doing the bidding of the branded pharmaceutical companies in trying to prevent the use of generics. Haddad blamed William Steiger, the US government's liaison to the transition working group that created the Global Fund, for trying to torpedo the use of generics by the Global Fund. At the 2003 Paris meeting, he confronted Secretary of Health and Human Services, Tommy Thompson:

At the Paris Global Fund meeting, I asked Secretary Thompson from the floor if the President continued to support the $300 generic. (As a Kennedy Democrat, I had called the Bush statement, courageous, faith-based and personal.) Thompson grew angry at me (and later perennially confronted me) but as chairman of the meeting that included most African Ambassadors, he angrily asked me what made me think the President would not stand by his word. (Haddad 2009)

Haddad suggested that the FDA approval process was a concerted effort by the branded pharmaceutical companies to delay the use of generics (Haddad 2004a).[26]

---

[25] See www.govtrack.us/congress/bill.xpd?bill=h108–1298.
[26] Similar concerns about the Bush administration and generics were summarized by Gross (2005).

Despite such criticism, the Bush administration continued to reiterate its goal of eventually using generics. In February 2004, Tobias restated these ideas in his remarks on the five-year strategy for PEPFAR:

What our policy will be, will be to buy drugs that are safe and effective at the lowest possible price. Now, if those happen to be drugs that are manufactured by generic companies, fine; if those are drugs that are manufactured by brand name companies, fine. But it's very important that there be some standards, some principles by which we can make those decisions. (Tobias 2004a)

Dr. Mark Dybul served as the deputy chief medical officer and would later succeed Randall Tobias as the US Global AIDS Coordinator. Like Tobias, he acknowledged the administration's "predilection is to use them [generics] if at all possible." He said that President Bush "had to have" meant generics in his State of the Union address, but "that doesn't translate automatically to use. You still have to consider quality, safety and efficacy" (quoted in Lueck 2004a).

Despite the assertions of openness to generic drugs, the United States rejected the adequacy of the WHO prequalification scheme. In May 2004 in testimony before Congress, Tobias, referencing the WHO prequalification website, noted "the WHO is not a regulatory authority and does not represent itself as such" (Tobias 2004b). He suggested that the WHO process was not equivalent to thorough review that the US FDA performs to assess the bioequivalence of generic drugs in the United States (Tobias 2004c).

The Bush administration raised advocates' fears by hosting a conference in March 2004 in Gaborone, Botswana, on the standards for Fixed-Dose Combination drugs (FDCs). FDCs were multiple drugs packaged in a multi-drug packet enabling patients to take fewer pills per day. Indian firms were among the first innovators of FDCs, packaging drugs (stavudine, lamivudine, and nevirapine) that were patented by three different firms (BMS, GSK, and Boehringer Ingelheim) in high-income countries into a single combination ('t Hoen et al. 2011). Activists from MSF and other organizations feared that the conference was designed to undermine the use of generic ARV drugs. A joint letter sent by 381 organizations to Ambassador Tobias raised concerns about the conference (CPTech 2004). They enlisted Democratic Congressman Henry Waxman as well as Senators Kennedy, McCain, and four others to write two separate letters in March to President Bush about the need to reverse course and authorize the use of generics (Kennedy et al. 2004). Waxman's stern letter opposed the onerous draft standards that had been circulated in advance of the gathering (Waxman 2004). The advocacy community was able to convince the European Agency for the

Evaluation of Medicinal Products (EMEA) not to send representatives to the conference, despite earlier involvement in planning the event.[27]

Bill Haddad had especially strong criticism of John Lange, Randall Tobias' deputy, for pushing an anti-generics agenda in Gaborone (Haddad 2004b). In a late March 2004 Council on Foreign Relations gathering, Richard Holbrooke, chairman of the Global Business Coalition on HIV/AIDS, chastised Lange in particular and the Bush administration for its unwillingness to support generics:

I am very disturbed by this. It's a big issue, and it's tearing apart all the good work that people are doing because there is a feeling that the United States is protecting the big [pharmaceutical companies]. (quoted in Nesmith 2004)

In May 2004, in an effort to quell the criticism about PEPFAR procurement, the Bush administration announced that it was developing a fast-track approval process for AIDS drugs through the FDA (Lueck 2004b). CHAI's Ira Magaziner suggested that former President Clinton may have had a hand in helping speed this initiative along. President Clinton had a meeting with President George W. Bush in early 2004, where President Clinton suggested PEPFAR was wasting money by not buying generics (Magaziner 2012).[28]

For his part, Dybul indicated that there were no voices of skepticism about the use of generic ARVs if quality could be assured. He said the "fact that the President put the generic price in the State of the Union address is as good an indication as any of interest and intent to purchase generics. Things don't accidentally get put in the State of the Union." He noted that every word is vetted. He reiterated the point that there was "no pushback from anyone in the administration at any point at any time. Most importantly, the President said we should get lowest price product as long as high quality was maintained" (Dybul 2012).

Although the WHO's prequalification scheme was respected and thought of as enormously beneficial for countries looking to the WHO for an imprimatur, Dybul noted that the WHO is not a regulatory authority. While Dybul suggested that PEPFAR officials had a good working relationship with the WHO, the WHO staff did not understand why the United States didn't just use their system. Dybul said the United

---

[27] For a variety of documents on the advocacy community's efforts, see www.healthgap.org/camp/pepfar.html.

[28] When President Clinton and President George H. W. Bush were appointed co-heads for tsunami relief later in 2004 they became friends, and after this President Clinton and President George W. Bush talked more frequently, and cooperation increased between the Clinton Foundation and the US government to expand AIDS care and treatment (Magaziner 2012).

States was not going to permit the use of products that they wouldn't give their own citizens. The Bush administration was sensitive to the notion that Africans were being used as guinea pigs. He suggested that there were "too many examples of that kind of system being abused and poor people suffering" (Dybul 2012).

After *The Washington Post* wrote a harsh piece criticizing the administration for not using the WHO's prequalification scheme, the "politicals" were more willing to move forward on generic drug purchases without some other quality check. The political types worried that "we are getting killed on this" and just wanted to "get the issue past us." Surprisingly, the scientific-medical types resisted and said that an additional quality review was necessary. Where old-line AIDS activists like Marty Delaney, who had fought for quality AIDS medicines in the United States, warned the Bush administration, "[D]on't dare back down on this," other activists strongly supported the swift use of generics (reported by Dybul 2012). In Dybul's view, many activists were misinformed about the administration's intentions, and their criticism perhaps hastened the Bush administration's embrace of the FDA's tentative approval process. That process already existed for drugs for the US market and was initially created so that as drugs came off patent, generic versions could swiftly come online. By using that process, Dybul suggested that not only were they able to extend generic versions internationally, but ARVs, including generic ddI and Gilead's Atripla, were able to get swifter approval for the US market (Dybul 2012).

The FDA, which has more staff and resources than the WHO, has a process similar to the WHO prequalification process, requiring applicants to provide information on the bioequivalence of the drugs. Where there are branded drugs still under patent protection in the United States, the FDA approval is listed as "tentative" rather than "full." In January 2005, the FDA announced that the first generic drugs were approved under its new process. The South African firm Aspen Pharmacare was approved for the co-packaged production of lamivudine/zidovudine and nevirapine, and the FDA waived the normal $500,000 fee, expediting the process in two weeks rather than the normal six months (McNeil Jr. 2005).

In the months following the Aspen approval, a number of other ARVs were also approved by the FDA. By 2008, the number of ARVs approved through the FDA tentative approval process had risen to 80, from 15 in 2005 (Holmes *et al.* 2011, 314). By July 2011, 131 ARVs had been approved through the FDA expedited review process (FDA 2011).

Despite these approvals, critics believed the FDA process to be an unnecessary duplication of the WHO prequalification scheme and charged that PEPFAR was still spending small proportions of money on generic drugs. The necessity of FDA approval can add both to the time and the costs involved, since the FDA may impose demands on manufacturers to repeat the bioequivalence tests they conducted for the WHO (Baker 2005). For example, Cipla's first drugs were not approved by the FDA until May 2006, four years after the drugs were initially prequalified by the WHO. Even though the Bush administration claimed that it only took two weeks to approve Aspen's application, critics charged that the paperwork and process leading up to the approval took months and months of work (Health GAP Coalition 2005). Initially, these fears about delays and procurement levels seemed to be substantiated. In FY 2004 and 2005, one study estimated that PEPFAR spent only 5 percent of its ARV treatment budget on generics (Ismail 2006). In FY 2006, generics accounted for about 27 percent of drug procurement spending in focus countries (Office of the US Global AIDS Coordinator 2007, 70).

Interestingly, in June 2005 some African governments – Nigeria, Uganda, Ethiopia, and Tanzania – rejected FDA approval for Aspen's drugs, suggesting that they would only accept drugs approved through the WHO process (Donnelly 2005). In response, the WHO and the FDA began to collaborate more (with an agreement to share confidential information signed in August 2005). FDA-approved drugs subsequently appeared on the WHO prequalified list. However, the reverse is not true. The SCMS can only purchase FDA-approved drugs on behalf of PEPFAR. The processes are similar, but not identical. According to Carmen Perez-Casas, a pharmacist with UNITAID and formerly the Global Fund and MSF, the dossiers are not fully comparable, because FDA reports do not contain all the same technical details found in WHO reports. Companies like Aurobindo and Encure that want to sell to PEPFAR have elected to apply only for FDA approval, withdrawing their dossiers from the WHO (Perez-Casas 2011).

The headline goal for PEPFAR, which helped reinforce to Congress the importance of the program, was the number of people on treatment. H.R. 1298 specified that 2 million people should be on ARVs through the help of the US government by the end of FY 2006. With drug quality concerns largely allayed by the FDA process, it became essential to stretch US appropriations farther by purchasing ARVs at the least cost. Generic drugs had and continue to have a significant cost advantage.

A January 2005 GAO study found that, compared to other AIDS treatment programs, the US government was potentially overpaying for drugs by buying branded drugs. The study found, based on prices quoted in June and July of 2004, that the price of 13 branded drugs ranged from costing $11 less per patient per year to $328 per patient per year more. At those costs, the GAO estimated that three of the four first-line regimens recommended by the WHO could be purchased for less by using generics, saving anywhere from $40 for ZDV + 3TC + EFV, to $343 for d4T + 3TC + NVP, to $368 less per person per year for ZDV + 3TC + NVP (the d4T + 3TC + EFV regimen cost the same for PEPFAR and other initiatives). The GAO estimated that by overpaying: "Such differences in price per person per year could translate into hundreds of millions of dollars of additional expense when considered on the scale of the plan's goal of treating 2 million people by the end of 2008" (GAO 2005). In April 2007, Henry Waxman, chairman of the House Committee on Oversight and Government Reform, would request detailed information on ARV procurement patterns from Mark Dybul, by then US Global AIDS Coordinator (Waxman 2007).

In light of these pressures, PEPFAR increasingly began to buy generic ARVs to meet its needs. By FY 2007, 73 percent of all PEPFAR-financed ARV drugs, including 93 percent of all drugs financed by its new supply chain management system, were generic (by volume) (Office of the US Global AIDS Coordinator 2008). This process was hastened when PEP-FAR began to pool procurement through the SCMS, a consortium of thirteen firms and NGOs that was created in late 2005 to handle ARV procurement and drug delivery for PEPFAR.[29] As shown in Table 6.5, PEPFAR's generic purchases increased dramatically between 2005 and 2008 (Holmes et al. 2011, 315). In a piece co-authored by Mark Dybul, Holmes et al. estimated generic drug purchases saved the US government more than $323 million in those three years alone (ibid., 313).

FDA rules clearly matter for producers of ARVs. A paradigmatic example is Ranbaxy, which the FDA found had quality-control issues at some of its plants in 2008 (Kaiser Health News 2008; InPharma 2012). As a consequence, PEPFAR suspended Ranbaxy ARVs from eligibility for procurement. A consent decree intended to lift the ban was finally signed at the end of December 2011/January 2012, but the ban had not been lifted at the time of writing (*The Economic Times of India* 2012).

The approval of generic drugs by the FDA and their increasing procurement through PEPFAR is the important story here. Together, these standards and the variety of procurement programs from the Global

---

[29] Participating institutions in the consortium include: Booz Allen Hamilton, Crown Agents USA, Inc. (CA-USA), i+solutions, JSI Research & Training Institute, Inc., Management Sciences for Health, The Manoff Group, MAP International, North-West University, Northrop Grumman, RTT, UPS Supply Chain Solutions, Voxiva, and 3i Infotech (SCMS Undated).

Table 6.5: *PEPFAR purchases of ARVs 2005, 2008*

	2005	2008
PEPFAR spending on ARVs	$117m	$202m
Generic as proportion of funding	9.17	76.41
Generic proportion by volume	14.8	89.33

Source: Holmes *et al.* 2011, 315.

Fund, UNITAID, PEPFAR, and other programs and organizations ultimately created a new competitive market landscape for the provision of ARVs. The legacy of these various interventions is the focus of the final section of this chapter.

Conclusions

The net effect of the changes in the financial, legal, and organizational environment described in this chapter has been a dramatically transformed market for ARVs, for both suppliers and recipients. With the advent of the Global Fund and PEPFAR, billions of dollars were made available for drug procurement. Within the context of the WTO TRIPS regime, pressure on branded pharmaceuticals companies to "back off" from pursuing their IPR created a more permissive legal and political context for developing countries to produce and trade in generic ARVs. The WHO's treatment guidelines provided medical practitioners and donors with guidance on what specific drugs should be bought. Both the WHO prequalification scheme and the FDA expedited process in turn specified what available drugs met international standards for quality. Together, the injection of financing and the changes in procurement rules created space for new providers, including generic ARV producers, to enter the market for ARVs, giving hope that a universal access to treatment regime could be achieved.

But what does the road ahead look like for the ARV market and access? While we provide a more thorough treatment in the concluding chapter, a brief discussion here can help set the stage. The landscape of ARV access has changed dramatically over the past decade. Although the need has only been partially met, the aspirations for universal access have helped transform the market from one characterized by low volumes and high mark-up to higher volumes with intense efforts to bring down prices. For many first-line therapies, drug prices have come down about as much as they can. The market has become more competitive, with a number of generics firms, particularly from India, producing most of the ARVs. The market has also become more complex, with strategic partnerships between generics firms and branded companies, as well as robust voluntary licensing agreements. Coupled with tiered pricing and large procurement orders from SCMS, UNITAID, and the Global Fund, the market for ARVs has been radically changed, oriented around extending access.

A number of concerns remain, not least of which are the stalled efforts to expand access in the face of tight foreign assistance budgets. Credible commitments of funds for procurement are becoming more uncertain, potentially leading firms to turn their businesses to other more lucrative opportunities. Shadlen has already warned that Indian firms were likely to do so in any case in the face of stronger patent protections for second-line drugs (Shadlen 2007). We return to this theme in the concluding chapter.

Other attributes of the market may also be undermining competition, and ultimately, innovation. While the WHO and FDA quality assurance programs expanded the number of approved suppliers for drugs between 2004 and 2008, Waning *et al.* worry that pooled procurement is leading to market concentration by a handful of buyers, and potentially a handful of suppliers (Waning, Kyle *et al.* 2010, 17). Disaggregated purchase orders in the early years of the Global Fund – with purchase orders from more than 100 countries – encouraged market entry, creating niche markets for manufacturers. They also worry that the benefits of pooled procurement may not materialize, since coordination across buyers involves some transactions costs, including the higher salaries and overheads that these initiatives cost. Indeed, they are concerned that one of the strengths of the Global Fund, encouraging local capacity building, might suffer, as pooled procurement fosters costly dependence on an international organization (Waning, Kyle *et al.* 2010, 16). As we discuss in Chapter 8, a persistent theme in our conversations with generic companies was the concern that pooled procurement had pushed prices so low that some companies were scaling-back their ARV business, and that few to no new companies were entering the market.

Broader issues may be as, or more important than, the distribution of Global Fund procurement money. Since 2005, Indian firms have been bound by global IPR rules; although possible to overstate, a number of second-generation ARVs are subject to patents, and thus Indian firms may be constrained by their ability to offer generic versions for some time to come. However, voluntary license programs by companies like Gilead have helped to ease this situation. With the persistent research findings that early ARV treatment can help prevent the spread of the HIV virus, there has been increased impetus to make treatment more widely available and at an early stage of the life cycle of the virus. Affordability of

ARVs becomes all the more critical in this context, particularly as foreign assistance budgets started to flat-line in 2009 and 2010 in response to the financial crisis. Persistent concerns about long-run affordability and access in light of India's gradual implementation of IPR rules prompted UNITAID to create the MPP in July 2008, a means for companies to share innovative ideas.[30]

We will return to these themes in the concluding chapter, as we discuss the future of access politics, both in terms of the case of HIV/AIDS drugs in particular, but also as a putative model for other issue domains in the health arena and beyond. In the following chapter, however, we see what lessons can be drawn from the AIDS treatment regime for market-transforming advocacy campaigns in a host of other domains.

---

[30] Headed initially by former MSF advocate Ellen 't Hoen, the Patent Pool became a separate entity in December 2009 and was funded for five years by UNITAID.

7 Lessons for other campaigns

> Regardless of the structure of the coalition, early work done to get all participants on the same page philosophically and strategically seems to be crucially important. Given enough time and mutual trust, a group can often find a way to converge around a rough policy agenda.
>
> Center for Nonprofit Studies report on *Lessons from Six Successful Campaigns*, including US advocacy that contributed to PEPFAR, 2005

Since the global AIDS treatment movement helped catalyze a dramatic increase in resources to fight the pandemic, advocates for other global causes have sought to learn from its success. In 2005, for example, the Center for Nonprofit Studies and the Aspen Institute issued a report of six successful campaigns that helped stimulate US engagement internationally on development and poverty, one of them being AIDS treatment mobilization (Chawla 2005). Likewise, in 2007, the US Coalition for Child Survival sponsored a report that sought to explain why advocates were successful in pushing for the creation of PEPFAR (McDonnell 2007).[1] As we will see later in this chapter, "malaria activists" have also sought to draw lessons from the HIV/AIDS campaign.

Indeed, movements for universal access to such goods as education have sought to emulate some of the specific organizational innovations wrought by AIDS treatment advocacy. In 2009, in a Brookings Institution paper, David Gartner, himself a former spokesperson for the Global AIDS Alliance, championed a funding mechanism for education, writing, "A Global Fund for Education should also draw on the successful experience of other innovative global development financing mechanisms. Among the most successful of these new organizations is the Global Fund to Fight AIDS, Tuberculosis, and Malaria (GFATM)." He credited the Global Fund with mobilizing billions of dollars for health and noted that "[o]ne of the keys to the GFATM's success in resource

---

[1] While less self-consciously systematic and academic in tone, these studies raise similar themes about the importance of framing and a common agenda.

213

mobilization has been the strong engagement of both civil society and developing countries as full partners with donors in its governance" (Gartner 2009b).

Moreover, advocates for other health causes were incredulous that AIDS seemed to command the resources it did. In a 2008 brief, "U.S. HIV/AIDS and Family Planning/Reproductive Health Assistance: A Growing Disparity within PEPFAR Focus Countries," Population Action International complained that money for reproductive health and family planning had stalled and even fallen, while funding for HIV programs increased dramatically (Population Action International 2008). Similarly, the consulting firm FSG has highlighted the disparity between funding for HIV/AIDS and the diarrheal diseases that are major killers of children, especially in Africa (FSG 2008). These kinds of concerns triggered a debate about whether HIV/AIDS was diverting money from other health causes (Shiffman 2006, 2008; Farmer 2007; Garrett 2007).

Scholars like Jeremy Shiffman have also sought to understand why AIDS generated the response it did while other health issues languished, applying such insights to the study of maternal mortality, newborn survival, and health systems strengthening (Shiffman and Smith 2007; Shiffman 2010; Hafner and Shiffman 2012; Shiffman and Quissell 2012). As he notes in a 2009 publication, "One reason for pursuing this question is that many global health analysts present evidence that material factors such as mortality and morbidity burden and the availability of cost-effective interventions may not explain the variance in the levels of attention health issues receive" (Shiffman 2009).

Rather than seek to explain differences in agenda-setting, we specified another, perhaps more ambitious task for ourselves: to understand why some campaigns for market transformation are more successful than others, using AIDS treatment advocacy as our model case study. Methodologically, the focus on a single-issue area poses challenges about "external validity" or the wider generalizability of our argument. Fortunately, our case possesses what social scientists refer to as "within-case" variation. Because some of the factors we identified as important in movement success changed over time, this before-and-after quality gives us more than a single observation to understand the success of AIDS treatment advocacy. For example, prior to cohering around access to treatment as its focal point, the nascent movement registered few successes. Once the movement articulated a clear ask for treatment and forged a strategy aimed at lowering drug prices, the movement was able to press its case more effectively. We have also shown how, as the US AIDS movement splintered over time, its policy influence diminished.

That said, the true test of our argument is still its ability to travel to other domains. This chapter makes the case that the AIDS treatment movement possessed a number of features that facilitated market transformation, and more importantly, these factors are germane to a set of other cases in the health arena and beyond. The first section outlines a typology of our five factors to understand the potential generalizability of our argument. We then apply the typology to a number of different cases, including malaria, maternal mortality, water/diarrheal disease, noncommunicable diseases, education, climate change, the ivory trade, sex trafficking, and abolition of the transatlantic slave trade, where we make predictions about the likely success of different movements.[2] The subsequent sections of the chapter develop mini-cases for each of these areas, which are meant to be illustrative and suggestive rather than definitive.

Applying our argument to other cases

How might our framework help us understand other cases? As we suggested, we see the following five factors – *a highly contestable market, a compelling frame, a coherent ask, low/favorable costs, and stabilizing institutions* – as being sequential steps in the advocacy process that can either hinder or facilitate advocacy success in transforming markets. Having favorable conditions on all five presents a most likely case for a long-run transformation of the market.

Other situations may not auger well for long-run stable market transformation and are at risk of backsliding to previous patterns of allocation or access. Specifically, if the first four forces are aligned in support of advocates' aims, but stabilizing institutions have not been created, then the new market structure in favor of access (or in support of campaigners' goals on other dimensions) may not endure. In other words, where advocates face a contestable market, have created a compelling frame, are unified in their demands, and have minimized the costs of their ask, but no institutions are in place to reinforce the new order, then the market transformation might not prove stable or durable.

Where advocates face markets that possess low contestability (either because the markets are very fragmented or the rules benefiting incumbents have a long history), then the road they face is harder. The chances of a market transformation are much less probable, but not impossible. Further, if campaigners fail to frame their case in a compelling way, their chances of success are diminished. Similarly, where advocates fail to

---

[2] Since some of these other issues like climate change are discussed in previous chapters, some cases receive more extensive treatment than others.

cohere on a common ask, they also reduce their likelihood of success. Finally, if the costs of their ask are high and/or campaigners cannot make inaction costly, then this, too, would reduce the likelihood of success.

While difficult to assess the relative weight of these different factors, we would assert that even where all the other factors are favorable but costs remain high, then this may pose a particularly challenging barrier to market transformation, in part because changing the costs of a market transformation may be the least tractable to human agency. Where advocates lack a compelling frame, for example, they can re-cast the issue. Where advocates have yet to reach consensus on a policy ask, they can organize and come together. But the immediate costs of market transformation may be substantial regardless of what advocates do, as with the case of climate change.

If we simplify so that each of our five factors takes on dichotomous properties (high/low market contestability, compelling/not compelling frame, coherent/incoherent ask, high/low costs, presence/absence of stabilizing institutions), then there are 2^5 or 32 possible combinations. However, more usefully, we can group possible outcomes on a continuum from most likely to least likely cases of market transformation. While we do not present all of the possibilities here in the text, we array some of the cells from the *most likely* as well as the *least likely* cases to give some intuitions about how these factors potentially conjoin (see Table 7.1).

In the next section, we apply these insights to a series of other cases, some of them related to global health (malaria, maternal mortality, water/ diarrheal disease, non-communicable diseases), but others like education, climate change, the ivory trade, and sex trafficking, in areas further afield from the health arena. These cases were chosen largely because they encompass some of the most important access campaigns and global problems of the early twenty-first century. In his guide to writing dissertations, Stephen Van Evera urges young scholars to select cases of "intrinsic importance" (Van Evera 1997, 87). We believe this is useful advice for older scholars as well. The cases in this chapter and the HIV/ AIDS case qualify, and we hope by selecting important cases with demonstrated utility in a wide array of cases that we can convince the reader that our theory of strategic moral action makes a major contribution. At least one additional case – abolition of slavery – was selected because it is a historical example that has been extensively examined in the literature on social movements and international relations (Nadelmann 1990; Keck and Sikkink 1998; Kaufmann and Pape 1999). If our framework can tell us something new about a case that is well known, we believe it can help us approach even well-trodden areas with fresh eyes.

Table 7.1: *Representation of continuum from most likely to least likely cases*

Most likely cases

Contestable	Frame	Coherence	Costs	Institutions	Prediction
High	Compelling	High	Low	Presence	**Most likely**
High	Compelling	High	Low	Absence	**Most likely** provided advocates can create institutions to reinforce the new market transformation
High	Not compelling	High	Low	Presence	**Most likely** provided advocates can overcome problems associated with a less than compelling frame
High	Compelling	Low	Low	Presence	**Most likely** provided advocates can cohere around a common ask
Low	Compelling	High	Low	Presence	**Most likely** provided advocates can identify/overcome obstacles posed by a non-contestable market
Low	Compelling	High	High	Presence	**Most likely** provided advocates can lower the costs of their ask or raise the costs of inaction

Least likely cases

Contestable	Frame	Coherence	Costs	Institutions	Prediction
Low	Not compelling	Low	High	Absence	**Least likely**
Low	Not compelling	Low	High	Presence	**Least likely** unless advocates can overcome low market contestability, re-frame the issue, cohere around a common ask, and lower costs
Low	Compelling	Low	High	Absence	**Least likely** unless advocates can overcome low market contestability, cohere around a common ask, lower costs, and create stabilizing institutions
Low	Not compelling	High	High	Absence	**Least likely** unless advocates can overcome low market contestability, re-frame the issue, lower costs, and create stabilizing institutions
High	Not compelling	Low	High	Absence	**Least likely** unless advocates can re-frame the issue, cohere around a common ask, lower costs, and create stabilizing institutions
Low	Not compelling	Low	Low	Absence	**Least likely** unless advocates can overcome low market contestability, re-frame the issue, cohere around a common ask, and create stabilizing institutions

Source: E. Kapstein and J. Busby.

For each of these cases, we seek to classify them on a continuum from most likely to least likely cases for market transformation, based on the configuration of the indicators at a particular point in time. Each case is represented by a line in the table, with our prediction about likely market transformation the final cell in the table. Some advocacy movements, like those promoting maternal mortality and climate change, have changed in important respects over time, providing what social scientists call "within-case variation." For example, in the case of maternal mortality, advocates initially were divided over the correct course of action but have increasingly rallied behind a common platform. The same might be said of advocates who are trying to bring a stop to sex trafficking. By contrast, climate advocates once were united behind a common approach of targets and timetables of binding emissions reductions. In the face of perceived high costs of action and political obstacles, however, the movement has become less united (see Table 7.2 for our list of cases).

The aim of these mini-cases is to demonstrate the potential generalizability of our argument to a series of important issue areas. The discussion for each is only cursory, and subject experts will undoubtedly find fault with our efforts to code individual attributes. Nonetheless, we believe that this extension of our argument to other domains should prove useful, both to scholars interested in the conditions under which social movements can succeed in transforming markets, but also advocates themselves as they seek to analyze why their efforts succeed or why they might be faltering.

Malaria: no more?

On April 1, 2011, *The New York Times* ran a remarkable article; one might almost have thought it an "April Fool's" joke if the topic were not so serious. It reported that "[a] few nonprofit groups have recently announced plans to wind down, not over financial problems, but because their missions are nearly finished. Most notable, perhaps, is Malaria No More, a popular nonprofit that supplies bed nets in malaria zones. Its goal is to end deaths from malaria, a target it sees fast approaching" (Strom 2011).

What made this commentary remarkable (and disconcerting) is the fact that malaria is still Africa's second-leading killer disease, following on the heels of HIV/AIDS. While malaria was largely eliminated on other continents through the active use of the DDT pesticide during the 1950s and 1960s, that method of eradication proved ineffective in Africa, where the disease and its mosquito-borne carriers were just too widespread (for useful background, see Gladwell 2001; Litsios 2002). For nearly

Table 1.2. *Application of our approach to other cases*

Case	Principle of market transformation	Contestable	Frame	Coherence	Costs	Institutions	Dependent variable	Prediction
ARVs/ AIDS	Universal access	High	Compelling	High	Low/Medium (declined over time)	Present (initially absent, Global Fund, PEPFAR, UNITAID)	Expanded numbers on treatment	**Most likely:** Stable market transformation (after costs declined, coherence achieved, and institutions built)
Malaria	Universal access	High	Compelling	High	High	Present (AMFm)	Expanded access to treatment/Reduction in malaria deaths	**Likely:** Possible transformation but only with lower costs
Maternal mortality	Universal access	Low	Compelling	High (used to be low)	Low	Present (Every Woman Every Child)	Reduction in maternal mortality/Expanded access to health clinics	**Mixed:** Possible transformation but market 'structure' difficult to influence
Water/ Diarrheal disease	Universal access	Low	Compelling	Low	High	Absent (World Water Forum)	Higher percentage of people with access/Lower incidence of diarrheal deaths	**Unlikely:** Unlikely transformation without a more focused ask
NCD/ Cancer/ Diabetes	Universal access	Mixed	Compelling	Low	High	Absent	Expanded numbers on treatment	**Mixed:** Possible transformation but difficult unless cohere on ask and bring costs down
Education	Universal access	Low	Not/Medium compelling	Low	High	Absent	Higher rate of participation in education/Improved educational outcomes	**Unlikely/Mixed:** Unlikely transformation unless advocates focus on structurally more concentrated areas; disruptive technologies provide a promising focal point for advocacy

Table 7.2: (*cont.*)

Case	Principle of market transformation	Contestable	Frame	Coherence	Costs	Institutions	Dependent variable	Prediction
Climate	Level playing field	Low	Not/Medium compelling	Low (used to be high)	High	Absent (weak, new institutions like ETS, CDM)	Reduced greenhouse gas emissions	**Unlikely:** Unlikely transformation without overcoming low market contestability, need for coherent ask and reduction of costs as well as stronger institutions
Elephant ivory trade	Prohibition	High	Not/Medium compelling	Low (used to be high)	High	Present (CITES)	Reduction in poaching	**Mixed:** Possible transformation if China can be convinced to use its market power to stop the trade
Sex trafficking	Universal elimination	Low	Compelling	Low (getting higher)	Low	Present (human rights treaties)	Reduction in numbers of people trafficked	**Mixed:** Difficult given market structure and absent a coherent policy ask
Abolition of Atlantic slave trade	universal prohibition	High	Compelling	High	High	Present (British Navy)	Blockage of importation of new slaves	**Mixed:** Possible transformation if British government is convinced to bear high costs

Source: E. Kapstein and J. Busby.

40 years, malaria was essentially a ticking time bomb, forgotten in the industrialized world until the late 1990s when its awful toll, especially on African children, again began to command public attention.

Given this renewed awakening about the malaria disease burden, a coalition of international agencies and health organizations came together in 1998 under the umbrella of the UN to form the "Roll Back Malaria" campaign, the objective of which was to cut malaria deaths in half by 2010. But according to the WHO, that objective was still far from being realized. Whereas the number of deaths from malaria reached between 1.1 to 1.3 million in 2000, that had fallen by only around 20 percent, to some 863,000, by 2008.[3] In fact, already in 2005 *The New York Times* had penned an editorial entitled "How Not to Roll Back Malaria," which criticized the campaign's management and strategy (*The New York Times* 2005).

It is an irony of history that contemporary strategic malaria advocacy would, to some degree, galvanize around the early failures of the Roll Back Malaria (RBM) campaign. In particular, the UN had decided to spend a "substantial proportion" of RBM's campaign funds on the purchase of various monotherapies that had long been used in malaria treatment, like chloroquine. But these monotherapies were "often ineffective in Africa because of parasite resistance" so malaria "activists" instead focused on getting artemisinin-based combination therapies (ACT) to sufferers from malaria (The *PLoS Medicine* Editors 2009). Unfortunately, these therapies were also considerably more expensive. Facing these high costs, some advocates would turn their attention to less-expensive anti-malaria solutions, like treated bed nets. In fact, providing these bed nets to malaria-plagued regions of Africa became the primary focus of the Malaria No More campaign.

But bed nets were only a partial solution at best, since they could not help treat those who were already sick. In thinking about how to roll out ACT to those who could not afford these drugs, malaria advocates drew lessons from what the AIDS movement had managed to achieve. A 2009 editorial in *PLoS Medicine* explicitly calling for greater "malaria activism" began as follows: "Probably no other disease in human history has been associated with social and political activism to the extent that the HIV epidemic has . . .. Such activism played a huge role in reducing the costs of antiretroviral drugs in developing countries." Similar political engagement, the editors said, is "needed to raise awareness of shortfalls in global

---

[3] For the latest data, see www.cdc.gov/malaria/. See also www.who.int/topics/malaria/en/.

efforts to control malaria." In particular, this new "wave" of malaria activism needed to focus on "ACT scale-up" (The *PLoS Medicine* Editors 2009).

What was the likelihood of successfully transforming the market for malaria treatment and prevention? In terms of market structure, like many drug markets in the developing world, "the anti-malarial market is huge in terms of those in need; it is small in terms of profit. By 1999, this had led to a virtually empty pipeline of new anti-malarial drugs" (Medicines for Malaria Venture 2012). A 2002 study documented that between 1975 and 1999 only four new malaria medications were approved as new chemical entities, and two more were approved shortly thereafter. This result, which was nonetheless better than other neglected diseases, constituted 0.3 percent of all the drugs approved during the same period (Trouiller *et al.* 2002, 2189). In the mid 1990s, malaria research received only $42 per fatal case, 80 times less than HIV/AIDS and 20 times less than asthma (ibid., 2191). By 2012, the WHO had prequalified only 25 medicines to treat malaria, from ten different suppliers. Compare this to HIV/AIDS, for which there were 299 different prequalified medicines (WHO 2012b). That mismatch between needs on the one hand and potential profits on the other is a leading cause of market failure in the global health arena. Here, the challenge was not so much that the market was diffused to a large number of suppliers, but that malaria sufferers in low-income countries, particularly children, did not generate enough demand to create much of a market to begin with. In the context of HIV/AIDS, when the first ARVs appeared on the market, the pharmas imagined a drug that was "low volume, high price," but given that there was a population with resources (or at least, with insurance and government support), there was enough incentive to create products to serve that market.

For malaria, until the creation of the Global Fund, that was largely not the case. In a sense, the market for malaria therapy was contestable, in that new producers could join the market, but there was not that much to contest. While we focus on market concentration and rules that reward incumbents, every market has its own particularities. This observation reminds us that advocacy in the world of pharmaceutical treatment must often focus on the challenge of how to change the way the drug market allocates its products.

In terms of the potential framing of this issue, advocates have a disease that kills large numbers of people, particularly children. Indeed, Malaria No More's basic motivation taps into that sentiment: "Malaria No More was born of a simple, startling insight: that ending malaria's death grip on Africa is the best humanitarian investment we can make in the world today" (Malaria No More undated). The disease, as our surveys suggested, is identified with death, although it is seen as a developing country problem that might complicate mobilization in countries where people are not affected by it. In part, it might be harder for people who lack familiarity with the disease to empathize with those affected, and it might also diminish their sense of the international transmission risk (though that might shift in the future if climate change extends the range of malarial mosquitoes).

Not surprisingly, malaria activists, like those in many other disease arenas, are divided between advocates of prevention and advocates of cure. In the particular case of malaria, the choice might be spending money on, say, bed nets and indoor spraying, versus spending money to buy drugs or for public health infrastructure such as sanitation systems. Perhaps the deepest source of division has been between advocates of eradication and those of control. In 2007, Bill Gates suggested that eradication of malaria might be possible, triggering a vigorous debate in the global health community. A number of other health experts, including Richard Feachem, the Global Fund's first executive director, as well as researchers associated with CHAI, worried that eradication, or even local elimination efforts would fail, like the previous efforts in the 1950s and 1960s (Tanner and de Savigny 2008; Bowdler 2010; Feachem et al. 2010; IRIN News 2010b; Kelland 2011). Feachem suggested that Gates' push for eradication constituted "a shock to the system for the malaria community, because for a couple of decades the 'E' words, eradication and elimination, were not used in polite company" (IRIN News 2010b). While some health experts were cautiously optimistic (Das and Horton 2010), others questioned whether the costs of elimination and eradication efforts might prove more costly than control (Sabot et al. 2010).

In terms of costs, some specific interventions are relatively inexpensive. Bed nets cost about $5–$10 per net. With the help of a Global Fund initiative described below, costs of ACT therapy have fallen by 80 percent, to between $0.46 cents and $1.67 (ReliefWeb 2012). That said, the net costs to donors might be fairly significant if the most aggressive efforts to expand the map of countries where malaria is eliminated are funded.

When the Global Fund was created, malaria had the fortune of being selected as one of the three diseases (along with AIDS and TB) that would be a core concern of the new organization. As a consequence, spending on malaria, like HIV/AIDS, would dramatically increase during the 2000s, by the Global Fund, the World Bank's Booster Program, as well as bilateral programs like US President George W. Bush's Malaria Initiative. Funding for malaria increased from less than $200 million in

2004 to nearly $1.8 billion in 2009. The WHO estimated that more than $6.1 billion would be needed in 2010 to implement the Global Malaria Action Plan (falling to nearly $3.4 billion in 2025) (WHO 2010e, 12). The incremental cost of mobilizing an additional $4 billion at a moment of economic turmoil and competition for foreign aid resources suggests that this cost might be a bridge too far.

More importantly, the estimates of lower long-run costs were contingent upon full funding in the early years that would lower treatment and control costs later on. Since the initiative by 2009 was already well off-track of these funding goals, then these savings may never be realized. It is worth emphasizing that part of the reason for the failure of the eradication effort in the 1950s and 1960s was a growing realization by governments that the costs were going to be much larger than they anticipated (Yekutiel 1981).

As we suggested, a major problem that advocates for enhanced malaria control faced was the absence of effective remedies. Many of the drugs that were available, like quinine and chloroquine, had increasingly become ineffective in the face of drug-resistant parasites. It was not until ACTs were approved in the late 1990s (beginning with Novartis's Coartem) that the international community had a potent tool to treat malaria and guard against drug resistance (Lite 2008).

Into this particular breach between human need and pharmaceutical markets stepped Nobel Prize-winning economist Kenneth Arrow, who had long been interested in the medical industry. In 2004 he urged the Institute of Medicine (IOM) of the National Academy of Sciences (NAS) to convene a committee that would address the drug shortage regarding malaria. The committee's recommendations were straightforward, at least in the economic sense of how a market failure in drugs might be most efficiently addressed. Specifically, Arrow's committee called for subsidization of the ACT market, stating that the industrialized world's foreign aid agencies, the World Bank, private donors and philanthropies (like the Gates Foundation), and international organizations like the Global Fund, should purchase ACT from the companies that manufactured the drug at negotiated prices. In turn, these agencies should sell the drugs at 90 percent off the negotiated price to developing world governments. Governments would thus be able to sell the drugs at a greatly reduced price (in the order of 20–50 cents per treatment) to those in need. This kernel of an idea was further developed by the World Bank, and by 2009 it was unveiled as the Affordable Medicines Facility for Malaria (AMFm), under the aegis of the Global Fund.

As a "Policy Brief" describing the AMFm put it, "The principle of the AMFm program is simple: it provides a co-payment to manufacturers covering a majority of the sales price for every ACT they sell to wholesalers. The wholesalers thus pay a lower price for ACTs and prices will fall throughout the supply chain, increasing affordability for the final consumer." The ACTs would then be sold over the counter in privately owned pharmacies and dispensaries; these subsidized drug supplies would thus "compete" to some degree with the public provision of the medications where (and when) they are available (a major issue in many developing countries with respect to medical care in general, and drugs in particular, is that there are two quite distinct markets, one private and one public. Public health insurance, however, is extremely limited, and often it is only the very poor who rely on publicly provided medical care; still, the presence of two different markets can create arbitrage opportunities). And with these lower prices for ACT, global health specialists also hope that excessive use of monotherapies will be reduced, because they are no longer effective against malaria and have become so cheap in Africa that they are often given to patients – especially children – instead of aspirin for common colds.

It should be noted that the creators of AMFm did not believe that its model would necessarily be limited to malaria; quite the contrary. They have argued, for example, that "within the global health space, the applicability for antibiotics should be explored, as these drugs face similar challenges of resistance and indiscriminate usage" (AMFm Policy Brief, March 2010). Indeed, AMFm's founders thought the model could potentially be rolled out to any drug which could benefit from a similar co-payment scheme. This was not, of course, the model applied to ARVs, where pharmaceutical companies were pressured to adopt differential pricing on the one hand, while drug companies in India were urged to enter the generics market on the other. In an important sense, then, there are different models for how drugs should be rolled out to the developing world, and these different models rely on different forms of subsidy, with one relying on taxpayers, the other relying on shareholders (although both could be fiscally equivalent).

Even though the AMFm as of this writing does not have a long track record, criticism of it has been forthcoming from various quarters. The US government, for example, initially expressed skepticism that the program will work "and that the limited money available to tackle malaria could therefore be better spent" (Jack 2009). And while the right answer in this particular case is that money almost certainly needs to be spent on both, a World Bank study usefully reminds us that "policymakers have to tradeoff between investments in AMFm and malaria prevention tools" (Laxminarayan, Klein, and Smith 2008). Further, the AMFm scheme requires careful monitoring of wholesalers and retailers, which is costly.

Wholesalers must be monitored to ensure that they really pass along the subsidy to retailers, and retailers must pass it on to consumers. How such monitoring could be carried out in a cost-effective manner in the African context remains to be seen. In addition, retailers must be educated about the new drug. One fear, for example, is that patients will end up taking both ACT for malaria and the existing monotherapies to treat fevers and colds, again pushing up resistance.

Since ACTs are derived from plants rather than from chemical synthesis, there are also lingering questions about how the price will evolve in the face of greatly increasing demand. If prices double, for example, what would that mean for the amount of ACT that could be subsidized? Apparently these sorts of questions still have not been answered. The AMFm ten-country pilot has already altered the market, driving prices down from about $6 to less than a dollar per dose, but the question is whether this market transformation is sustainable. As Amy Maxmen noted in *Nature Medicine*, "But some global health coordinators voice concerns about how dramatically the initiative has altered the supply chain and funneled ACTs into just a handful of the countries that need them" (Maxmen 2012). Sixty percent of global ACT orders have been routed through the AMFm, and stockouts and delays quickly became the norm. In 2011, Novartis, the company that initially patented combination therapy, announced that it could not fulfill a major order.

One result of the AMFm process was a shift from local drug wholesalers to AMFm-approved vendors, only one of which is located in Africa. As James Tibenderana of the Uganda-based Malaria Consortium notes: "ACT manufacturers outside of the AMFm are moving on to making other drugs, leaving fewer companies in the market. So if AMFm comes to an end, the only players that will be capable of providing ACTs are the ones who had been included in the program" (quoted in Maxmen 2012). With a major review of AMFm pending at the end of 2012 (and some suggestion that the United States may be hostile to it), whether or not the experiment of the AMFm proves to have lasting effects on the market for malaria medicines remains up in the air at the time of writing (Fan 2012). With the selection of Mark Dybul to lead the Global Fund in November 2012, the Global Fund Board also appeared to signal that the AMFm experiment would end as a stand-alone program and be integrated in broader grant-making efforts (Butler 2012; *The Economist* 2012).

What is clear from this case study is that malaria advocates have yet to converge on a strategy for how best to advance the objective of "Malaria No More." Should dollars be allocated toward bed nets or to new drugs? Eradication or control? The openness of the market to new providers, the deadliness of the disease, and financial support from a variety of donors has made the malaria market transformable.

However, it is unclear if the strategy itself will ultimately bear fruit in terms of a long-term reduction in malaria deaths and eradication of the disease itself. Without a coherent strategy aimed at cost reduction and market stability, let alone the biological imperatives of battling the malaria parasite, malaria advocates may be disappointed to find that they are making less progress than hoped in conquering this disease.

Maternal mortality

Advocates concerned about maternal mortality seek universal access to health services for women to prevent deaths before, during, and after childbirth. In terms of the market for maternal mortality services, the notion of a "market" may be somewhat strained when the expectation is that such services should be provided by the state. In some countries private providers, either health clinics or midwives, are present to assist in childbirth. The central point to emphasize here is that even where there are markets for maternal care, there is no homogenous universal product that a few firms provide that would change the delivery of service if only a movement materialized to push in that direction. There is no pill or nutritional supplement that a few firms might provide for a woman to take to ensure a safe and healthy birth. Transforming service delivery could only be a piecemeal process at the national level that would require transforming health systems as well as local service provision.

In terms of frames, maternal mortality advocates have a compelling moral frame: medical services to ensure safe childbirth are necessary for life. Potential challenges to this frame are that the problem, even though ostensibly universal, may be perceived as exclusively a developing country issue, and also disproportionately salient to women. International support by rich countries might be needed to fund a healthy motherhood initiative. Because most women in Western countries have access to such services, they might be taken for granted to the extent that it is more difficult to envision a context in which those services are lacking, dampening the salience of a putative appeal. Given that many decision-makers are men, this, too, might diminish the resonance of a maternal mortality campaign. That said, the necessity of these services for life gives them the potential for universal resonance. However, as Shiffman and Smith argue, maternal mortality advocates, at least through the mid 2000s, were divided on what the appropriate policy "ask" should be. It was only when advocates converged on a common solution – expansion of community care services coupled with more skilled clinical services in the event of an emergency – that the maternal mortality movement began to gain traction.

Such services, particularly the training and deployment of community workers, could be done relatively inexpensively. Malawi, for example, was able to successfully deploy health workers at the community level and help address maternal and infant health despite being a very poor country (Dugger 2009). Because many poor countries lack established health clinics in the first place, it is not clear whether there are incumbent service providers, like doctors or nurses, who might resist this move to protect their business, although in some countries this could happen. The upshot of this observation is that costs to donors and costs to firms to achieve significant reductions in maternal mortality might not be especially onerous. That said, the implementation costs of extending services in remote, rural areas might be more costly.

In 2010, Ban Ki-Moon launched an initiative on women and children's health, dubbed Every Woman and Every Child, and attracted commitments of $40 billion over five years. A portion of those funds were to be directed to support access to family planning, as well as other women's health issues (WHO 2010d). By 2012, supporters claimed that it had successfully mobilized $20 billion in two years and disbursed $10 billion (UN 2012c). Since the effort encompassed expenditures on other issues like HIV/AIDS, it is unclear how much of that total was specifically for maternal mortality. That said, as noted in Chapter 4, thanks to increasing unity among advocates, funding for maternal and child health had already increased from $563 million in 2003 to more than $1.2 billion in 2008 (in constant dollars). A 2012 report by the UN Commission on Life-Saving Commodities for Women and Children identified thirteen commodities that could be procured to support the Every Woman and Every Child initiative, including such drugs as oxytocin for post-partum hemorrhages, contraceptive implants, and oral rehydration therapy to treat infant diarrhea. The commission estimated that $2.6 billion over five years would be sufficient to avert 6 million deaths, including 230,000 maternal deaths, suggesting that significant gains could be had at relatively low costs (UN 2012d).

In terms of institutions, Shiffman and Smith's initial view was that "[w]ith respect to actors, the global policy community has been fragmented, no powerful institutions have emerged to guide the initiative, and organisational rivalries have persisted throughout its history" (Shiffman and Smith 2007, 1377). They contrasted that with other issues like child survival (UNICEF), family planning (UNFPDA), and technical advice (WHO), where a single organization took charge over these issue areas (ibid., 1374). An Inter-Agency Group for Safe Motherhood created in response to a 1987 conference was not regarded as successful, given its exclusive membership and low-level technical officers of important agencies. No organization owned this issue to really drive the process (ibid.). The MDGs process established reduction of maternal mortality by three-quarters as a core goal (UN 2012b). Shiffman and Smith pointed helpfully to the emergence of the Partnership for Maternal, Newborn and Child Health with the 20-year anniversary of the first initiative on the topic potentially yielding major progress (Shiffman and Smith 2007, 1378). The Every Woman and Every Child effort created in 2010, as of this writing, had the strong support of the Secretary General, but it is unclear what new institutional structures might be needed to make good on the 2012 recommendations from the Commission on Commodities.

To date, progress on this issue has been meager. The World Bank reported: "Of all the MDGs, the least progress has been made on the maternal health goal – worldwide, the maternal mortality ratio declined at less than 1% from 1990 to 2005." A 2010 study estimated that only 23 of 181 countries were on track to meet the goal to reduce the maternal mortality ratio by three-quarters (Hogan *et al.* 2010). A 2011 study suggested that only 11 countries would meet that goal (Lozano *et al.* 2011).

Thus, this particular issue possesses a mix of favorable attributes for successful market transformation. The structural fragmentation of health service delivery is perhaps the most difficult challenge, given that there are so many providers whose behavior would have to be influenced in the event of a major push for change. At the same time, the absence of markets in this space, the expectation of state provision but the paucity of clinics, doctors, and nurses, might prove to be a second formidable challenge, even if the ultimate price tag and absence of incumbents might not. The centrality of maternal survival bodes reasonably well for finding a compelling frame, and the lack of a coherent policy ask appears to have been overcome. Institutionally, the portents of a coordinating body suggested that this issue might be increasingly ripe for a successful market transformation, at least at the end of the 2000s before the financial crisis hit.

Clean water and diarrheal disease: a right to water?

In the wake of mobilization to address HIV/AIDS, campaigners for other issue areas, like clean water access, have sought to emulate the success of treatment advocates. A number of organizations emerged to press for expanded access to clean water with significant implications for water-borne diseases like diarrhea. Examples include the European effort Right

2 Water,[4] a Canadian effort Blue Planet Project,[5] the Right to Water campaign from Green Cross International,[6] the Global WASH campaign (Global Water, Sanitation and Hygiene for All) from the Water Supply & Sanitation Collaborative Council,[7] and the End Water Poverty coalition.[8]

Like maternal mortality, water provision is fragmented among many different service providers, even if, in some countries, there may be a national water authority that has responsibility for providing access. A handful of private water companies have begun to have multinational responsibility for water systems and infrastructure in different countries (and have become prominent targets of advocacy in countries like Bolivia, where water services have been privatized). However, by and large water is still fragmented into national, or even municipal systems of provision, with many local services providers. In many poor countries, again despite an expectation of state provision, clean water services are often lacking, forcing people to rely on for-profit vendors of water services, often small-scale entrepreneurs. Like maternal mortality, this problem cannot be addressed with a single product or technological innovation that a handful of providers can make available. Sanitation systems, water infrastructure, behavioral change, as well as procurement and billing systems, are all needed.

That said, the necessity of clean water to life bodes well for successful framing, as our surveys suggest. A specific emphasis on diarrheal disease, too, could be linked to survival in ways that are compelling, although our survey evidence suggests that US survey respondents do not appreciate the potential severity of diarrhea as a leading cause of death, particularly of children, in developing countries (on this point, see FSG 2008). This might make it more difficult to elevate the problem's significance from being perceived merely as an inconvenience. Addressing the broader problem of infant death rather than diarrhea per se might be a more productive strategy. Indeed, advocates have sought to fuse concerns about maternal and child mortality through the UN-supported Every Mother Every Child initiative, launched in 2010 as part of the UN Millennium Development Goals Summit (UN 2012a).

As for water, given the fragmented structure of the market, it is not particularly clear what the specific ask of this emerging movement might

[4] www.right2water.eu/.
[5] www.blueplanetproject.net/RightToWater/human_right.html.
[6] www.watertreaty.org/index.php.
[7] www.wsscc.org/wash-advocacy/campaigns-events/global-wash-campaign.
[8] www.endwaterpoverty.org/.

be. In 2012, campaigners pressed governments to label access to water as a human right (Provost 2012). Some potential examples might include a global fund for water. The MDG process established improvement of access to clean water and reduction of diarrheal deaths as goals. In March 2012, the WHO announced that the MDG goal to halve the number of people who lacked access to safe drinking water had been reached in 2010, five years ahead of schedule, meaning that 89 percent of the world's population had access to "safe," or at the very least, improved water sources (Ford 2012). That said, movement coherence demands more than a normative goal, but some indication of a strategy for realizing those ends.

In terms of costs, it is not clear, given the lack of specificity regarding the policy ask, how much it would cost to provide clean water universally. Certainly, measures to prevent deaths from diarrhea through oral rehydration therapy cost pennies, but the broader goal of universal access to clean water is a much more ambitious one. If provision of clean water demands the extension of modern piping and sanitation systems, then the costs to governments might be quite high. One 2010 estimate put donor support for water and sanitation at $8 billion annually (Provost 2012). In some countries, if extending access required privatization of national water systems, regulation, or even re-nationalization of private sources, then these actions might trigger incumbent resistance. Certainly, efforts to privatize water delivery in some countries, such as Bolivia, triggered massive protest movements in the 2000s (Malkin 2006). Further, privatization has not always succeeded, as governments then balk at giving the utilities the price adjustments they require in order to be profitable while making huge capital investments.

Clean water is an under-institutionalized area. While there are national systems that support universal access, particularly in wealthy countries, there are not clear rules to incentivize providers to reward access, particularly in under-served countries. Although the triennial World Water Forum has been meeting since 1997, it is unclear what leverage this particular body might have beyond agenda-setting. As a consequence, this area appears somewhat less favorable than maternal mortality for a successful market transformation, since the structure of the market, such as it is, is highly fragmented. The nascent movement has a compelling issue but lacks a coherent policy ask. Further, whatever the movement asks for may prove costly to provide and will require institutional development to reinforce and stabilize a new market structure. Again, even where countries have engaged, for example, in water sector privatization, the results have often proved disappointing, as governments were unable to put in place the necessary regulatory structures that gave these utilities an acceptable level of profit.

Non-communicable diseases: the next big thing in global health?

In September 2011, the UN hosted a high-level meeting on non-communicable diseases (NCDs), diseases that include cancer, heart disease, diabetes, and chronic respiratory disease. The meeting concluded with a General Assembly resolution declaring that the UN would seek to "address the prevention and control of non-communicable diseases worldwide" (Fan and Khan 2012). This was only the second health meeting of this stature that the UN hosted, the last comparable meeting being the 2001 General Assembly meeting on HIV/AIDS.

While historically such diseases were identified largely with conditions of affluence and aging populations in Western countries, rising prosperity and changing diets and lifestyles have made NCDs among the most deadly killers in middle-income, and increasingly lower-income countries, killing 57 million annually (WHO 2011d; Fan and Khan 2012). As Bollyky notes, 80 percent of NCD deaths are in low- and middle-income countries, up from 40 percent in 1990 (Bollyky 2012).

By most accounts, the 2011 meeting, coming at a time of acute weakness in the global economy generally and the EU in particular, produced few concrete results. As Sheri Fink and Rebecca Rabinowitz noted, "[T]he U.S., Canada and the European Union – along with several other developed countries – generally opposed setting immediate targets for reducing the prevalence of NCDs and resisted explicit calls for taxation on unhealthy products, industry regulation, and patent exemptions to lower drug prices" (Fink and Rabinowitz 2011). In spring 2012, the World Health Assembly did adopt a global target of a 25 percent reduction in premature mortality, but it is unclear what that will mean in practice (Fan and Khan 2012).

Given the diversity of industries and diseases covered, there is no single market that would be transformed by an NCD campaign. Tobacco, drug, beverage, and food companies could all be subject to some "anti-corporate" actions depending on the agenda of particular movements. At present, these agendas are rather diffuse, although a clearer set of priorities and targets may be emerging. Thus, whether or not these markets are contestable might depend on the affected industry and the policy ask.

On the pharmaceutical side, some drugs, like for diabetes and asthma, are off-patent and open to generic competition (Bollyky 2012). For other diseases like a number of cancers, the treatment technologies are produced by only a handful of companies that enjoy patent protection, the industrial structure making a market transformation possible, but the patent rules shielding incumbents from competition by new entrants.

In this context it is intriguing that contestation over cancer drug patent rights was at the heart of legal disputes between Western companies Novartis, Bayer, and Roche, and Indian generic companies in 2012 (Ahmed and Sharma 2012; Chatterjee 2012). Though Indian patent courts decided in favor of generics in these cases, the rules over IP both for and against generic competition remain very much in question.

Since NCDs are now among the leading killers in low- and middle-income countries, a campaign for universal access to treatment has some chance of universal resonance. As our surveys suggested, while some of these diseases are seen as arising from lifestyle choices, cancer broadly was regarded as a disease that affects people through no fault of their own. Furthermore, these NCDs are generally viewed as widely affecting everyone around the world. Given these results, a campaign for access likely has some resonance.

As Bollyky noted, "NCDs that are preventable and treatable in developed countries are often death sentences in the developing world." It is not too hard to imagine an effective campaign drawing attention to access to the vaccine against the human papillomavirus and cervical cancer, the leading cause of death for women in sub-Saharan Africa and South Asia (Bollyky 2012). Indeed, former President George W. Bush made just such a connection on World AIDS Day 2011 when he announced a new initiative, Pink Ribbon Red Ribbon, as part of his work as a former president to extend breast and cervical cancer screening and treatment to women. He made the case for why such an effort was important: "It is heart-wrenching to save a woman from AIDS, only to watch her die from cervical cancer, which is more prevalent in women with HIV" (Bush 2012).

However, advocates for addressing NCDs were only united in their demand that the issue get on the global agenda; unfortunately, they lacked consensus on their policy ask, or what needed to be done. One of the leading campaign groups, the NCD Alliance, is made up of diabetes, heart, cancer, and lung disease advocacy federations. Supported by a dozen major pharmaceutical and medical device companies, the NCD Alliance opposed easing patent protection, whereas a block of 132 low- and middle-income countries had a different view (Fink and Rabinowitz 2011). As Bollyky notes, health campaigners also clashed over other issues. Some advocates complained that mental health was not included in the agenda. The Gates Foundation, for its part, worried that the focus on NCDs could divert attention and support away from other health measures (Bollyky 2012). This disagreement suggests that advocates concerned about NCDs have not united on a common ask, and until they cohere on a common agenda, they are likely to struggle.

In terms of developing a strategy for meeting the costs associated with greater access to treatment of NCDs, advocates face a number of challenges. First, the timing of the issue's emergence is not fortuitous, given the parlous state of the global economy and foreign aid budgets. In any event, the net costs to governments might be quite large. The WHO estimated that a range of measures to address the four major risk factors (tobacco, alcohol use, physical inactivity, and unhealthy diet) would cost $11.4 billion a year in developing countries (Bollyky 2012). Nils Daulaire, Director of the Office of Global Affairs at the US Department of Health and Human Services in the Obama administration, expressed the view of donor governments: "We don't feel there should be cuts for maternal and child survival, AIDS, immunization programs, or the control of pandemic diseases. The US Congress has made it crystal clear: Budgets will not be increased, they will be reduced" (quoted in Fink and Rabinowitz 2011). Further, some of the incumbent industries that would be affected by measures to address NCDs, such as tobacco and alcohol, will see potential existential threats to their industries and oppose them strongly. Since these industries also happen to be large tax revenue generators for developing world governments, their concerns will likely be taken quite seriously.

These circumstances led Fink and Rabinowitz to conclude that "[b]y all indications, the breathtaking advances made in AIDS treatment in developing countries are unlikely to be replicated here" (Fink and Rabinowitz 2011). Bollyky was more optimistic, but he cautioned that advocates needed to change strategy and focus on the most important risk factors. He suggested that the meeting would have likely been a failure even in good economic times. Failure was a result of "poorly conceived collective action" and that "trying to address these diseases as a single class and on a global level broadened opposition and diffused support for effective action." By lumping all these health conditions together, Bollyky notes that otherwise "disconnected industries" including agriculture and pharma companies, all came together to oppose targets and actions against various risk factors. He also argues that a broad agenda made it harder to mobilize sufferers since the benefits for any particular affected constituency are unclear (Bollyky 2012). In this sense, NCDs face a classic collective action problem in terms of organizing those who would benefit from greater access to treatment.

Citing tobacco as a key risk factor, Bollyky emphasizes that the existing WHO Framework Convention on Tobacco Control provides a possible model of an institutional platform that is seeking to address taxation, advertising, and overall consumption of that product. This raises the question of how broadly applicable the tobacco convention is to other

NCDs. If it provides a "focal point" for the NCD campaign, it could help advance this movement's agenda and chances for success. Conversely, until advocates focus their efforts on contestable industries, and articulate a clear, narrower policy ask, they are likely to engender significant opposition from donors worried about the costs (and governments worried about lost tax revenues) of the initiative, as well as the industries whose profits will be affected.

Education for all

Like the campaign for universal access to clean water, education advocates, inspired in part by the ARV treatment access movement, have emerged to press for wider access to schooling. Also like maternal mortality and clean water, the education goal received some institutional backing through the MDGs process. Specifically, MDG 2 called for universal access to primary schooling by 2015.

Here, too, an education campaign may suffer from some of the same weaknesses that likely will affect both maternal mortality and clean water. To begin, the structure of the market for education differs enormously from one country to the next. Even in countries where education is virtually a state monopoly, for example, multiple organizations may influence the curriculum and who controls the classroom. In France, for example, where the state exercises control over most education at all levels (even influencing the curriculum of private and parochial schools), teachers' unions continue to be extremely powerful. In other cases, one finds a mix of public and private educational establishments, with entry into the market being relatively easy. Today, "online" or internet-based education may be a "disruptive technology" that will change market structures. The important point is that unlike pharmaceuticals, where a handful of firms produces drugs for a given health problem, there are few global brands in education whose behavioral change would unilaterally transform the market. This factor alone makes a structural transformation in the market unlikely.

That said, there may be pieces of the market where transformation of products related to education could be said to be more concentrated and thus more contestable, given the demand for high-quality instructional software and the related hardware. For example, a number of firms dominate the laptop and software markets. An effort has emerged to produce low-cost laptops for less than $100 (Fildes 2007), associated with the One Laptop Per Child campaign.[9] A former Amazon executive

---

[9] http://one.laptop.org/.

also started an effort in 2010 to distribute free e-books or electronic readers to children in developing countries (Stone 2012).

One could imagine that some software applications would be subject to pressure for universal access, whether for word processing, spreadsheets, bibliographic resources, or language translation. Linux-based collaboration among computer programmers was intended to overcome the proprietary restrictions of fee-based operating systems. Indeed, freeware programs like Zotero, a bibliography-building program, offer some scope for expanded access to those who cannot afford to buy programs like EndNote.

Another example hits closer to the scholarly home. Academics have started to grumble about the proprietary, fee-based access to scholarly journals that places much of their work behind a pay-wall, restricting access to universities with extremely expensive subscriptions, and keeping their readership lower than it otherwise might be (Gusterson 2012; Nexon 2012). This movement for open-source publications could have more success, since a handful of publishing houses are responsible for academic journals, making market entry by new open-source publications a potential new equilibrium or focal point, or if the incumbent journal publishers themselves feel the need to provide more access. The appropriate business model will remain a challenge. Perhaps these firms will experiment with differential pricing across different classes of academic institutions, if they have not already done so. Some of the challenges associated with pharmaceutical drugs will surely be of concern here as well, with the possibility of copyright violations and re-importation of scholarship from low-income markets to wealthier markets through email or web-based file-sharing services. Google, for example, ran into precisely this kind of trouble and resistance from publishers when it tried to offer books through Google Books on-line (Gross 2012; Reuters 2012a).

Another example may also have some promise to revolutionize access. Stanford and Harvard Universities, for example, have begun to offer on-line courses in a handful of subjects for free, part of an initiative called edX (Associated Press 2012; Lewin 2012). Two Stanford computer scientists also launched a competing for-profit venture called Coursera, which has agreements with a wider set of universities (Lewin 2012). Such courses may in time, given the stature of these two universities (and the schools that make up Coursera), create pressures for mimicry from other institutions, but also challenge some of the fee-based degree programs at other incumbent universities. While other on-line university programs exist, the more prestigious universities are uniquely capable of resisting market entry by new rivals, as they are global brands with a pedigree.

Indeed, one might question why a student from Bangalore would want to pay money to get a degree in computer science from an American state university if s/he could get a certificate of completion from Stanford or Harvard.

In terms of a compelling frame, our survey evidence in Chapter 3 suggested that the issue, while regarded as important, might potentially be more salient in poorer than rich countries. Though education is universally seen as desirable, people in advanced industrialized countries may be as preoccupied by their own access needs and those of their children before being able to imagine much scope for global generosity. Primary education, which already has more universal coverage in rich countries, may be an exception. Seeing young children, particularly young girls, lack schooling and educational opportunities can be evocative as individual campaigns. Note the ubiquitous late-night television commercials from actress Sally Struthers on behalf of the Christian Children's Fund and, more recently, Alyssa Milano on behalf of UNICEF.

In terms of a coherent policy ask, we would argue as outsiders to this movement that it is unclear if one has emerged. As we noted, some advocates favor a global education fund, modeled on the Global Fund for AIDS, TB, and Malaria. Though this model may potentially inspire, its function and purpose would likely have to be further specified to generate real support. Despite interest from the Obama administration in a fund, the results have been "disappointing," according to Desmond Birmingham, who notes, "The high-level U.S. political commitment has eroded, partly because of a lack of clear vision in the education community on how best to use potential support" (Birmingham 2010).

As we suggested, there are a variety of other goals that, given the fragmentation of the market, might possess more latent potential for market transformation. Some of them, like campaigns for one laptop per child, already exist. Still, we believe that the policy ask is in need of further refinement. For example, since 2002, the advocacy NGO, RESULTS, has championed the Education for All campaign, and in 2012 focused its advocacy on a specific ask, targeting the World Bank and its apparently failed 2010 pledge to provide $750 million for education over five years (RESULTS 2012).

While this demand has a specific price tag (and a fairly expensive one), it is difficult to evaluate the costliness of the broader call for universal education access in the absence of a clear policy ask. Many of the likely measures to extend educational access, for example, would likely entail significant costs, particularly if they involved construction of new schools and funding for more teachers. Gartner's Global Fund for Education imagined an organization capable of disbursing $7 billion a year, a rather sizable figure (Gartner 2009b). Again, new technologies could bring down substantially the costs associated with greater access to education, and it might behoove advocates to focus on such opportunities.

As for institutions to support global access to education, obviously these are either non-existent or, if built on the back of existing organizations, then woefully under-funded. In a sense, the campaign would already have to have succeeded in putting global education access front and center on the agenda of the international community. Yes, organizations like UNESCO exist, but the point about institutions is that they have the authority to create and sustain the rules of the market in a way that they do not today in the education space. The MDG process has put education access on a long list of important items for development, but the education-related goal of universal access to primary education is unlikely to be achieved by 2015 as initially intended (UN 2012b). The process of goal-setting on its own is unlikely to create lasting incentives for access in the absence of more significant institutionalization.

In 2011, the Global Partnership for Education was launched in Copenhagen, a renaming of the Fast-Track Initiative, a process that started in 2002 and which over ten years mobilized a modest $2 billion (Pfeifer 2011). At that meeting, the World Bank reaffirmed its funding commitment of $750 billion over five years, while other donors pledged about $1.5 billion (Oxfam 2011). In 2012, the UN Secretary General launched another new initiative on education, called Education First, appointing former British Prime Minister Gordon Brown to lead it.[10] It remains to be seen if these efforts, re-branded and re-cast, will be successful, given the modest progress made in the previous decade.

Still, given the fragmentation of the market for education, the structural obstacles for market transformation are perhaps the first barrier that advocates have to overcome, as identifying tractable pieces of the education market will likely shape the frame and policy ask that campaigners ultimately deploy. These, in turn, will shape the perceived costliness of these initiatives both to governments and incumbent providers. Disruptive technologies, however, could radically alter the education landscape, especially if prestigious institutions begin to offer certificates of completion (if not yet degrees) for courses of study. Advocates who wish to promote greater access to education globally might well focus their efforts on working with these "new" entrants.

---

[10] See http://globaleducationfirst.org/.

Climate change: how about changing the market, too?

The advocacy movement to address climate change, unlike access campaigns, has largely sought to forestall a global public bad. Nonetheless, the metaphor of market transformation applies. Where the treatment campaign sought expanded access to ARVs largely through changes in the price mechanism, climate activists wish to generate incentives for the replacement of carbon-intensive dirty energy with lower and/or zero carbon resources. While this could in theory be achieved in a variety of ways, through regulation, prices, and subsidies, the challenge fundamentally is to increase the price on carbon and make it more attractive for incumbents to shift to cleaner energy sources and/or to encourage market entry by cleaner energy sources. One could conceive of the climate campaign in terms of universal access, access to clean energy, or protection from a global public bad.

Looking at our framework, we can anticipate the expected success or failure of climate change advocacy. In terms of market structure and contestability, there are diverse sources of greenhouse gas emissions that come from different market activities, some from the production of energy primarily for electricity, others from the transport sector, still others from emissions that emerge from agriculture and land-use changes. Emissions come from different energy sources – coal, oil, natural gas, burning trees, dung, etc. – as well as from different chemical compounds in the case of hydrofluorocarbons (HFCs) that, in addition to their contribution to the ozone hole, are also potent greenhouse gases. Transforming the market therefore requires a simultaneous transformation in multiple domains, in multiple markets, with there being few concentrated points along the way.

Internationally, some sectors, like oil, may be relatively concentrated, but the number of firms, between multinational oil companies and national oil companies, still is large and disaggregated. The same could be said of the number of car companies. Some areas, like electric power production, may be controlled by a limited number of companies at the national level (in some cases controlled by a national power company), but internationally, the number of producers is quite large. In terms of the fluidity of the rules, the climate rules that exist are of recent creation and are thus contestable; they are, in fact, the very rules that are meant to encourage a transition to clean energy, like the Kyoto Protocol, the EU emissions trading scheme, and the taxes on airline travel in the EU. Where rules are more stable and durable, they tend to be national ones that subsidize the advantages of incumbent fossil fuel firms.

Climate change, while increasingly implicated in the deaths of individuals from increased exposure to climate-related hazards, is not so closely identified with survival (however, in some low-lying island countries, climate change is certainly regarded as an existential threat). Nonetheless, advocates have struggled to identify a compelling frame. Its master frame, climate change framed as a global crisis, in some cases has had demobilizing effects, as the severity of the problem reinforced the notion that the problem was intractable (FrameWorks Institute 2001; Obelisk Seven Blog 2010; Busby 2010a; Busby and Albertson 2011). As climate change becomes increasingly identified with local effects (that is, geographically proximate effects on people's nearby surroundings), then appeals by advocates may prove more compelling, though this would imply a universal strategy of emphasizing local effects rather than global ones.

As we argued in Chapter 4 on movement coherence, climate change advocates were united around a common ask of binding emissions reductions and targets and timetables, but as that effort proved contentious and unsuccessful in enlisting important countries like the United States, the movement has fractured into a less united force.

In terms of costs, incumbent firms, including producers of carbonintensive energy sources and electric utilities, have vigorously fought to defeat policies that would raise their costs. While advocates have tried to downplay both the aggregate costs to countries of transitioning to a clean energy future, many incumbent firms, particularly producers of coal and oil, regard climate policies as costly and antithetical to their business (Busby 2008; 2010a). Governments, asked to pay for the transition costs of their own countries, also see the price tag as costly. While a true cost–benefit analysis would compare the costs of action to inaction,[11] the upfront costs to a clean energy transition have proven more salient than avoiding the long-run costs of climate damage.

Finally, the institutional edifice in support of clean energy as suggested above is largely absent and where it exists, the rules are new, contested, weak, and only provide partial coverage to some countries (with the United States, China, India, and others either by choice or by design excluded from having obligations). The strongest rules are present in the EU, but like its new aviation tax, are strongly contested (Busby 2010b).

---

[11] The Stern Report for the UK government represents one such controversial effort to assess the long-run costs and benefits of addressing and failing to address climate change. Its findings are contested, in part because of assumptions about the discount rate and how to treat the future costs of climate change. The Stern Report assumes a low discount rate, which weighs future costs more heavily than traditional cost–benefit analysis, which typically discounts that future more heavily, potentially skewing analysis to weigh present costs more heavily over future benefits (HM Treasury 2006; Nordhaus 2006).

Thus, from this perspective, chances of market transformation appear unlikely. Unless advocates can find a structural handle of concentrated activity, identify a more compelling frame, cohere on a common demand, lower the costs of action, and institutionalize policies that reward clean energy activity, the chances of market transformation remain slim. Of course, a crisis might generate a transformation in some of these dynamics, making the existing order seem less defensible, but such an external event may only emerge when it is too late to do much to avoid the problem.

As Victor *et al.* point out, some short-lived but potent greenhouse gases like black carbon, methane, lower atmospheric ozone, and HFCs, might be more susceptible to swift reduction and market transformation. They suggest that technologies already exist to realize deep emissions reductions from these sources, and that, importantly, addressing these emissions could yield a favorable benefit–cost ratio: "[C]ontrolling these pollutants would actually serve the immediate interests of developing countries, where pollutants such as soot and ozone damage vital crops and cause respiratory and heart diseases" (Victor, Kennel, and Ramanathan 2012). Similar efforts to identify lower-cost emissions savings from Reducing Emissions from Deforestation and Degradation have a similar potential to transform the timber sector and provide important benefits in averted emissions (World Bank 2007; Butler 2012). Advocates will have to be creative in identifying favorable opportunities for action in an arena that otherwise looks like an unlikely case for market transformation.

The elephant ivory trade: a market transforms and a movement loses ground

Throughout 2012, a series of stories about poaching of endangered elephants and rhinos appeared about record numbers of both animals slaughtered, mostly in Africa, but also remnant populations in Asia (Christy 2012; Gettleman 2012; Revkin 2012). For many observers, the decimation of elephant and rhino populations was shocking by the speed with which it was unfolding. In 2011, 38.8 tons of illegal elephant ivory (equivalent to about 4,000 elephants) was seized around the world, a record amount since data began to be kept in 2002. Since this figure likely reflects a fraction of the amount actually traded, the numbers of elephants killed could be high as 25,000 to 30,000 (out of a population that perhaps was between about 500,000 and 700,000) (Christy 2012; Gettleman 2012). Through the first nine months of 2012, more than 400 rhinos were killed in South Africa alone, more than 250 of them in the heart of the country's magnificent Kruger National Park (Cota-Larson 2012). The killings of elephants and rhinos undermined what had been earlier conservation movement successes. Indeed, a market *had been* successfully transformed, but now things were moving in the opposite direction. What happened?

To understand the recent turn of events, we focus on the market for elephant ivory. At the urging of Western conservation groups like the NGO, TRAFFIC, and its parent organization, the World Wildlife Fund (WWF), among others, the ivory trade had initially been outlawed in 1989 with apparent success through the Convention on the International Trade in Endangered Species (CITES). After a decade in which as many as 600,000 elephants were killed, the United States unilaterally banned ivory imports in 1989, and Kenya burned 13 tons of ivory in the same year. The CITES ban went into effect in 1990, although Zimbabwe, Malawi, Namibia, Botswana, and Zambia entered reservations and remained outside the ban (Christy 2012). CITES has long been considered one of the most successful international environmental agreements, enforced through national legislation and international collaboration through Interpol.

While African state weakness is an important part of the story why rhinos and elephants are vulnerable, the biggest change that has imperiled wildlife is increasing Asian demand, particularly in China, where rising wealth and consumerism are allowing people to afford items once the preserve of the wealthy. Gettleman explains:

The vast majority of the illegal ivory – experts say as much as 70 percent – is flowing to China, and though the Chinese have coveted ivory for centuries, never before have so many of them been able to afford it. China's economic boom has created a vast middle class, pushing the price of ivory to a stratospheric $1,000 per pound on the streets of Beijing. (Gettleman 2012)

Christy makes a similar point, "For the first time in generations many Chinese can afford to reach forward into a wealthy future, and they can also afford to look back into their own vibrant past" (Christy 2012). A US State Department official put the argument starkly: "China is the epicenter of demand. Without the demand from China, this would all but dry up" (quoted in Gettleman 2012).

There are a number of important loopholes that have gradually undermined the sticking power of this ban. First, ivory bought prior to the ban can still be traded within countries, making it easy for people to claim their ivory items are "pre-ban." Moreover, some countries like Thailand, which has its own domestic elephant population, have rules that allow the trade in ivory from elephants that died of natural causes or where the tips of tusks of living elephants have been cut off. Corrupt customs and wildlife officials who turn a blind eye to the ivory trade, or themselves take part in it, are also part of the problem (Christy 2012).

Most importantly, in the face of rising elephant and rhino numbers, some countries like Zimbabwe that have collected ivory from culled animals or from those that had died from natural causes, sought a means to gain revenue from the sale of such ivory in exchange for their participation in the CITES ivory ban. In the 1997 meeting of the conference of parties of the CITES regime, an occasional sale of ivory was approved, beginning with a 1999 sale to Japan that yielded 55 tons for $5m. In 2004 and 2005, China, along with Japan, petitioned for another sale. In July 2008, the CITES regime approved the sale of 115 tons of ivory by Botswana, Zimbabwe, South Africa, and Namibia to Japan and China. This set the stage for the massive efforts to kill elephants and stockpile ivory in the late 2000s and early 2010s. What was the intent of the sale and how did it go awry?

Revkin suggests that the Chinese government "has cornered the ivory market" and "by raising prices, intensified poaching pressure on elephants." The initial idea of the sale was to "flood the market and drop prices, stifling the illicit trade" (Revkin 2012). However, as Christy reports, the 2008 auction process was gamed by the Japanese and Chinese, who colluded to keep prices low but then, in China's case, turned around to sell the ivory at high prices. The Japanese buyers noted that they preferred "primarily medium-size, high-quality tusks," while the Chinese preferred "either large, whole tusks for big sculptures or small pieces for decorative touches." With each country bidding on different types of ivory, they kept the sales price low (Christy 2012).

Though Japan and China were able to obtain ivory at relatively low prices ($67 a pound compared to the previous black market price of $386 a pound), the Chinese ended up keeping the price of legal ivory high at more than $500 a pound. Again, Christy provides the details:

Instead the Chinese government did the unexpected. It raised ivory prices. Through its craft association, CACA, the government charged entrepreneur Xue Ping $500 a pound, a markup of 650 percent, and imposed fees on the Beijing Ivory Carving Factory that brought the company's costs to $530 a pound for Grade A ivory. China also devised a ten-year plan to limit supply and is releasing about five tons into its market annually. The Chinese government, which controls who may sell ivory in China, wasn't undercutting the black market – it was using its monopoly power to outperform the black market. (Christy 2012)

The result of this market scarcity is actually encouraging ivory traders to try to kill elephants and hoard more ivory, based on the expectation that possessing ivory from extinct species might be very lucrative. As one Thai-based conservationist put it, "Ivory traders are stockpiling. Since CITES has a history of relaxing trade bans, they feel it's a safe gamble" (quoted in Christy 2012). In the parlance of our argument, we are witnessing how a concentrated market structure, characterized by a monopoly buyer, can swiftly transform a market.

While advocates have historically framed the argument in terms of saving endangered species for their own sake, this argument has had difficulty convincing cash-strapped governments in Africa that sales of ivory are shortsighted. To be sure, efforts to support eco-tourism have attempted to create value in live elephants, but the lucrative possibilities of the ivory trade were hard to resist. With elephant populations recovering, the thinking was that the sale of already seized ivory could potentially marry conservation and commerce. Such logic was certainly compelling to a number of African governments, though many, if not all, conservation groups opposed the lifting of the ban for the auction. Indeed, this suggests that if a ban is to be successful, advocates of species conservation must convince countries that possess the animals also to support the ban. Importantly, both TRAFFIC and WWF endorsed the 2008 auction (Christy 2012). Ivory and elephant conservation, including requests from Tanzania for a new sale of ivory, were on the CITES agenda in the lead-up to its 2013 "conference of parties," the meeting of the convention's members that occurred every three years (*The Guardian* 2012) but were ultimately dropped.

With ivory prices in 2012 twenty times the price paid in Africa, Christy argued: "[t]he genie cannot be returned to her bottle: The 2008 legal ivory will forever shelter smuggled ivory." Any policy to help restore elephant herds depends in part on convincing consumers to change their habits. Former NBA basketball player, Yao Ming, embarked on a summer 2012 tour to try to draw attention to the Chinese role in poaching. Christy noted that large amounts of ivory have been implicated in religious trinkets and encouraged Catholic and Buddhist religious leaders to change norms. In Christy's view, the only thing that could work is a return to a ban: "[a]n ivory ban is the only thing we've seen that's worked. When there was a ban in place, elephant populations recovered. They relaxed the ban and poaching has soared" (quoted in Revkin 2012).

With the CITES conference of parties meeting in March 2013, the institutional edifice to address the trade remains in place but the secretariat appears to have limited capacity for oversight. Christy reported that until 2011, CITES had only one enforcement officer and depended on the outside support of groups like TRAFFIC to monitor the trade. That said, with the ivory trade concentrated in China and largely controlled by the Chinese government, the potential to transform the market still exists.

However, whether or not the Chinese will feel compelled to rein in the ivory trade may well determine the fate of the world's elephant population.

Sex trafficking and modern slavery*

No global market would seem to be more in need of transformation than the market for sexual services, which involves the trafficking of women and girls across borders. Human trafficking is, in essence, a modern form of slavery, and when most people think about slavery – if they think about it at all – they probably assume that it was eliminated during the nineteenth century. Unfortunately, this is far from the truth; in fact, it is likely that more people are being trafficked across borders against their will now than at any point in the past (this section draws in part on Kapstein 2006b).

What does "market transformation" mean in the case of human trafficking? Would it mean the elimination of prostitution? Would it mean the end of women crossing borders to provide sexual services? Or would it just focus on the *coercive, transnational* aspects of the sex trade? Coming to agreement on these questions has prevented the international community, including governments and NGOs, from cohering around a unified set of policies. Further, the very structure of the market makes transformation quite difficult. Providers of slaves are not very concentrated, and the demand is equally diffuse. Thus, targeting the market on the demand and supply sides is challenging (and of course, those who demand sexual services are unlikely to be convinced that it should be terminated).

The modern global slave trade generally involves the use of deception and coercion to induce victims to cross national borders in search of new jobs; once the target has arrived in a foreign country, she (for it is usually a she) is then forced into some form of labor bondage. Although hard figures are difficult to obtain, the US government estimates that some 600,000–800,000 people are subjected to such treatment each year. Approximately 80 percent of today's slaves on the global market are female, and up to 50 percent are under the age of 18. Most of the slaves come from countries such as Albania, Belarus, China, Romania, Russia, and Thailand, while the most frequent destinations for traffickers are in Asia, followed by the advanced industrialized states of Western Europe and North America, and a number of states in the Middle East (including Israel).

Slavers typically recruit poor people in poor countries by promising them good jobs in distant places. A recruiter will then offer a victim a generous loan – at an exorbitant interest rate – to help with travel

---

* Reprinted and adapted by permission of *Foreign Affairs*, November / December 2006. © 2006 by the Council on Foreign Relations, Inc. www.ForeignAffairs.com.

arrangements, papers, and locating a job in the new community. On arrival, the promised job never materializes, and thus the large debt – up to several thousand dollars – can never be repaid. The victim is then stripped of all travel documents, given a false identity, and forced into a job. He or she – and his or her family – are threatened with disfigurement or death should the slave try to alert the authorities or escape. Girls and women in the sex trade are also often compelled to take drugs, and the cost of these is added to their debt.

As a result of low entry costs of the modern slave trade, the business is characterized by numerous criminal gangs instead of one large mafia. These gangs are mainly from Asia, Eastern Europe, and Latin America. Besides easy profits, the slave trade offers another advantage to criminals: the risks of arrest are low and the penalties are relatively light. In the United States, for example, drug traffickers generally face much stiffer sentences than do those who traffic in humans.

Slavery is widely recognized as the most abhorrent violation of a person's liberty, and the practice runs counter to the entire modern history of human rights, suggesting that framing the issue in these terms would very likely be quite effective. However, advocates are not unified on what should be done. In both the United States and Western Europe, numerous NGOs and media outlets are concerned with this issue (*The New York Times* columnist Nicholas Kristof, for example, has often written about sex trafficking), and many celebrities (such as the actress Demi Moore) now speak out regularly against human trafficking. These groups have had some success in criminalizing human trafficking, particularly in the United States (including in individual American states). Outside the industrialized world, such nongovernmental forces play a much smaller role, and the situation for women and girls is often much worse as a result. In Thailand, for example, traders who bring in Burmese women for prostitution are rarely prosecuted. In Russia, government officials show little concern over the plight of young women trafficked into or out of their country. And in the Persian Gulf, the use of slaves remains widespread, even though it has been illegal since the 1960s.

Washington and its allies in the industrialized world have traditionally taken the position that, rather than target governments, they should focus their efforts on the demand and supply sides of the slavery problem. But Western countries and NGOs that focus on this problem disagree about what those steps should be. Many European officials, for example, argue that it would suffice to tackle the demand side of slavery by legalizing prostitution in the industrialized world, which would supposedly reduce human trafficking by curbing the demand for slaves; conversely, it is also asserted that the supply side should be addressed by promoting economic development and growth in poor countries. For their part, UN officials generally focus on the need to strengthen the 2000 protocol, for example, by educating police officers and prosecutors about its content.

The weakness of these differing solutions is evident by contrasting the positions taken in the Netherlands and Sweden. The Dutch government has explicitly stated that its legalization of sex work was meant to facilitate "action against sexual violence and abuse and human trafficking." The idea was that once brothels were permitted and regulated, the police would be better able "to pick up signs of human trafficking" and prevent it. But the Dutch strategy has not achieved much. Sex slaves have continued to enter the black market, providing their services at lower prices than those charged by prostitutes in the officially sanctioned red-light district. The slaves work in areas such as railroad stations and on those streets that are off-limits to legal prostitutes, and they attract clients who are too poor to pay official prices. The police, meanwhile, have proved no more able than in the past to stop such practices.

Interestingly, Sweden – a country usually known for its relaxed attitudes toward sexuality – has taken the opposite tack, criminalizing the buying of sex. Since 1999, when this new law was introduced, some 750 men in Sweden have been charged with seeking to purchase the services of a prostitute, a crime punishable by up to six months in jail. The Swedish government claims that this policy has greatly reduced the number of prostitutes working the country's streets, although some analysts claim that the law has merely driven Sweden's prostitutes and their clients deeper underground. Some states have alternatively focused on acts committed by their citizens while abroad. France, for example, has played a leading role in prosecuting "sex tourists," who seek pleasure in countries such as Thailand.

The differing positions of governments are mirrored by the absence of clear asks on the part of the relevant NGO community. The websites of such American-based groups as the Polaris Project and the Human Trafficking Project suggest that their focus is on educating the public about sex trafficking and calling for tougher state laws aimed at combating this trade. In Europe, however, there are efforts to draw distinctions between "prostitution" – which at least some NGOs seem to accept, or even support – and sex trafficking, which most groups seek to stop, even though there are disagreements about which policies would be most effective. Echoing this view was Noy Thrupkaew, whose 2012 *New York Times* opinion piece called the punitive Swedish-style advocacy efforts to "end-demand" a "misguided moral crusade," suggesting that:

[t]he best law-enforcement strategy to prevent trafficking into forced prostitution is not an end-demand campaign that harms current sex workers. What's needed

instead is a commitment to seriously investigate and prosecute traffickers and impose harsh punishment on those who rape and assault sex workers. (Thrupkaew 2012)

Depending on the policy ask, the costs of addressing modern slavery may vary greatly. A strategy devoted to criminalizing the sex trade and stifling demand may run into major implementation costs. While sex workers themselves are a weak political constituency, their employers have more power, if only through their ability to steer some profits toward the buying off of law enforcement officials.

In order to thrive, the slave trade requires the direct or indirect involvement of national governments, at both the source and the destination. For example, in a September 2005 memorandum to Secretary of State Condoleezza Rice, President Bush stated that the Cambodian government had "failed to address the trafficking complicity of senior law enforcement officials" in that country and that the Myanmar military was "directly involved in forced labor." Bush also singled out a number of other governments – including those of Ecuador, Kuwait, Saudi Arabia, and Venezuela – for failing to "show a serious commitment" or to devote "sufficient attention" to stopping human trafficking in their countries. Thus, efforts to shut down the slavers will be resisted, but it is unclear how expensive efforts to curtail the trade would be.

Institutionally, this area has a number of international treaties on its side. One of the UN's first acts after its establishment was to pass the Convention for the Suppression of the Trafficking in Persons, which the General Assembly approved in 1949. That convention updated international agreements from 1904 and 1910 on the "suppression of the white slave trade." Although it dealt largely with prostitution, the 1949 treaty was far more ambitious in certain respects than anything that has been proposed in more recent times. In fact, the convention's blanket condemnation of all forms of prostitution and brothels looks almost quaint by today's standards, given the number of governments (such as, most famously, that of the Netherlands) that have since legalized the sex trade.

The most authoritative modern international agreement aimed at the slave trade is the "Protocol to Prevent, Suppress, and Punish Trafficking in Persons, Especially Women and Children," which was approved by the UN General Assembly in 2000. Unlike earlier slavery treaties, the protocol does not mention prostitution; instead, it aims to serve as the "universal instrument that addresses all aspects of trafficking in persons." Also in 2000, the United States passed the ambitious Trafficking Victims Protection Act (TVPA), which was signed into law by President Bill Clinton and re-authorized and strengthened by President Bush in

2003. The TVPA, which is widely regarded as a model for other countries, establishes a more precise definition of what constitutes human trafficking, imposes stronger penalties than had previously existed, and allocates funds for compensation to the victims of human trafficking and for cooperation with foreign countries.

Since the passage of the TVPA, the United States has charged nearly 200 individuals with sex trafficking, up from only 34 during the five years before the law came into effect. Federal prosecutors have won 109 convictions in these cases, up from 20 in the preceding period. Sentences have ranged from 16 months to 23 years. The US government has also charged 59 defendants with labor trafficking (two major cases involved 24 of these individuals). These cases led to, among other things, the first-ever extradition of Mexican citizens to the United States to face labor-trafficking charges.

Most other governments, however, have not made combating the slave trade as high a priority as Washington. This includes many Western European governments, which (with a few notable exceptions, such as in Sweden and the Netherlands), have done little to stop the flow of slaves from Eastern Europe. As a result, ever-increasing numbers of young women and girls are being forced to work the streets of France, Germany, and Italy.

Although the United States has sought to cooperate with foreign governments in combating the slave trade, it has rarely punished a country for failing to act against human trafficking. It is probably no coincidence that the lists of non-compliant states include important oil producers (such as Kuwait and Saudi Arabia), key allies in Washington's war on terror (such as Uzbekistan), and great powers (such as China, India, and Russia). Under US law, the president has the authority to impose economic sanctions on states that fail to combat the slave trade by blocking foreign aid and military assistance. Unfortunately, this is rarely a useful tool, since most of the countries in question either do not receive US aid or are of such compelling importance to national security that the president is unwilling to crack down on them. The Bush administration, like its European counterparts, seemed to feel that a few slaves should not be allowed to get in the way of high politics.

That attitude may have started to change. In 2012, at the Clinton Global Initiative, President Obama made human trafficking a priority, announcing a series of measures that would punish government agencies and contractors for any involvement in the trade (Feller 2012). At the same time, more anti-trafficking movements are cohering around the policy ask of tougher penalties aimed at those engaged in the sex trade.

Drawing from our analysis of what features of a social movement are most likely to promote a market transformation, we would argue the following with respect to those who wish to advance the cause of eliminating the global traffic in women and girls: first, as noted above, focusing on a clear ask of criminalizing human trafficking (where US-based groups have probably had their greatest success in lobbying state governments); second, and related, an effort to raise the costs associated with trafficking by (a) demanding tougher sentences on those who are prosecuted for this crime, and (b) "naming and shaming" governments that continue to allow the trade to flourish (perhaps by holding demonstrations when officials from such countries visit Washington or European capitals). We are under no illusions, however, that the end of human trafficking will occur anytime soon.

Abolition of the transatlantic slave trade

How might our framework help us explain historic cases of market transformation by principled advocacy movements? One example is the Atlantic slave trade, highlighted in scholarship by Kaufmann and Pape as one of the rare exemplars of costly moral action (Kaufmann and Pape 1999). What features of the slave trade made it amenable to attack by an organized campaign that ultimately succeeded in its effort to halt the traffic? Or, put a little differently, what questions would we need to answer to be able to definitively assess the likelihood of market transformation (meaning the abolition of the Atlantic slave trade) and advocacy success?

First, we would need to know something about the structure of the market. We would want to know how many shipping companies were involved in the practice. Was the slave trade highly concentrated among a few entrepreneurs, or was it quite diffuse? In other words, how easy was it to target those who supplied shipping services? On the demand side, we do know that there were points of control that aggregated demand geographically through ports. The slave trade was one in which a handful of largely UK-based ports – first London, then Bristol, and later surpassed by Liverpool – were responsible for sending slaves between Africa and the New World (Nadelmann 1990). This concentration suggests a source of leverage, because controlling the trade through these ports could disrupt the entire practice, provided no substitute ports could be established.[12] Initially, the rules gave monopoly power to the city of

---

[12] Barrett makes the same argument with respect to controlling the fur seal trade that also was controlled through a single port in the UK (see Barrett 2003, Ch. 2).

London as the country's unique slave port. This was later contested by other ports, including Bristol and Liverpool, which wanted to profit from the slave trade themselves. Later, in response to mobilization by the abolitionist movement, the rules that shaped the buying and selling of slaves were changed to outlaw the practice altogether.

Next, we would want to know about the relevant frames. While universal campaigns might need to draw on globally resonant themes like the sanctity of life, this was an era before true transnational mobilization by advocacy movements took place (although it is true that American and British abolitionists were in regular contact). Indeed, this case is more akin to one where locally resonant frames were more important than global ones, since the Royal Navy alone could determine the Atlantic trade's fate.

Given that there was a dominant power in the world that possessed the ability to exercise unilateral control over the slave trade, there was less need for a truly universal movement for abolition. Interestingly, the "frame" used to shape the battle against slavery did not make use of the phrase "human rights" or invoke man's cruelty to his fellow man. As Kaufmann and Pape point out, abolitionists focused instead on the corrosive nature of the political corruption associated with slavery, namely, the financial hold that slavers had on British politicians, and it was this frame that helped agitate the broader public for reform.

In addition to information on market structure and framing, we need to know something of the movement's coherence to assess the likelihood of market transformation. The London Committee for the Abolition of the Slave Trade, founded in 1787, was the main vehicle for coordinating abolition groups in the country. As Kaufmann and Pape note, while abolition of slavery was the ultimate goal, advocates focused on a particular market transformation as their primary policy ask: abolition of the slave trade. The British movement came to be led by the charismatic William Wilberforce, and after more than two decades of struggle, campaigners from the Society for Effecting the Abolition of the Slave Trade successfully convinced the British Parliament to ban the trade in two pieces of legislation in 1806 and 1807. The 1807 legislation banned the imports of slaves into the West Indian colonies, forbade citizens from engaging in the slave trade, and banned foreign slavers from using British ports (Kaufmann and Pape 1999, 649).

Fourth, we need to understand the costs of this policy ask. Kaufmann and Pape suggest that the costs to the British government in the form of lost soldiers' lives and extra costs of sugar, lost exports, etc., amounted to less than 2 percent of the nation's annual income each year for sixty years (ibid., 637). Still, that is a substantial sum for a single policy action. By this metric, the abolition of the slave trade poses a hard case for us, and one where, just looking at costs, we would not have predicted a favorable outcome. It should also be noted that abolishing the trade took sixty years, well beyond the time horizon of most economic agents.

However, the slave trade had other characteristics that made it susceptible to transformation, namely, the concentration of the trade through British ports and, most important from an institutional perspective, the backing of a hegemonic power and its navy. These structural and institutional features of the traffic in humans made abolition more likely to achieve once the British state adopted this cause. The important point here is that the British government made a persistent effort at gunpoint (it took many decades to bring a halt to the trade) to change the incentives of slavers. These institutional incentives reinforced the principle that the slave trade had no place in modern society.

Still, the abolition case poses a tough test for our argument. Favoring market transformation, some aspects of the Atlantic slave trade were concentrated through the port structure in the UK. While the freedom of the individual could have been a globally resonant frame, the centrality of Britain, both to the trade itself and the pre-eminent economic position of the country more generally, made locally resonant frames more important from an advocacy standpoint. While *ex post*, we can understand how anti-corruption frames resonated, it is harder to claim that we could have predicted that such a frame would have resonated *ex ante*. Further, the biggest barrier we would have expected advocates to face was the sheer cost of the enterprise and the time it took for the campaign ultimately to succeed. Sixty years of effort, considerable lost revenue to the national treasury, and the costs of human lives lost in the struggle, make for a relatively tough case in favor of market transformation.[13]

---

[13] As one of us has argued in a previous work, where financial costs and social values are in conflict, governments will be more likely to support the moral-based claims of advocacy movements if the country's "gatekeepers" or decision-makers ultimately believe that the pursuit of those values is important. This has a structural component to it, as it depends on the number of gatekeepers and the spread of their views. Where there are a few gatekeepers with decision-making authority who share the view that values are important, a government is more likely to support the movement's position. In countries with more gatekeepers with diverse views, policy change is less likely. The British parliamentary system, with strong party discipline, is thought to have few gatekeepers (Busby 2010a; gatekeepers theory is inspired by foundational work on veto players by Tsebelis 2002).

Conclusions

These short case studies are hardly comprehensive, and we recognize that each may engender discussion and debate among subject experts. While some of the cases, like climate change and sex trafficking, are close to our substantive areas of research, our judgments and coding of the other cases are largely based on our reading of the secondary literature. We encourage scholars of these cases to critique and expand the arguments put forward here.

While we sought to ensure that the application of our argument did not on its face do violence to the historical record, the most important question is not whether our argument is factually correct in all particulars, but whether it is useful.[14] We believe that our theory of strategic moral action passes that test. The attention our argument brings to market structure, resonant frames, movement coherence, the costs of the policy ask, and stabilizing institutions individually and together provide important guides to assess the likelihood of market transformation and advocacy success in a variety of areas.

For advocates themselves, we also believe our analysis bears close examination. To some extent, our theory may be seen as a "checklist" that can guide movements as they seek to influence particular issue-areas. By asking whether industry structures are contestable, frames are compelling, policy asks are coherent and relatively low-cost, and institutions are present, traps may be avoided and strategies recalibrated. And while these variables may not cover the waterfront of all the issues that advocates face (we have, for example, paid little attention to the internal workings of social movements, which are a focal point of much of the earlier literature), we do think that our comparative analysis indicates the potential of the approach we have adopted.

Our theory of strategic moral action is useful for another reason, in that it can be viewed in sequential terms, allowing us to see where movements are placed in terms of their "life cycle." If the market structure that advocates face is difficult to contest (e.g. because of excessive fragmentation on the supply or demand sides), movements may never really gain traction. Next, in the absence of a compelling frame, advocates may have trouble generating much interest about their issue from the media or the wider public. Even with a compelling frame, unless and until movements cohere around a common ask, we would expect them to have difficulty convincing target actors to listen to them. Even where they are able to

---

[14] For a similar argument about the role of theory, see Waltz (1979).

overcome this obstacle, they may face an uphill battle to win meaningful policy changes if the costs of their "ask" are too high. Finally, in the absence of institutions that help stabilize the market around a new principle of access, the commitments that advocates have won may not endure. In the face of such difficulties, a movement may fracture and backslide to an earlier stage.

Along these lines, one piece of unfinished business that we must now confront concerns the "inter-temporal" problem of social movements, or their long-run influence and how deeply institutionalized the principles of transformation actually become in a given market. Slavery, for example, was abolished in most countries many years ago, but by some accounts it is still thriving today. With respect to HIV/AIDS, our main concern in this book, experts have been raising red flags in recent years with respect to donor exhaustion and the approaching limits of the universal access regime. Does this mean that the AIDS treatment "model" may be more limited in its applicability than we have implied, even in the global health arena? Since the social science literature often asserts that, once established, institutions are "sticky" and not prone to change without powerful exogenous shocks, it is also important from a theoretical perspective to revisit that conceptualization from the perspective of a longer time-horizon or what the French call the "longue durée." It is to those themes we now turn in our concluding chapter.

8   Conclusions: implications for research and policy

> Now what?
>
> Former New York State Governor Eliot Spitzer, reflecting on the Occupy
> Wall Street Movement (quoted in Sorkin 2012)

For its 2011 "Person of the Year," *Time Magazine* named "the protester."
In so doing, this venerable media institution celebrated the "Occupy Wall
Street Movement," launched in September of that year, alongside the Arab
Spring, which had brought down long-standing dictators in Tunisia, Egypt,
and Libya. Unlike the Arab Spring, however, the Occupy Wall Street
Movement has had few meaningful repercussions. Its vague incantation
"We are the 99 percent" was not accompanied by any robust policy plat-
form. As columnist Andrew Ross Sorkin wrote dismissively, the movement
was nothing more than "a fad" (Sorkin 2012).

Why did the Occupy Wall Street Movement fail to reform America's
banking system, much less tackle its growing level of income inequality?[1]
That question brings us back to the heart of this book, which was motivated
by our interest in why some advocacy campaigns succeed, while others
wither. In our effort to address that question, we elaborated a theory of
strategic moral action and a related set of hypotheses, which emphasize
market structure, framing, movement coherence, costs, and institutional
frameworks. We provided some preliminary "tests" of that theory beyond
the AIDS case in the previous chapter. In this concluding chapter we return
to the issue of movement success but examine it from an inter-temporal or
forward-looking perspective. That is, we seek to understand the extent to
which even "successful" advocacy movements, like the one for universal
access to AIDS treatment, become embedded as "permanent" features of
the global economic landscape, transforming markets in fundamental ways.

We begin the chapter by trying to assess the future of the AIDS
treatment regime. This discussion is not only important because of the
scale of this particular disease, but because it may provide us with

---

[1] For one analysis which emphasizes the vagueness of the Occupy movement's demands,
see Gitlin 2012.

insights into the future of global health funding and capacity-building. Unfortunately, we are not altogether sanguine about either the future prospects of the global AIDS regime or about the extension of the universal access concept to health care more generally. While there are some promising signs that advocates, governments, and industry are seeking cooperative solutions to extending access, the high costs associated with funding that effort – especially in light of the 2008 financial crisis and industrialized world economic slowdown – make it a difficult "sell," given other demands on scarce fiscal resources.

Beyond global health and from a more theoretical perspective, the AIDS case may also teach us something of value with respect to the concept of institutions and institutionalization. In the political economy literature, it is generally assumed that, once established, institutions become "sticky"; since institutions are seen as an equilibrium position, they can only be dislodged by some exogenous or external shocks. We thus have a relatively impoverished conceptualization of institutional evolution (or devolution) and change over time. In our discussion of the AIDS regime, in contrast, we try to be attentive to the *internal* contradictions and tensions, as well as the *external* forces, which could upend the institutions that now support universal access to treatment. In short, we hope our analysis will stimulate those with a more general interest in the institutions literature to advance our academic understanding of the institutional life cycle.

We then ask whether differential pricing of "essential" medicines has become a new principle of global drug access and allocation, beyond the AIDS case. If differential or subsidized pricing has indeed become the new norm for pharmaceuticals, does it represent the "leading edge" of a broader global movement that is demanding universal access to health care? Given the growing role of pharmaceutical expenditures in the health care sector, the link between the two is hardly far-fetched.

After reflecting on these questions, we then provide some thoughts on future research. Just as this book draws on several disciplines, so we call for more research that uses a variety of tools and methods in approaching the questions that we have raised but only partly answered. In particular, we hope to see the creation of more publicly available data sets that make it easier for scholars to conduct quantitative analysis. While we do not view quantitative research as the "be all and end all" of scholarship, we do believe that more work along these lines could enable all those interested in the role of advocacy in the global economy – including advocates themselves – to gain a deeper appreciation of movement success factors. This type of analysis, of course, should continue to be complemented by careful case study research.

Whither the AIDS regime?

As we pointed out in the preceding chapter, the AIDS treatment regime faces a number of severe challenges as it looks beyond the "success" it has enjoyed to date. That success, however, should not be minimized. Mead Over of the Center for Global Development, for example, has estimated that the "percentage of those needing and receiving treatment increased from less than 5 percent in 2003 to about 36 percent in 2009" (Over 2011, 81). By 2011, UNAIDS provided an even higher number, stating that 54 percent of those sick enough under 2010 guidelines to warrant treatment were receiving it, an incredible statistic given the relatively short history of the universal access regime (UNAIDS 2012a).[2] Global spending on AIDS rose from $300 million in 1999 to over $10 billion per annum by 2009 (Bonnel *et al.* 2009, 161). This record of gains led advocates to start talking about an "AIDS-free generation" during the 2012 International AIDS Society conference, held in Washington DC.

We note, of course, that 54 percent is a far cry from 100 percent. In this sense, the "universal access" to treatment campaign remains aspirational rather than fully realized. One does not hear about HIV/AIDS that it is now time to fold up that proverbial tent and move on to other diseases. The gap between what has been achieved and what is needed does, however, pose some stark questions. Most grimly, one might wonder whether there will be adequate funds available to maintain the current 54 percent – *the current 8 million people* – on ARV treatment for the rest of their lives, much less to expand that number. Related, what are the chances for a technological breakthrough, like a vaccine, that could greatly reduce the future costs of this disease burden?

With respect to the durability of the current regime, experts are not sanguine. Despite all the recent talk about an AIDS-free generation and the end of the AIDS pandemic, Laurie Garrett strikes a more pessimistic tone, flagging a $7 billion gap between what is being spent on AIDS and what experts think is needed:

[L]et's be clear: The end of HIV is not in sight. Even if that $7 billion and political commitment can be conjured, and the best-available treatment and prevention tools are implemented, the world will still witness some 1 million new infections every year, well into the 2020s. (Garrett 2012b)

---

[2] Until 2010, WHO treatment guidelines recommended that people get on treatment when the CD4 count dropped below 200. In 2010, the guidelines were revised to 350, meaning that people should get on treatment earlier, before their CD4 count drops still further.

For his part, economist Rene Bonnel, in a 2009 World Bank study, concludes "that the current 'business' model is unsustainable" for two reasons (Bonnel *et al.* 2009, 160). First, funding levels are simply failing to keep pace with rising financial demands (again, think of the gap between how many are receiving treatment today and the objective of universal access, a target that keeps shifting as more cases of AIDS develop). Second, the funding that is available is, in Bonnel's words, "fragmented," meaning that various donors, both public and private, are spending scarce funds in a variety of different ways, not all of which are complementary. Mark Dybul, Peter Piot, and Julio Frenk provide support for this position:

> As an example, within the UN system alone, and in spite of the existence of UNAIDS, eleven organizations are engaged in HIV/AIDS; the Global Fund provides 24 percent of external funding and the U.S. government 45 percent. Other bilateral institutions are in the game, as are large contributors like the Bill and Melinda Gates Foundation. (Dybul, Piot, and Frenk 2012)

Bonnel argues that greater coordination among these donors is essential if the international community is to maintain people on treatment, much less expand their numbers.

Over is similarly pessimistic about the robustness of the current regime, but for some additional reasons beyond the funding picture. Indeed, he is pessimistic even if current funding levels for AIDS treatment are maintained, which, of course, is a big "if." Regarding present funding levels, Over calls AIDS treatment the first global "entitlement" program, meaning that once people are being funded for treatment, it becomes extremely difficult to drop them from the rolls. Will voters in the United States and other industrialized countries continue to support this entitlement program as its costs rise over time? And those costs will most certainly rise, short of a technological breakthrough. Over estimates that the price tag associated with a program approaching universal access would be in the order of $50 billion per annum in 2009 dollars (Over 2011, 100).

But then Over goes on to ask, suppose they *do* continue to fund access to treatment programs? Is that all to the good? He suggests that the consequences may not be totally benign, because it is likely that financing treatment means less money for other AIDS programs like prevention, much less for other foreign assistance programs, like funding for education and improving health systems, that can be viewed as indirect prevention schemes. Over's analysis indicates that we might be "damned if we do and damned if we don't." As a consequence, he lays out a comprehensive program for "achieving an AIDS transition" which allocates funds between treatment and prevention in such a way as to reduce the number of new infections (we note that the WHO and UNAIDS have united around a similar "Treatment 2.0 Program" with the objective of getting 15 million people on treatment by 2015). The relative complexity of Over's program and Treatment 2.0, however, pose the question of political and economic feasibility. How likely is it that the different actors who would have to be involved in such a program can coordinate around the Over transition or the UN proposal? Again, we are reminded of Bonnel's concern about donor fragmentation, or donors "doing their own thing," rather than rallying around a common program and allocating financial and programmatic responsibilities based on comparative advantage.

From our perspective, the rising costs associated with the AIDS treatment regime alone are worrisome. As we hypothesized in Chapter 1, movements succeed in part by lowering the costs associated with achieving a market transformation. In the AIDS case, it was the promise of "cheap" ARVs in the context of low-cost implementation strategies (like the one pioneered by Paul Farmer and Partners in Health in Haiti) that made the universal access to treatment regime appear as if it could be realized. In contrast, climate change advocates have never convinced relevant stakeholders (including incumbent firms) that the costs of reducing greenhouse gases could be greatly reduced; to them, it is an expensive proposition in terms of lost profits and adaptation costs.

With the emphasis on getting more and more people on treatment, a well-known but under-reported problem also persists: the so-called "loss to follow-up." By some accounts, treatment programs have trouble locating between 15 and 40 percent of their patients from one-to-three years after initially getting them on treatment (Miller et al. 2010; Tuller 2010; Alamo et al. 2012; we note that some studies even put the number of those lost to follow-up at a higher percentage). These patients may have moved, stopped treatment altogether, changed providers, or died. What this finding means is unclear, but it suggests that the statistic of 8 million people on treatment may be misleading, as this number may actually reflect the number of people who have ever started treatment. To be sure, many lives have been extended with ARVs, but we may not have an accurate portrait of the true numbers of people who are alive today and remain on treatment. While fewer people on treatment lowers the long-run costs associated with the initiative, it also means that the effort has been less successful than advertised, and it raises potentially terrifying questions about disease resistance. Should this loss to follow-up problem persist and become more widely known, it could undercut the rationale and political support for treatment provision.

While fears of drug-resistant strains of HIV have not proven as severe as many analysts initially feared, we remain concerned by the possibility of a "new wave" of HIV/AIDS that could be even more difficult to treat than the current strains. In order to be effective, PWAs must maintain their commitment to treatment for their entire lives. If they stop treatment and then have unprotected sex, HIV could continue its spread in a much more virulent form, since more people could find the current treatment regime ineffective. This means that new regimens must be constantly introduced, at greater and greater cost. For these reasons, we believe that adherence to treatment is a crucial area for further study.

Despite these challenges, new innovations in treatment coupled with partnerships between branded and generic firms may extend developing country access to second- and third-line technologies in the near future. In August 2012, for example, the US FDA approved the so-called Quad, Gilead's first four-drug ARV formula that consisted of two drugs, emtricitabine and tenofovir, that already form part of existing multi-drug combinations (namely, Atripla, Complera, and Truvada) and two other new drugs, elvitegravir and cobicistat (elvitegravir is part of a new type of drugs called integrase inhibitors that block production of an enzyme the virus uses to insert its DNA into a host cell, and cobicistat is a drug that helps the body metabolize elvitegravir). The Quad was set to retail at $28,500 per patient in the United States, drawing negative attention from US AIDS activists, even as the drug promised fewer side-effects than some other drugs (Pollack 2012). At the same time, Gilead prepared the way for swifter rollout of the drug in developing countries through a voluntary licensing agreement with Indian generic companies.

As former Global Fund Executive Director Richard Feachem told us, this decision was potentially momentous. With Gilead working with Aurobindo, Matrix, Ranbaxy, and other companies through voluntary licensing agreements, their fast-track applications to the FDA are likely to be approved, in his words, "thick and fast." He noted that Atripla, Gilead's triple-drug combination, was available in developing countries like Malawi, twenty-four months after it was available in San Francisco. In the past, developing countries tended to lag behind the industrialized world by ten-to-fifteen years in access to the latest drugs. With the Quad, the hope is that the time from US availability to developing countries will be in the order of 18 months. The important point to note is that the groundwork for technology transfer to India started months before the Quad received FDA approval for the US market (Feachem 2012).

With all this emphasis on access to treatment and delivering low-cost ARVs, there are worries that a focus on making markets for particular treatment technologies misses the mark with respect to the general challenge of global health and the particular one of HIV/AIDS. Writing about UNITAID, Victoria Fan and Rachel Silverman posed the question, "More provocatively: has UNITAID's approach of using 'innovation [to] make markets work for the neediest' devolved into a hammer in search of an innovative, market-based nail?" They suggested that perhaps UNITAID's emphasis on "value for money" potentially "conflates strategy with mission" by looking for impacts on markets for medicines rather than how to make the largest contribution to improvements in human health (Fan and Silverman 2012). Timberg and Halperin raise similar issues about the current AIDS regime in their recent book, *Tinderbox*, expressing concern that the emphasis on technological breakthroughs like pharmaceutical treatments and vaccines has displaced the promise of indigenously developed prevention strategies (Timberg and Halperin 2012; for a similar perspective, see Epstein 2007).

Moreover, with policy-makers focused on demonstrable and measurable results, a focus on treatment emphasized the collection of a single metric – the number of people on treatment – which has glossed over more difficult-to-measure issues like their long-run survival, the loss to follow-up, and the overall quality of care. We can see these pressures to simplify and quantify in this anecdote Mark Dybul told about a conversation with White House chief of staff Josh Bolten in the early days of PEPFAR:

One of the things I remember is that Josh would ask the most important questions. There was one meeting, six months into PEPFAR, and he asked, "What is the single most important marker in PEPFAR?" I said, well, we have prevention, care and treatment, and the reduction in infections is most important. And Josh said, "No, what is the most important marker." I said it is the number of people on treatment because we can show success rapidly. Josh asked, "How many are on treatment?" I said 25,000 in the first six months. He said, "That's not very much." (Donnelly 2011)

Thus, the number of people on treatment became and remains the headline goal for both advocates and policy-makers, even as the number of new infections makes it clear that a treatment only, or at least treatment-centric agenda, would fail, as the mass of new infections swelled the ranks of PWAs ultimately in need of treatment. The point here is that a focus on market interventions to bring down the price of AIDS drugs and get more people on treatment potentially misses the wider mark of needing to address other aspects of the problem, like prevention, that may or may not be amenable to market-based solutions.

Advocates are aware of the challenge, and scientific discoveries related to treatment have bolstered the view that early treatment can disrupt the chain of transmission of the virus (Brown 2011; Cohen *et al.* 2011). Indeed, the "treatment as prevention" agenda that emerged in 2011 and

2012 has become part of the new push for an "AIDS-free generation," as celebrated at the 2012 International AIDS conference in Washington DC (Knox 2012; Sun 2012). On the basis of these findings, the WHO revised its treatment guidelines, suggesting that treatment should be available to the partner with HIV in so-called "serodiscordant couples," whatever their CD4 count (WHO 2012d). Under these guidelines, an additional 4 million people should have access to treatment, meaning that only 42 percent of those who are eligible for treatment actually had access (UNAIDS 2012a, 126).

Of course, such programs would necessarily entail greater short-run costs of extending treatment to far more people, even if the long-run costs are greatly reduced (Busby 2009; Granich *et al.* 2009). That agenda would require a transformation in how the disease is currently dealt with. The current system practices a sort of triage, putting people on treatment when they are already showing some signs of illness, when their CD4 counts have already dropped to a level below 350. Catching people early in their infections and getting them on treatment immediately would require more robust universal testing programs, possibly even mandatory ones.

At the same time, funding would have to be found to treat both the people who already show signs of illness, as well as those who are otherwise asymptomatic but are HIV+. Beyond the logistical challenges associated with this enterprise, the problem is funding. Identifying additional resources in an era of constrained foreign assistance budgets has become a central challenge. Affected nations are increasingly picking up the tab for funding their own treatment programs. For example, South Africa, the country with the largest number of PWAs, dramatically increased spending on HIV/AIDS under the leadership of Jacob Zuma, and by 2011 had assumed more than 80 percent of the costs of its treatment program (UNAIDS 2012b). However, treatment as prevention has to be part of a wider set of prevention strategies that includes a greater reliance on male circumcision and programs to encourage fewer sexual partners. Treatment alone will not be sufficient, and additional donor resources will be required for this expanded agenda to succeed. Where such funds would come from, for example on a proposed financial transactions or "Tobin" tax, remains to be seen as of this writing (these issues are discussed in more detail in Busby 2012; 2012a).

Complicating the picture still further are other developments in the global health arena, including the renewed push for strengthening of national health systems versus vertical, disease-specific interventions. One persistent criticism of the AIDS response was that it helped create separate facilities and programs for AIDS to the detriment of wider health systems capacity. Put starkly, if you had a broken leg or faced some other illness, you might not get access to services or treatment (Garrett 2007). To be sure, some practitioners like Paul Farmer disputed the assertion that AIDS funding necessarily came at the expense of wider health systems. Some evidence suggested that the facilities and experience associated with HIV/AIDS created positive spillovers for other areas (Farmer et al. 2007).

Nonetheless, siloed or vertical disease-specific interventions in the 2000s proliferated, creating a panoply of funding sources, programs, and reporting requirements, leading to a complex uncoordinated health space of multilateral donors, NGOs, private providers, among others (Fidler 2007; 2010). Despite efforts to simplify programming and coordinate, such as the "Three Ones" initiative among African countries, the United States, UK, and UNAIDS,[3] and the so-called H8 meeting of top health organizations,[4] the health arena has become too inefficient and duplicative in Dybul, Piot, and Frenk's view. They make a plea for a health systems-centric approach that would add coherence to the diverse landscape of health systems: "[W]e believe it is likely that an integrated approach focused on the health of a person and community is more cost-effective than a silo approach focused on a specific disease or health threat" (Dybul, Piot, and Frenk 2012). They call for greater coordination of programming and integration of external funding streams. What this means in practice, however, remains unclear.

Alongside this renewed questioning of vertical disease interventions, we see some turmoil surrounding the leading institution behind such interventions, namely, the Global Fund. In 2011, for example, the Global Fund experienced a severe reputational crisis among its donors, who discovered a relatively small amount of fraud in its programming – some $34 million out of a $20 billion portfolio. The revelation of this problem triggered a more vigorous internal investigation of management, leading to a report that suggested broader systemic problems with the Fund's operations (Barclay 2011). As a consequence, then Executive Director Michel Kazatchine was forced to share power with a general manager, leading Kazatchine to resign in January 2012 (McNeil Jr. 2012a).

The upheaval at the Fund inevitably led to some handwringing about its future. While the Fund's own reputational fortunes rebounded, its

---

[3] UNAIDS 2004.
[4] The H-8 is an informal group of eight organizations (GAVI, Bill & Melinda Gates Foundation, the Global Fund, UNAIDS, UNICEF, WHO, World Bank, and UN Population Fund) that have met annually to discuss priorities in the health arena (Gorman 2008; Doughton 2009).

future remained in flux as a new director was selected at the end of 2012.[5] Former PEPFAR director Mark Dybul was tapped by the Board to lead the Global Fund through this transition (Busby 2012; McNeil Jr. 2012b). In this context of organizational change and renewed budgetary pressures, especially since the financial crisis of 2008, pursuit of a new approach to health in developing countries will almost certainly have major implications for AIDS treatment.

As for the specific threat posed by HIV/AIDS, technological break-throughs remain possible that could dramatically alter its future course and those of the institutions that surround it. Yet over the past decade or more, the headlines have been full of promising approaches, from vaccines to scores of prevention techniques. How one allocates funds between current treatment and future technology is, of course, an issue of major significance. That issue also points to the question of where the incentives are pointing for the actors in the AIDS space. Are pharmaceutical firms motivated to pursue an AIDS vaccine, or are they focusing on new treatments? Indeed, are they still motivated to pursue new drugs in this space when they are likely to have no choice but to "voluntarily" license their IP to generics manufacturers, donate it, or price it at something close to marginal cost?

These questions lead us to ask about the future access to essential medicines more generally. Is there a new global principle of how such drugs ought to be sold around the world? Have essential medicines been transformed into merit goods, which everyone should have access to, no matter where they live or what they earn? If so, what are the implications of this norm for access to health more generally?

New norms for global health

Writing of the AIDS treatment regime, political scientist Jeremy Youde has suggested that "[t]he emergence of universal ARV access enriches our understanding of how and why the international community embraces certain norms" (Youde 2008, 436). Comparing AIDS treatment to an earlier, failed attempt at fostering a global norm on universal access to primary health care (the so-called Alma-Ata or "Health for All" Declaration of 1978), Youde finds three factors that explain much of the difference in the two cases: *first*, he credits AIDS advocates with political and economic savvy, crafting a feasible roll-out strategy that appealed to

---

[5] As difficult as the Fund's position was, the WHO's financial position was perhaps even worse in the wake of the financial crisis, with its $5.4 billion 2006–7 biennial budget slashed by more than $1.5 billion by 2012–13 (Garrett 2012a).

different constituencies. *Second*, timing: the Alma-Ata Declaration was announced in the midst of the Cold War, when trans-national and global cooperation was more difficult to pursue, while AIDS programs grew during a time when the global economy was relatively open and strong (and when technology like the internet facilitated communication between AIDS advocates). *Third*, successful framing of ARV treatment brought out the life-or-death nature of access to these medicines and the unfairness of forcing people (mainly in the developing world) to accept a preventable death sentence because of an inability to pay for medication. While we have not emphasized the specific timing dimension so much in this book, we find that much we have written here is in agreement with his analysis.

While few would disagree that a norm regarding access to AIDS treatment has clearly emerged in the international system over the past decade, what are the implications for "essential medicines" more generally? Should we expect many if not most drugs on countries' formulary lists to be made available at differential prices, meaning high prices for industrialized world consumers and low prices for developing nation consumers? Will drugs for cancer and diabetes be allocated in the future like drugs for AIDS today?

These questions are especially pertinent, given that pharmaceutical companies had originally hoped to "ring-fence" differential pricing for antiretrovirals and did not view AIDS as a precedent for how the industry would respond to developing world disease burdens and drug markets more generally (Devereaux 2004, 14). For the pharmaceutical companies, differential pricing caused at least two long-run concerns: first, "reference pricing" of drugs, and second, "parallel imports." Reference pricing referred to the fear that industrialized countries' health systems would use developing world drug prices as their reference point, putting pressures on the pharmaceutical firms to reduce what they charged wealthy consumers, thus making it difficult to recoup their investments. Parallel imports meant that countries that acquired drugs cheaply, as in the developing world, might resell them to richer nations at a profit. For big pharma, putting a lid on these potential challenges was absolutely essential to making the AIDS treatment regime work. Again, one way to make that happen was to frame that regime as an exception rather than the rule when it came to drug access.

At the same time, they also recognized that developing countries' health ministries would face pressures to bring in cheap generic substitutes or engage in compulsory licensing (with likely encouragement from development-related advocacy campaigns) for one drug after the other, especially if the branded firms did not respond to their health needs.

As Merck's then Chairman Raymond Gilmartin said in 2001, "If we don't solve the drug access problem, then our intellectual property is at risk" (cited in Devereaux 2004, 14). The pricing of drugs for the developing world, therefore, became a major business policy concern, even if some of these markets remained small in global terms.

At first glance at least, there are some promising signs that the drug companies are trying to institutionalize the differential pricing regime across their portfolio of medications, suggesting that cross-subsidization from rich to poor is really working at the global level. Examine, for example, the following statement from GSK regarding its pricing policies:

Pricing is one factor that impacts access to medicines and vaccines. We are adopting a range of innovative pricing models that reflect our commitment to work with governments and other stakeholders to deliver our medicines and vaccines to as many of the people who need them as possible ... Being flexible in our pricing can help to build our business in emerging markets by increasing the overall volume of products we sell. However, our ability to offer not-for-profit or highly preferential prices in the world's poorest countries is only sustainable if we can continue to make an adequate return on our medicines and vaccines in better-off markets ... We seek to price medicines fairly in these countries and at a level that reflects their value to patients and payers. (GSK 2011, 13)

This assertion of an explicit pricing policy that subsidizes developing world consumption through profits from industrialized world consumers certainly sounds like the basis for a new norm of universal drug access. In October 2012, GSK, after having been fined $3 billion three months earlier for safety issues, went a step further and pledged to make the results of its clinical trials available to other researchers as well as its library of tuberculosis-related medicines (following a similar move for malaria drugs in 2009) (Reuters 2012b).

Yet if this norm rests on a "bargain" in which property rights are protected in return for preferential pricing, it may be a fragile one, as actions by firms and governments make plain. On the corporate side, having "lost" the TRIPS battle over public health – to the extent that developing country claims that the health needs of their people trumped the property rights of the firms – the pharmaceutical corporations turned their attention from the multilateral setting of the WTO to the bilateral and regional settings of inter-governmental "free trade agreements" (FTAs). While the United States and EU have proved willing to promote the cause of "TRIPS-plus" in these bilateral agreements, they have also caused substantial controversy within the developing world, and legal challenges to pharmaceutical patents, particularly in India, suggest that the rules in this arena remain fluid and open to interpretation.

These "TRIPS-plus" provisions or protections of pharmaceutical property rights are generally stronger than those found in the WTO accord. As noted above, the United States has signed such agreements over the past decade with Jordan, Singapore, Chile, Central America, the Dominican Republic, Australia, Morocco and Bahrain. The EU and Switzerland have similarly focused on FTAs featuring TRIPS-plus provisions in the 2000s (for a review, see Morin 2006). The features of such agreements include "extending the term of a patent longer than the twenty-year minimum or introducing provisions that limit the use of compulsory licenses or that restrict generic competition." Among the most contested of these provisions is so-called "data exclusivity." This allows pharmaceutical companies to maintain exclusive rights over, for example, the results of clinical trials for some period of time, perhaps five to ten years (on one advocacy group's perspective on TRIPS-plus, that of MSF (see MSF 2011)).

What does TRIPS-plus mean in practice? Not surprisingly, there is debate surrounding that question. Former USTR Mickey Kantor, for example, admits that while some FTAs contain *additional* IP protections beyond those seen in TRIPS, he argues from a *legal standpoint* that "characterizing these provisions as TRIPS-plus is misleading ... because these provisions are, in fact, fully compliant with the framework established by TRIPS" (Kantor 2005). From a medical perspective, however, groups like MSF view TRIPS-plus as a way of limiting generic competition (since generics manufacturers would have to replicate clinical trial results in order to secure approval for their drugs) and the conditions under which compulsory licensing can take place. In 2012, MSF and other groups remained concerned that pending regional and bilateral agreements such as the Trans-Pacific Partnership and a proposed EU–India agreement would further limit the abilities of generic drug firms from developing countries to produce low-cost medications (Baker 2012; Boseley 2012).

Debates over TRIPS-plus provisions have already spilled into courtrooms in the developing world, most prominently in India. In September 2012, for example, an Indian appellate board rejected a demand by Bayer to prevent the issuance of a compulsory license for one of its drugs used for liver and kidney cancer treatment (Chatterjee 2012). Several other cases are now being heard in Indian patent courts pitting multinational firms against local generics producers.

Beyond the ongoing legal skirmishes over TRIPS provisions, there are other reasons why pricing offers like that of GSK may, in fact, be of limited consequence. *First*, unlike the early 1990s, when the great success of the emerging and frontier markets was still a glimmer in the eye, these economies are now world-beaters in terms of economic development and growth. Giving away drugs in the world's fastest-growing economies may not seem like a sensible or low-cost proposition to most pharmaceutical executives. *Second*, as the cost of health care rises in the industrialized world, the possibility of "blow-back" or reference pricing from low-priced drugs in developing countries may prove irresistible, as GSK implies in its access statement. It is one thing for AIDS drugs to be distributed globally at low cost; it's another for cancer drugs, which in the more common cases afflict very large numbers of individuals around the world. *Third*, even with differential pricing the cost of most drugs will remain out of reach for developing world consumers, suggesting that some PEPFAR or Global Fund-like mechanism would ultimately be needed for a much wider range of diseases, including such industrialized world afflictions like cancer and diabetes. The outlook for such a broader fund, however, seems bleak. *Finally*, to the extent that a "cosmopolitan" sensibility is spreading globally to the detriment of a "statist" one, meaning a sensibility which takes the individual as the unit of analysis rather than the state, even when it comes to the world economy, firms among other agents may increasingly seek health care regimes in which individuals pay according to their incomes, rather than according to the country they live in (thus forcing wealthy people who live in poor countries to pay full freight for their medications). This kind of screening is, of course, quite expensive at present, but the mobilization of new technology in this direction could allow health ministries and pharmaceutical manufacturers to achieve differential pricing at a much more fine-grained level than that of average per-capita incomes at the national level. In fact, at least some branded pharmaceutical firms now have "drug access teams" that work on developing patient targeting along income lines (Interview with pharmaceutical executive who works on drug access issues 2012).

In the realm of HIV/AIDS, both firms and advocates continue to wrestle with the possibilities and problems associated with this emergent access norm. Even as the prices of first-line therapies were driven about as low as they possibly could, concerns remained about access to drugs for those who need second-line and third-line therapies. Here, there are contradictory forces at work. On the one hand, some branded pharmaceutical companies like Gilead have joined the Medicines Patent Pool (MPP), a project that started under the auspices of UNITAID in 2009, to share IP and/or have signed voluntary licensing agreements with Indian generic firms to produce low-cost versions of their drugs for developing country markets, as noted in the previous section (Hirschler 2011; McNeil Jr. 2011; Gilead 2012). On the other hand, other companies like Abbott and BMS have pursued exclusive patent rights for their ARVs in India. The Indian patent office rejected the patent applications from Abbott (for Kaletra) and from BMS (atazanavir) on the grounds of insufficient innovation (Mukherjee 2011). In this context, we note that Kaletra was Abbott's second-best seller in 2009, generating $1.37 billion for the company, suggesting that the company is not yet prepared to give up those profits (Boseley 2011).

The ongoing contestation by branded firms of India's IPR rules and the continued pursuit by industrialized countries of TRIPS-plus type agreements raise difficult questions about the appropriate strategy that advocates of expanded drug access should develop going forward. As we previously discussed, in the early years of the global treatment advocacy movement, campaigners from Health GAP, MSF, TAC, and CPTech often used strategies of protest and contestation to raise the costs for incumbent firms and politicians who failed to support that goal or otherwise aggressively pursued protection of branded pharmaceuticals patent rights. Given that advocacy movements frequently have difficulty sustaining their mobilization as well as media and public interest for long periods of time (Downs 1972), campaigners often gradually pursue strategies of collaboration that move them from outsiders at the gates of official authority to insiders, potentially creating tensions within the movement between radicals and more moderate elements. This is the story at the heart of ACT UP's fragmentation in the early 1990s as some activists reached an accommodation with such US government agencies as NIH and CDC on strategies to develop clinical trials for new AIDS drugs (these struggles are documented in *How to Survive a Plague*, as well as in the ACT UP archive of interviews with leading activists (Gould 2009; France 2012)).

From a firm-level perspective, however, constant battles with advocates over access to their products could also prove costly from both a reputational and even financial standpoint, to the extent lawsuits over patent rights and shareholder activism are involved. Both advocates and firms in the global health space might therefore benefit from a "truce" of sorts and an effort to find common ground on drug access. This type of cooperative logic, for example, has informed the efforts to create certification schemes for forest products, apparel, and other areas (Bartley 2007). Indeed, as we have suggested, there are some examples of such logic now at work in the medical field as well.

The MPP, for example, represents in some respects a collaborative effort to enlist the support of incumbent firms, competitors, government labs, international organizations, as well as activists in a new model of drug development. Indeed, the first head of the patent pool was none other than Ellen 't Hoen, the former MSF campaigner who then went "inside" to UNITAID. As discussed in Chapter 4, some of the same kinds of cleavages between advocates have emerged with respect to the patent pool.

The back and forth between advocates on whether or not to support the patent pool is quite intriguing from a strategic viewpoint. At their core, the issue that divides the advocacy community comes down to whether or not the compromises made to get Gilead to sign on to the agreements to share their intellectual property are worth it. Jamie Love, for example, who was among the first to advance the linkage between pharmaceutical patents and human lives, ironically defended the Gilead agreement with the MPP against even more radical detractors, such as the New York based group I-MAK, an organization supported by activists from ACT UP Paris and the International Treatment Preparedness Coalition (ITPC) (ITPC 2011).

While Love tangled with Gilead as recently as 2007 over its voluntary license before the US Federal Trade Commission, on the MPP licensing agreement with Gilead, he wrote:

In theory, the licenses could have been better, and indeed, Gilead may agree to further amendments – for example, to allow products from some countries outside of India. However, the sweeping changes in the licenses that are set out the petition, while desirable, were not about to happen, and I think, won't happen, without something more substantial changing the negotiation. People can set the bar higher – but setting the bar too high means no licenses at this point. (Love 2011)

In this context, it is difficult to know how Gilead's leadership regarded the petition efforts to cancel the patent pool agreement. We note that some companies like Johnson & Johnson, after being invited by the patent pool to join discussions, publicly declined to do so (New 2012). As the firm-level literature on boycotts suggests, companies that have an interest in sustaining a good international reputation are more likely to be targeted for action. Thus, while Johnson and Johnson might be the target of advocacy pressure in the short-run, they, like Exxon Mobil on climate policy, may be able to shoulder bad press if they just ignore it and focus instead on other issues which it believes have greater resonance with the public.

What all this suggests is that while a new norm for global health provision, based around differential pricing and greater access to medical breakthroughs, may be under development, it is far from being institutionalized; and some advocates would view TRIPS-plus as a definite step backwards in terms of such a norm. We should also emphasize that even if the international community backed such a norm more vigorously, it would still have to be implemented at the national level by willing governments.

At this level, the policies of at least some governments would seem to be contrary to the goal of more broad-based access to essential medicines. Tariff policy in many countries, for example, leads to high prices on imported medicines, which is not surprising if we assume that governments consider these products to have relatively inelastic demand curves. A study from the American Enterprise Institute, for example:

> finds a negative association between access to essential medicines, as measured by the United Nations, and the degree to which countries inflate the price of medicines. If the relationship is as causal as we suspect, this means that for countries with high tariff rates such as Nigeria (20 percent), Uganda (10 percent), Kenya (10 percent), Tanzania (10 percent), Congo (8.8 percent), and Zimbabwe (7.5 percent), many tens of millions more people could afford access to valuable medicines if all tariffs were removed. (Bate and Tren 2006)

What are the implications of the essential medicines "debate" for global health more generally? Our analysis leads us to some skepticism that a movement today is in any better position to advance such a goal than it was at the time of the 1978 "Health For All" declaration. Such an effort would likely confront most of the problems that ultimately trip up advocacy movements, including incoherence, high costs, and an absence of credible institutions. While a "health for all" norm provides a compelling frame, it also hides the strategy that would put this into effect. Would such a norm emphasize maternal mortality and health care for infants and children, or would it focus on deadly, non-communicable diseases? It is in part because the advancement of such a broad-based health norm is so difficult to achieve in practice that advocates may continue to focus their energies on the pharmaceutical firms and the "essential medicines" they provide as a "second-best" approach to improving global public health.

Market transformations and social movements: thoughts on further research

As we noted in Chapter 1, the role of social movements in influencing corporate strategy has drawn increasing attention from the academic world. That literature has begun to have the hallmarks of a meaningful research program, with important, policy-relevant questions being framed in terms of testable hypotheses that make use of various datasets.

We hope that our book has contributed to such an evolving research project, by elaborating a theory of strategic moral action that takes into account the role of industry structure, frames, policy coherence, costs, and institutions, in shaping the conditions underlying movement success. Our approach may also be valuable to scholars and practitioners alike as they use the sequential logic of strategic moral action to see where movements are in their "life cycle" and their likelihood of success.

Still, there is much work to be done. We are the first to admit that this book, for example, could have benefited greatly from some of the datasets that scholars have already developed, so that we could have engaged in quantitative analysis of our theory and its related hypotheses. Though a few datasets related to anti-corporate social movements have been developed in recent years, they have not yet been placed in the public domain by their authors. Beyond making the existing data available, most of which focus on the United States, the construction of new datasets on transnational social movements and their impacts remains a major task. For example, while some scholars have examined the effects of social movements on US stock prices, this type of work could be extended to other global markets as well.

Beyond data gathering, there are many other tasks that await ambitious researchers in the fields of "contentious" and "private" politics. First, with few exceptions, scholars have focused on *firm-level* rather than *industry-level* characteristics that make targets amenable to advocacy attack. Thus, the research to date has emphasized the role of leading firms and prominent brands in anti-corporate campaigns, the idea being that these firms have the most goodwill to lose (along with the most available resources to meet advocacy demands) and are therefore most likely to negotiate over advocacy grievances. Research on which industries are most likely to be on the receiving end of a campaign, however, is much less well developed. Are heavily regulated industries, for instance, more or less likely to be targeted by advocates? Are concentrated industries more likely to be targeted than competitive industries? How do product characteristics influence which industries will be targeted?

Second, and related, we still know very little about the conditions under which advocacy campaigns succeed. Obviously, we have advanced some hypotheses in this book and provided several comparative cases, but additional qualitative and quantitative research here is essential. Further, more refined definitions of success are a crucial accompaniment to this exercise, especially taking into account the inter-temporal dimension. We have noted, for example, that success at time t0 may appear as a failure at time t1.

Third, ever since the introduction of David Baron's pioneering work on corporate social responsibility, scholars have drawn a distinction between advocates' pursuit of "private politics" that focuses on firms and "contentious politics" that focuses on government policy. Underlying this division is a view that transnational social movements face high costs at the international level, especially if their objective is to change the policies of many different governments around the world. A much lower-cost strategy is to target multinational firms, which can change their own global policies – and perhaps those of an entire industry – at the stroke of a chief executive's pen. But it is clear that advocacy movements deploy both private and contentious politics, and more research is needed on that mix. What is the "optimal" campaign strategy, meaning how are scarce resources allocated to public and private sector targets? From a normative perspective, one might ask, how *should* scarce resources best be allocated? How do firm and industry level characteristics influence the split between public and private politics? Very little work to date has addressed these important questions.

Fourth, and from a more general political economy perspective, one issue that intrigues us concerns the conceptualization of advocacy movements. Are advocates an "interest group" like any other, or do they act more like "social planners" who promote the general welfare? As we noted in the introduction to this book, there is at least an implicit inference in much of the relevant literature that advocacy movements are "good" or morally superior to other organized groupings. Indeed, the very names used to describe what advocates do, like "moral action," suggest such ethical superiority. Related, we have suggested that advocates may, at least incidentally, serve to make markets more contestable by changing the terms of entry for potential competitors. That, of course, is not a morally superior act, but rather, one that is welfare-enhancing. Again, the question of how best to conceptualize advocates and their social role is one that deserves further analysis. This work is also important from a modeling perspective, so that the "objective function" of advocates is most accurately depicted.

On a related note, one important question for analysts of advocacy movements to ponder is the right balance between "outsider" protest strategies versus "insider" efforts, and indeed this very debate helped pull apart the US-based AIDS movement ACT UP. In some sense, this is the same kind of challenge the civil rights activist Bayard Rustin wrote about in his 1964 essay, "From Protest to Politics." Rustin wrote of the challenge activists have as their movements mature: "But the difference between expediency and morality in politics is the difference between selling out a principle and making smaller concessions to win larger ones. The leader who shrinks from this task reveals not his purity but his lack of political sense" (Rustin 1964).

Along these lines, the social movements literature has long popularized the notion of the "radical flank effect" (Haines 1995; McAdam,

McCarthy, and Zald 1996, 14). In some cases, the efforts by radicals produce positive results, by bringing attention to the issue, by making the moderates look more reasonable, or by creating crises that enable moderates to successfully press their demands. However, as Haines notes, the radical flank effects are not always positive. Their actions can de-legitimate the movement through the media and the wider public, endanger access to decision-makers and funding, and possibly trigger a repressive backlash against the movement (Haines 1995).

While we are convinced that advocates need to be united in their strategic direction, we are less convinced that they need to agree on a common set of tactics, at least in the movement's early stages. Here, it may be useful to let "a thousand flowers bloom" in order to determine the mix of tactics that is most efficacious. That said, judging whether or not radicals at a given moment are helpful or hurtful to the cause depends greatly on the situation and the perceived willingness by the target actor to engage moderate forces and whether more radical oppositional tactics help or undermine the position of reformers within target organizations. Again, this raises the question of the "optimal mix" of campaign tactics as a movement seeks to engage its target.

Fifth, beyond the movements themselves, social scientists are also deeply interested in the role of institutions in economic and political life, and the "opportunity sets" and incentives they provide to various agents within a society. From an economics perspective, institutions represent an equilibrium position, though whether that equilibrium is the outcome of the interactions between contending social forces (the "pulling and hauling" of such forces, to use Dahl's famous terminology) or simply represents the dominant interest's preferences about how the world should operate, remain contested. In any case, it has long been assumed that once institutions are created they are difficult to change, and that a society's choices become "path-dependent" as a result.

In this book, we have charted the rise of new institutional arrangements that helped to stabilize the market transformation that occurred in the case of AIDS drugs. We admittedly have less to say, however, about the durability of these institutions. As noted above, it is generally supposed in the literature that institutions are sticky; our analysis, however, leads us to believe that this view is worth reconsidering. Researchers need to ask hard questions about the conditions under which new institutions emerge and the durability of institutions both old and new.[6] We believe that a great

---

[6] A related important literature on institutional design may provide some insights on their durability (Koremenos, Lipson, and Snidal 2001).

deal of useful work needs to be done in this area, in part through case studies that trace the rise and fall of different institutional structures.

Further, the "domestic" and "international" literatures on institutions need a deeper engagement. Are international institutions more or less sticky than domestic ones? Some scholars might answer in the affirmative, to the extent they believe that such institutions are more "removed" from domestic politics. Is their life cycle driven by similar internal contradictions and external pressures? Here, the role of world politics and the changing balance of power must be taken into account. Overall, this kind of comparative analysis could prove useful to scholars of domestic and world politics alike as they try to further understand how institutions rise and fall.

Finally, the business literature on corporate strategy could also profit from a deeper analysis of advocacy movements. To date, the strategy literature has focused rather narrowly on the competitive landscape, meaning the structure of the industry and the nature of the firms within it. Very little work in strategy has examined the role of public policy in shaping (or tilting) that landscape, much less on how social movements can influence the competitive terrain. In short, the strategy literature needs to bring in actors beside firms as it tries to understand why executives act the way they do.

Concluding remarks

About 30 years ago, a mysterious disease began to afflict the gay communities of New York and San Francisco. That disease would become known as AIDS, and its cause – the HIV virus – would be discovered a few years later. By the late 1980s, the first ARV drug, AZT, became available, and a decade later the "triple cocktail" that turned AIDS from a death sentence into a chronic condition entered the marketplace.

Over the next few years, however, the international community seemed to dither in its response to the spreading AIDS pandemic. Few politicians would speak openly about the disease and the need for public programs to combat it. Global health officials emphasized other priorities, especially in the context of developing world health systems with limited resources and capabilities. And AIDS advocates themselves were divided over whether treatment or prevention should be the focus of an anti-AIDS campaign.

Despite these unpromising background conditions, by the early years of the new millennium the international community had dedicated itself to the creation of an unprecedented entitlement program, promising everyone with AIDS access to ARV medications, no matter their incomes or their place of residency. This "global access" regime transformed the market for ARV drugs, from one that had been "low volume, high price" to one based on an access principle of drugs for all. How that remarkable transformation occurred has been the subject of this book.

Yet, as consequential as this single market transformation has been in terms of lives saved, we have not been content to focus on this one case alone. It is our hope and belief that the AIDS example provides lessons for other advocacy movements in terms of what it takes to make a fundamental shift in market logic possible. We have been motivated to extend our argument by the many other challenges that the world now faces, including climate change, modern slavery and sex trafficking, and a host of other deadly diseases that particularly afflict women, children, and other vulnerable groups.

If advocates are to help bring about market transformations, they must overcome a successive set of hurdles. These include the need to understand the market structures they face, the development of a compelling frame and coherent ask, a feasible cost–benefit strategy, and a set of institutions to stabilize any new market arrangements.

References

Abbott, Kenneth W., and Duncan Snidal. 1998. "Why States Act Through
Formal International Organizations." *The Journal of Conflict Resolution* 42 (1)
(February 1): 3–32.

Abelson, Reed. 2003. "Glaxo Will Further Cut Prices Of AIDS Drugs
to Poor Nations." *The New York Times*, April 27, www.nytimes.com/
2003/04/28/business/glaxo-will-further-cut-prices-of-aids-drugs-to-poor-
nations.html.

Acharya, Amitav. 2004. "How Ideas Spread: Whose Norms Matter? Norm
Localization and Institutional Change in Asian Regionalism." *International
Organization* 58 (1): 239–75.

Ahmed, Rumman, and Amol Sharma. 2012. "Novartis Fights India for Cancer
Pill Patent." *Wall Street Journal*, August 19, http://online.wsj.com/article/
SB10000872396390444233104577594973786074692.html.

Alamo, Stella T., Robert Colebunders, Joseph Ouma, Pamela Sunday, Glenn
Wagner, Fred Wabwire-Mangen, and Marie Laga. 2012. "Return to
Normal Life After AIDS as a Reason for Lost to Follow up in a Community-
based Antiretroviral Treatment Program." *Journal of Acquired Immune
Deficiency Syndromes* (1999) (March 14), www.ncbi.nlm.nih.gov/pubmed/
22421744.

Alter, Karen J., and Sophie Meunier. 2009. "The Politics of International
Regime Complexity." *Perspectives on Politics* 7: 13–24.

Altman, Lawrence K. 2003. "Clinton Group Gets Discount for AIDS Drugs."
The New York Times, October 23, www.nytimes.com/2003/10/24/health/
24AIDS.html.

and Donald G. McNeil Jr. 2004. "U.N. Agency Drops 2 Drugs for AIDS Care
Worldwide." *The New York Times*, June 15, www.nytimes.com/2004/06/16/
world/un-agency-drops-2-drugs-for-aids-care-worldwide.html.

AMFm (Affordable Medicines Facility for Malaria). 2010. "'Saving Lives,
Buying Time': Lessons in Good Subsidy Design." Policy Brief, March 8.

Angell, Marcia. 2004. *The Truth About the Drug Companies: How They Deceive Us
and What to Do About It.* 1st edn. New York: Random House.

Annan, Kofi. 2001. "The Secretary-General Address to the African Summit on
HIV/AIDS, Tuberculosis and Other Infectious Diseases," www.cptech.org/
ip/health/abuja/annan04262001.html.

Arno, Peter, and Karyn L. Feiden. 1992. *Against the Odds: The Story of AIDS
Drug Development, Politics And Profits.* 1st edn. New York: HarperCollins.

277

Associated Press. 2012. "Now Free Online Classes from Harvard, Stanford."
   The Times Of India, August 5, http://articles.timesofindia.indiatimes.com/
   2012–08–06/education/33064199_1_edx-mit-s-computer-science-free-
   online-classes.
Attaran, Amir. 2004. "How Do Patents And Economic Policies Affect Access
   To Essential Medicines In Developing Countries?" *Health Affairs* 23 (3)
   (May 1): 155–66. doi:10.1377/hlthaff.23.3.155.
   and L. Gillespie-White. 2001. "Do Patents for Antiretroviral Drugs Constrain
   Access to AIDS Treatment in Africa?" *JAMA: The Journal of the American
   Medical Association* 286 (15) (October 17): 1886–92.
   and Jeffrey Sachs. 2002. "Defining and Refining International Donor Support
   for Combating the AIDS Pandemic." *The Lancet* 357: 57–61.
Avant, Deborah D. 1994. *Political Institutions and Military Change: Lessons from
   Peripheral Wars*. Ithaca, NY: Cornell University Press.
Axelrod, Robert. 1984. *The Evolution of Cooperation*. New York: Basic Books.
Bach, David, and David Allen. 2010. "What Every CEO Needs to Know About
   Nonmarket Strategy." *MIT Sloan Management Review*, http://sloanreview.
   mit.edu/the-magazine/2010-spring/51301/what-every-ceo-needs-to-know-
   about-nonmarket-strategy/.
Backman, Gunilla, Paul Hunt, Rajat Khosla, Camila Jaramillo-Strouss,
   Belachew Mekuria Fikre, Caroline Rumble, David Pevalin *et al*. 2008.
   "Health Systems and the Right to Health: An Assessment of 194 Countries."
   The Lancet 372 (9655) (December 10): 2047–85. doi:10.1016/S0140–6736
   (08)61781-X.
Baker, Brook. 2005. "US FDA Approves South African Generic ARV (2),"
   www.essentialdrugs.org/edrug/archive/200501/msg00104.php.
   2011. "Inside Views: Corporate Self-Interest and Strategic Choices: Gilead
   Licenses to Medicines Patent Pool," www.ip-watch.org/2011/07/21/
   corporate-self-interest-and-strategic-choices-gilead-licenses-to-medicines-
   patent-pool/.
Baker, Dean. 2012. "The Pacific Free Trade Deal That's Anything but Free."
   The Guardian, August 26, www.guardian.co.uk/commentisfree/2012/aug/27/
   pacific-free-trade-deal.
Barclay, Eliza. 2011. "Global Health Fund Finds Some Fraud, Recoups Losses:
   NPR." *NPR.org*, www.npr.org/blogs/health/2011/01/24/133188263/global-
   health-fund-finds-some-fraud-recoups-losses.
Barnett, Michael N., and Raymond Duvall, eds. 2005. *Power in Global
   Governance*. Cambridge University Press.
Barnett, Michael N., and Martha Finnemore. 1999. "The Politics, Power, and
   Pathologies of International Organizations." *International Organization* 53
   (4): 699–732.
Baron, David P. 2005. *Business and Its Environment*. 5th edn. Englewood Cliffs,
   NJ: Prentice Hall.
Barr, David. 2007. "Interview." ACT UP Oral History Project. MIX – The New
   York Lesbian & Gay Experimental Film Festival, www.actuporalhistory.org/
   interviews/images/barr.pdf.
Barrett, Scott. 2003. *Environment and Statecraft*. Oxford University Press.

Bartley, Tim. 2007. "Institutional Emergence in an Era of Globalization: The Rise of Transnational Private Regulation of Labor and Environmental Conditions." *American Journal of Sociology* 113 (2): 297–351.

Barton, John H. 2004. "TRIPS and The Global Pharmaceutical Market." *Health Affairs* 23 (3) (May 1): 146–54.

Basheer, Shamnad. 2008. "USPTO Rejects Gilead's Patents Covering Key HIV Drugs," http://spicyipindia.blogspot.com/2008/01/uspto-rejects-gileads-patents-covering.html.

Bate, Roger, and Richard Tren. 2006. *The WTO and Access to Essential Medicines.* AEI Health Policy Outlook. American Enterprise Institute, www.aei.org/article/health/the-wto-and-access-to-essential-medicines/.

Baumol, William J. 1982. "Contestable Markets: An Uprising in the Theory of Industry Structure." *American Economic Review* 72 (1): 1–15.

Becker, Gary S. 1974. "A Theory of Social Interactions." *Journal of Political Economy* 82 (6) (November 1): 1063–93.

Behrman, Greg. 2004. *The Invisible People: How the U.S. Has Slept Through the Global AIDS Pandemic, the Greatest Humanitarian Catastrophe of Our Time.* New York: Free Press.

Benn, Christoph. 2010. "Personal Communication," November 8.

Berinsky, Adam J., Gregory A. Huber, and Gabriel S. Lenz. 2012. "Evaluating Online Labor Markets for Experimental Research: Amazon.com's Mechanical Turk." *Political Analysis* (March 2), http://pan.oxfordjournals.org/content/early/2012/03/02/pan.mpr057.

Berle, Adolph A., and Gardiner C. Means. 1932. *The Modern Corporation and Private Property.* New York: Harcourt Brace.

Berman, Daniel. 2012. "Interview," May 30.

Berndt, Ernst R. 2002. "Pharmaceuticals in U.S. Health Care: Determinants of Quantity and Price." *Journal of Economic Perspectives* 16 (4): 45–66.

Biermann, Frank, and Bernd Siebenhüner. 2009. *Managers of Global Change: The Influence of International Environmental Bureaucracies.* Cambridge, MA: MIT Press.

Birmingham, Desmond. 2010. *Reviving the Global Education Compact: Four Options for Global Education Funding.* Center for Global Development, www.cgdev.org/content/publications/detail/1423802/.

Bob, Clifford. 2005. *The Marketing of Rebellion: Insurgents, Media, and International Activism (Cambridge Studies in Contentious Politics).* New York: Cambridge University Press, www.loc.gov/catdir/toc/ecip052/2004024987.html.

Bollyky, Thomas J. 2012. "Developing Symptoms." *Foreign Affairs*, May 1, www.foreignaffairs.com/articles/137536/thomas-j-bollyky/developing-symptoms.

Boneberg, Paul. 2012. "Interview," July 24.

Bonnel, Rene, Elizabeth Lule, Richard Seifman, and Antonio C. David. 2009. "The Financial Architecture of the Response to the HIV Epidemic: Challenges and Sustainability Issues." In *The Changing HIV/AIDS Landscape*, 161–95. Washington DC: World Bank, www.cabdirect.org/abstracts/20093306557.html;jsessionid=22E49D9DC67EE98BA1798C82AC3DF986.

Boseley, Sarah. 2007. "Paul Hunt: UN Special Rapporteur on the Right to Health." *The Lancet* 370 (9585) (August 4): 381, doi:10.1016/S0140–6736(07)61179–9.

2011. "Drug Company's Loss Could Be Africa's Gain." *The Guardian*, January 3, www.guardian.co.uk/society/sarah-boseley-global-health/2011/jan/04/aids-pharmaceuticals-industry.

2012. "Does EU/India Free Trade Agreement Spell the End of Cheap Drugs for Poor Countries?" *The Guardian*, February 9, www.guardian.co.uk/society/sarah-boseley-global-health/2012/feb/10/hiv-infection-pharmaceuticals-industry.

Bowdler, Neil. 2010. "Beating Malaria 'Impossible' Now." *BBC*, October 29, sec. Health, www.bbc.co.uk/news/health-11643868.

Brenner, Carl Noakes. 2003. "Agency, Institutions, and the Enduring Pattern of American Civil-military Relations." Ph.D. thesis, Georgetown University.

Brown, David. 2011. "HIV Drugs Sharply Cut Risk of Transmission, Study Finds." *The Washington Post*, May 12, www.washingtonpost.com/national/hiv_drugs_sharply_cut_risk_of_transmission_study_finds/2011/05/12/AFmFdV1G_story.html.

Brundtland, Gro Harlem. 1998. Speech of the WHO Director-General, at the World Health Assembly Meeting of the WHO, Geneva, October 13.

Buckley, Cara. 2011. "Occupy Wall Street Organizers Consider Value of Camps." *The New York Times*, November 15, www.nytimes.com/2011/11/16/nyregion/occupy-wall-street-organizers-consider-value-of-camps.html.

and Colin Moynihan. 2011. "Occupy Wall Street Protest Reaches a Crossroads." *The New York Times*, November 4, www.nytimes.com/2011/11/06/nyregion/occupy-wall-street-protest-reaches-a-crossroads.html.

Burkhalter, Holly. 2004. "Trick or Treat?" *Foreign Affairs*, October 27, www.foreignaffairs.com/articles/64228/holly-burkhalter/trick-or-treat?page=2.

Busby, Joshua. 2008. "The Hardest Problem in the World: Leadership in the Climate Regime." In *The Dispensable Hegemon: Explaining Contemporary International Leadership and Cooperation*, Stefan Brem and Kendall Stiles, eds., 73–104. London: Routledge.

2009. "Global AIDS Policy in the Age of Obama." *Journal of HIV/AIDS & Social Services* 8 (2): 120–6.

2010a. *Moral Movements and Foreign Policy*. Cambridge University Press.

2010b. "After Copenhagen: Climate Governance and the Road Ahead." *Council on Foreign Relations*, www.cfr.org/publication/22726/after_copenhagen.html.

2010c. *Moral Movements and Foreign Policy*. Cambridge University Press.

2012. "World AIDS Day 2012: A Moment for Optimism?" *Duck of Minerva*, www.whiteoliphaunt.com/duckofminerva/2012/12/world-aids-day-2012-a-moment-for-optimism.html.

2012a. "The Duck of Minerva: An AIDS-Free Generation? HIV Is Not A Fad." *The Duck of Minerva*, http://duckofminerva.blogspot.com/2012/07/an-aids-free-generation-hiv-is-not-fad.html.

2012b. "An AIDS-Free Generation? HIV Is Not A Fad – Joshua Busby." *Global Health Governance*, http://blogs.shu.edu/ghg/2012/07/25/an-aids-free-generation-hiv-is-not-a-fad-joshua-busby/.

and Bethany Albertson. 2011. "Hearts or Minds? Persuasive Messages on Climate Change." Paper presented at the 2010 Western Political Science Association Conference, San Francisco, April 1–4.

Bush, George W. 2003. "Address Before a Joint Session of the Congress on the State of the Union." *The American Presidency Project*, www.presidency.ucsb. edu/ws/index.php?pid=29645.

2010. *Decision Points*. New York: Crown.

2012. "Extend the Success Against AIDS to Other Devastating Diseases." *The Washington Post*, July 23, www.washingtonpost.com/opinions/george-w-bush-extend-success-against-aids-to-other-devastating-diseases/2012/07/22/gJQAxs042W_story.html.

Butler, Declan. 2012. "Malaria Programme Gets Kiss of Death from Global Fund." *Nature*, November, http://blogs.nature.com/news/2012/11/malaria-medicines-venture-gets-kiss-of-death-from-global-fund.html.

Butler, Rhett. 2012. *REDD*. Mongabay, http://rainforests.mongabay.com/redd/.

Cahill, Sean, and Lyndel Urbano. 2009. "The Christian Right: Wrong on AIDS." *TheBody.com*, www.thebody.com/content/art56485.html.

Cameron, C. Daryl, and B. Keith Payne. 2011. "Escaping Affect: How Motivated Emotion Regulation Creates Insensitivity to Mass Suffering." *Journal of Personality and Social Psychology* 100 (1): 1–15.

Carpenter, R. Charli. 2011. "Vetting the Advocacy Agenda: Network Centrality and the Paradox of Weapons Norms." *International Organization* 65 (01): 69–102.

CDC (Centres for Disease Control). 1981. "Mortality and Morbidity Weekly Report," June 5, www.cdc.gov/mmwr/previews/mmwrhtml/june_5.htm.

2010. *AIDS Surveillance – Trends (1985–2010)*, www.cdc.gov/hiv/topics/surveillance/resources/slides/trends/index.htm.

CFR (Council on Foreign Relations). 2010. "A Conversation with Michel Kazatchkine, Executive Director of the Global Fund to Fight AIDS, Tuberculosis and Malaria," www.cfr.org/publication/22589/conversation_with_michel_kazatchkine_executive_director_of_the_global_fund_to_fight_aids_tuberculosis_and_malaria.html.

CHAI (Clinton Health Access Initiative). Undated. "What We've Accomplished," www.clintonfoundation.org/what-we-do/clinton-health-access-initiative/what-we-ve-accomplished.

2008a. "Clinton HIV/AIDS Initiative – Procurement Consortium List (September 2008)," www.clintonfoundation.org/download/?guid=8261818e-ca75–102b-81f3–00304860f676.

2008b. "Antiretroviral Price List," www.clintonfoundation.org/download/?guid=62e82ddc-98de-102b-be34–001143e0d9b6.

2010. "CHAI Drug Quality Policy."

2011. "Antiretrovrial (ARV) Ceiling Price List," www.clintonfoundation.org/files/chai_arv_ceilingPriceList_201105_english.pdf.

Charity Wire. 2003. *Focus on the Family Applauds Passage of Global AIDS Bill*, www.charitywire.com/charity63/03879.html.

Chatterjee, Patralekha. 2012. "India: Balancing Public and Private Interests in the Intellectual Property Regime". *Intellectual Property Watch*, September 17, www.ip-watch.org/2012/09/18/india-balancing-public-and-private-interests-in-the-intellectual-property-regime/.

Chawla, Purnima. 2005. *Advocacy for Impact: Lessons from Six Successful Campaigns*. Center for Nonprofit Strategies, www.connectusfund.org/resources/advocacy-impact-lessons-six-successful-campaigns.

Checkel, Jeffrey T. 1999. "Norms, Institutions, and National Identity in Contemporary Europe." *International Studies Quarterly* 43 (1): 84–114.

Chien, Colleen V. 2007. "HIV/AIDS Drugs for Sub-Saharan Africa: How Do Brand and Generic Supply Compare?" *PloS One* 2 (3): 1–6.

Chong, Dennis, and James N. Druckman. 2007. "A Theory of Framing and Opinion Formation in Competitive Elite Environments." *Journal of Communication* 57 (1): 99–118.

Chorev, Nitsan. 2012. "Changing Global Norms Through Reactive Diffusion: The Case of Intellectual Property Protection of AIDS Drugs." *American Sociological Review* 77 (5): 831–53.

Christy, Bryan. 2012. "Ivory Worship – Pictures, More From National Geographic Magazine," October, http://ngm.nationalgeographic.com/2012/10/ivory/christy-text?source=religious_ivory_news.

Cohen, Myron S., Ying Q. Chen, Marybeth McCauley, Theresa Gamble, Mina C. Hosseinipour, Nagalingeswaran Kumarasamy, James G. Hakim *et al.* 2011. "Prevention of HIV-1 Infection with Early Antiretroviral Therapy." *New England Journal of Medicine* 365 (6) (August 11): 493–505.

Cohen, Richard E., and Peter Bell. 2007. "Congressional Insiders Poll." *National Journal*, http://syndication.nationaljournal.com/images/203Insiderspoll_NJlogo.pdf.

Comanor, William S. 1986. "The Political Economy of the Pharmaceutical Industry." *Journal of Economic Literature* 24 (3): 1178–217.

Condliffe, Kate. 2012. "Interview," March 8.

Cooper, Helene, Rachel Zimmerman, and Laurie McGinley. 2001. "AIDS Epidemic puts Drug Firms in a Vise: Treatment Vs. Profits." *The Wall Street Journal*, March 2.

Coriat, Benjamin, ed. 2008. *The Political Economy of HIV/AIDS in Developing Countries: TRIPS, Public Health Systems and Free Access*. Cheltenham: Edward Elgar Publishing.

Cortell, Andrew, and James W. Davis. 2000. "Understanding the Domestic Impact of International Norms: A Research Agenda." *International Studies Review* 2 (1): 65–87.

Cota-Larson, Rhishja. 2012. "Rhino Crisis Round Up: 430 Rhinos Killed in S Africa & More." *Jetpack by WordPress.com*, http://jetpack.wordpress.com/jetpack-comment/.

CPTech (Consumer Projection Technology). 1999a. *Activities for NGO Representatives Thursday March 25, 1999*. Geneva, Switzerland, www.cptech.org/march99-cl/mar25agenda.html.

1999b. "August 1, 1999 Open Letter to Vice President Al Gore, Signed by 307 Public Health Experts and Concerned Persons, Regarding US Trade Pressures on South Africa Efforts to Obtain Access to Essential Medicines," www.cptech.org/ip/health/sa/goresignon.html.

1999c. "Sign the Open Letter to the WTO Member States Regarding Access to Medical Technologies," www.cptech.org/ip/health/wto-99-signon.txt.

1999d. *Amsterdam Statement to WTO Member States on Access to Medicine*. Amsterdam, Holland, www.cptech.org/ip/health/amsterdamstatement.html.

2002a. "Joint Letter from Consumer Project on Technology, Essential Action, Médecins Sans Frontières, Oxfam International, Health GAP Coalition, and the Third World Network to the World Trade Organization's TRIPS Council," www.cptech.org/ip/health/art30exports.html.

2002b. "Sign-on Letter to U.S. Trade Representative Zoellick Circulated by Health GAP and Médecins Sans Frontières," www.cptech.org/ip/wto/p6/signon12192002.html.

2004. "Generic Medicines and U.S.-initiated Conference on Fixed-Dose Combinations," www.cptech.org/ip/health/aids/fdc/signon03292004.html.

2006. "Sign-on Letter to State and USTR Regarding Pressures on Thailand for Issuing Compulsory License," www.cptech.org/ip/health/c/thailand/2riceschwabthaicl.html.

Crossette, Barbara. 2001. "U.S. Drops Case Over AIDS Drugs in Brazil." *The New York Times*, June 25, www.nytimes.com/2001/06/26/world/us-drops-case-over-aids-drugs-in-brazil.html.

d'Adesky, Anne-christine. 2004. *Moving Mountains: The Race to Treat Global AIDS*. New York: Verso.

and Ann T. Rossetti. 2005. *Pills Profits Protest: Chronicle of the Global AIDS Movement*. New York: Outcast Films.

Dance with Shadows/Pillscribe. 2010. "Cipla's Generic HIV Drug Tenofovir Receives USFDA Approval," www.dancewithshadows.com/pillscribe/ciplas-generic-hiv-drug-tenofovir-receives-usfda-approval/.

Danzon, Patricia M. 1996. "The Uses and Abuses of International Price Comparisons." In *Competitive Strategies in the Pharmaceutical Industry*, Robert Helms, ed. Washington DC: AEI Press.

2001. "Differential Pricing for Pharmaceuticals: Reconciling Access, R&D and Patents." The Wharton School, University of Pennsylvania, http://hc.wharton.upenn.edu/danzon/html/CV%20pubs/commissionedit12.15.01.pdf.

and Adrian Towse. 2003. "Differential Pricing for Pharmaceuticals: Reconciling Access, R&D and Patents." *International Journal of Health Care Finance and Economics* 3: 183–205.

Das, Pam, and Richard Horton. 2010. "Malaria Elimination: Worthy, Challenging, and Just Possible." *The Lancet* 376 (9752) (November): 1515–17.

Daschle, Tom, John McCain, and Ted Kennedy. 2003. "Letter from Senators Daschle, McCain and Kennedy to the GAO Requesting a Cost Study of HIV/AIDS Drugs," www.cptech.org/ip/health/aids/senate06132003.html.

de Soto, Hernando. 2000. *The Mystery of Capital: Why Capitalism Triumphs in the West and Fails Everywhere Else*. 1st edn. New York: Basic Books.

Deitelhoff, Nicole. 2008. "Isolated Hegemon: The Creation of the International Criminal Court." In *Cooperating Without America: Theories and Case Studies of Non-hegemonic Regimes*, Stefan Brem and Kendall Stiles, eds., 142–72. London: Routledge.

2009. "The Discursive Process of Legalization: Charting Islands of Persuasion in the ICC Case." *International Organization* 63 (01): 33–65.

Demeritt, Jacqueline. 2012. "International Organizations and Government Killing: Does Naming and Shaming Save Lives?" *International Interactions* 38 (5): 597–621.

Devereaux, Charan. 2004. *International Trade Meets Public Health: TRIPS and Access to Medicines*. Cambridge, MA: Kennedy School of Government, Harvard University.

Robert Z. Lawrence, and Michael D. Watkins. 2006. *Case Studies in US Trade Negotiation, Volume 1: Making the Rules.* Washington DC: Institute for International Economics.

Dietrich, John. 2007. "The Politics of PEPFAR: The President's Emergency Plan for AIDS Relief." *Ethics and International Affairs* 21 (3): 277–92.

Donnelly, John. 2001. "Prevention Urged in AIDS Fight: Natsios Says Fund Should Spend Less on HIV Treatment." *Boston Globe*, June 7.

2005. "AIDS Drugs Hit Roadblock In Africa," http://lists.essential.org/pipermail/ip-health/2005-June/008035.html.

2011. *Dybul on PEPFAR: "The Sky Was the Limit".* Science Speaks: HIV & TB News. Center for Global Health Policy.

2012. "The President's Emergency Plan for AIDS Relief: How George W. Bush and Aides came to 'Think Big' on Battling HIV." *Health Affairs* 31 (7) (July 1): 1389–96.

Dorow, Heidi. 2007. "Interview." ACT UP Oral History Project. MIX – The New York Lesbian & Gay Experimental Film Festival, www.actuporalhistory.org/interviews/images/dorow.pdf.

Doughton, Sandi. 2009. "Global-health Stars Converge on Seattle," http://seattletimes.nwsource.com/html/health/2009348027_healthdavos17m0.html.

Douste-Blazy, Philippe. 2011. "UNITAID: Innovative Financing for Health and Development," www.unitaid.eu/images/NewWeb/documents/UNITAID_in_2011/UNITAID_in_2011_EN_June13.pdf.

and Daniel Altman. 2010. *Power in Numbers: UNITAID, Innovative Financing, and the Quest for Massive Good.* New York: PublicAffairs.

Downs, Anthony. 1972. "Up and Down with Ecology: The 'Issue Attention' Cycle." *The Public Interest* 28 (Summer): 38–50.

Drahos, Peter. 2007. "Four Lessons for Developing Countries from the Trade Negotiations over Access to Medicines." *Liverpool Law Review* 28: 11–39.

Drezner, Daniel. 2007. *All Politics Is Global.* Princeton University Press.

Druckman, James. 2001. "The Implications of Framing Effects for Citizen Competence." *Political Behavior* 23 (3): 225–56.

Dugger, Celia W. 2006. "Clinton Makes Up for Lost Time in Battling AIDS," www.aegis.org/news/nyt/2006/NYT060823.html.

2009. "Child Mortality Rate Declines Globally." *The New York Times*, September 10, sec. World, www.nytimes.com/2009/09/10/world/10child.html.

Dunlap, David W. 1995. "Different Faces of AIDS are Conjured up by Politicians." *The New York Times*, July 8.

Dunlap, Riley E. 2008. "Partisan Gap on Global Warming Grows," www.gallup.com/poll/107593/Partisan-Gap-Global-Warming-Grows.aspx.

Dybul, Mark. 2009. "Personal Communication," December 3.

2012. "Interview," September 24.

Peter Piot, and Julio Frenk. 2012. *Reshaping Global Health.* Policy Review. Hoover Institution, www.hoover.org/publications/policy-review/article/118116.

Economic Times of India, The. 2012. *Ranbaxy Hires Consultants as Part of Consent Decree with USFDA*, http://economictimes.indiatimes.com/news/news-by-industry/healthcare/biotech/pharmaceuticals/ranbaxy-hires-consultants-as-part-of-consent-decree-with-usfda/articleshow/13481989.cms.

Economist, The. 2012. "Heal Thyself." *The Economist,* www.economist.com/news/science-and-technology/21567054-grappling-controversial-malaria-programme-heal-thyself.

Eesley, Charles E., and Michael Lenox. 2006. "Secondary Stakeholder Actions and the Selection of Firm Targets," http://papers.ssrn.com/sol3/papers.cfm?abstract_id=1926944.

Eigo, Jim. 2004. "Interview." ACT UP Oral History Project. MIX – The New York Lesbian & Gay Experimental Film Festival, www.actuporalhistory.org/interviews/images/eigo.pdf.

Elliott, Kimberly, and Carsten Fink. 2008. *"Tripping Over Health: U.S. Policy on Patents and Drug Access in Developing Countries (White House and the World Policy Brief)."* Center for Global Development, www.cgdev.org/content/publications/detail/967265.

Ellison, Sara Fisher, and Catherine Wolfram. 2006. "Coordinating on Lower Prices: Pharmaceutical Pricing under Political Pressure." *The RAND Journal of Economics* 37 (2) (July 1): 324–40.

Entman, Robert M. 1993. "Framing: Toward Clarification of a Fractured Paradigm." *Journal of Communication* 43 (4): 51.

Epstein, Helen. 2007. *The Invisible Cure: Africa, the West, and the Fight Against AIDS.* Vol. I. New York: Farrar, Straus and Giroux.

Epstein, Steven. 1996. *Impure Science: AIDS, Activism, and the Politics of Knowledge.* University of California Press.

essentialdrugs.org. 2001. "GSK Licenses ARVs to South African Generic Manufacturer," www.essentialdrugs.org/edrug/archive/200110/msg00023.php.

Fan, Victoria. 2012. "A Global Health Mystery: What's Behind the US Government Position on AMFm? Global Health Policy." Center for Global Development, http://blogs.cgdev.org/globalhealth/2012/09/a-global-health-mystery-whats-behind-the-us-government-position-on-amfm.php.

Fan, Victoria, and Laura Khan. 2012. "One Year Later: What Happened to Non-Communicable Diseases? Global Health Policy." Center for Global Development, http://blogs.cgdev.org/globalhealth/2012/09/one-year-later-what-happened-to-non-communicable-diseases.php.

Fan, Victoria, and Rachel Silverman. 2012. "Should UNITAID Rethink its Raison d'Être?" Center for Global Development, http://blogs.cgdev.org/globalhealth/2012/09/should-unitaid-rethink-its-raison-detre.php.

Farmer, Paul. 2007. "From 'Marvelous Momentum' to Health Care for All," www.foreignaffairs.org/special/global_health/farmer.

Jeffrey Sachs, Alex de Waal, Roger Bate, Kathryn Boateng, and Laurie Garrett. 2007. "How to Promote Global Health." *Foreign Affairs,* January 23, www.foreignaffairs.com/discussions/roundtables/how-to-promote-global-health.

FDA (Food and Drug Administration). 2011. "President's Emergency Plan for AIDS Relief – Approved and Tentatively Approved Antiretrovirals in

Association with the President's Emergency Plan," www.fda.gov/
InternationalPrograms/FDABeyondOurBordersForeignOffices/
AsiaandAfrica/ucm119231.htm.

Feachem, Richard G. A. 2012. "Interview," September 11.

Allison A. Phillips, Geoffrey A. Targett, and Robert W. Snow. 2010. "Call to
Action: Priorities for Malaria Elimination." *The Lancet* 376 (9752)
(November): 1517–21.

Fearon, James, and Alexander Wendt. 2003. "Rationalism v. Constructivism:
A Skeptical View." In *Handbook of International Relations*, Walter Carlsnaes,
Thomas Risse-Kappen, and Beth A. Simmons, eds., 52–72. London,
Thousand Oaks, CA: Sage Publications.

Feddersen, Timothy J., and Thomas W. Gilligan. 2001. "Saints and Markets:
Activists and the Supply of Credence Goods." *Journal of Economics &
Management Strategy* 10 (1): 149–71.

Feller, Ben. 2012. "Clinton Global Initiative: Obama Outlines Steps to Fight
Human Trafficking." *Huffington Post*, September 24, www.huffingtonpost.
com/2012/09/25/obama-human-trafficking-cgi_n_1913051.html.

Fidler, David. 2007. "Architecture Amidst Anarchy: Global Health's Quest for
Governance." *Global Health Governance* 1 (1): 1–17.

    2008. "After the Revolution: Global Health Politics in a Time of Economic
Crisis and Threatening Future Trends." *Global Health Governance* 2 (2):
1–21.

    2010. "The Challenges of Global Health Governance," www.cfr.org/
publication/22202/challenges_of_global_health_governance.html.

Fildes, Jonathan. 2007. "'$100 Laptop' to Sell to Public." BBC, September 24,
http://news.bbc.co.uk/2/hi/technology/6994957.stm.

Fink, Carsten. 2005. "Intellectual Property and Public Health: The WTO's
August 2003 Decision in Perspective." Richard Newfarmer, ed. World
Bank, http://siteresources.worldbank.org/INTRANETTRADE/Resources/
Internal-Training/6_Carsten_Health15_Pubhealth.pdf.

    2008. "Intellectual Property and Public Health: An Overview of the Debate with
a Focus on US Policy, Working Paper Number 146." Center for Global
Development, www.cgdev.org/content/publications/detail/16228/.

    and Kimberly Elliott. 2008. "Tripping over Health: U.S. Policy on Patents
and Drug Access in Developing Countries." In *The White House and the
World*, Nancy Birdsall ed. 215–40. Washington DC: Center for Global
Development, www.cgdev.org/content/publications/detail/16560/.

Fink, Sheri, and Rebecca Rabinowitz. 2011. "The UN's Battle With NCDs."
Foreign Affairs, September 20, www.foreignaffairs.com/articles/68280/sheri-
fink-and-rebecca-rabinowitz/the-uns-battle-with-ncds.

Finnemore, Martha, and Kathryn Sikkink. 1998. "International Norm
Dynamics and Political Change." *International Organization* 52 (04):
887–917.

Fleet, Julian, and Bechir N'Daw. 2008. "Trade, Intellectual Property and Access
to Affordable HIV Medicines." In *The HIV Pandemic: Local and Global
Implications*, Eduard J Beck, Nicholas Mays, Alan W. Whiteside, and Jose
M. Zuniga, eds., 660–73. Oxford University Press.

Fligstein, Neil. 2002. *The Architecture of Markets: An Economic Sociology of Twenty-First-Century Capitalist Societies*. Princeton University Press.

2008. "Fields, Power, and Social Skill: A Critical Analysis of the New Institutionalisms." *International Public Management Review* 9 (1): 227–53.

Flynn, Matthew. 2008. "Public Production of Anti-Retroviral Medicines in Brazil, 1990–2007." *Development and Change* 39 (4): 513–36.

Ford, Liz. 2012. "Millennium Development Goal on Safe Drinking Water Reaches Target Early." *The Guardian*, March 6, www.guardian.co.uk/global-development/2012/mar/06/water-millennium-development-goals.

Ford, Sarah. 2000. "Compulsory Licensing Provisions under the TRIPs Agreement: Balancing Pills and Patents." *American University International Law Review* 15 (4): 941–74.

FrameWorks Institute. 2001. *FrameWorks Toolkit on Talking Global Warming*. Washington DC.

France, David. 2012. *How to Survive a Plague*, http://surviveaplague.com/.

Franke-Ruta, Garance. 2007. "Interview." ACT UP Oral History Project. MIX – The New York Lesbian & Gay Experimental Film Festival, www.actuporalhistory.org/interviews/images/ruta.pdf.

Friedman, Monroe. 1999. *Consumer Boycotts: Effecting Change Through the Marketplace and Media*. London: Routledge.

Frist, Bill. 2009. *A Heart to Serve: The Passion to Bring Health, Hope, and Healing*. Hachette Digital, Inc.

Frontline. 2006. "Interview: Peter Piot." *The Age of AIDS*, www.pbs.org/wgbh/pages/frontline/aids/interviews/piot.html.

FSG. 2008. *Diarrheal Disease Advocacy: Findings from a Scan of the Global Funding and Policy Landscape*, www.fsg.org/Portals/0/Uploads/Documents/PDF/Diarrheal_Disease_Advocacy.pdf?cpgn=WP%20DL%20-%20Diarrheal%20Disease%20Advocacy.

Fuller, Thomas. 2007. "Thailand Takes on Drug Industry, and May Be Winning." *The New York Times*, April 10, www.nytimes.com/2007/04/11/world/asia/11iht-pharma.4.5240049.html?pagewanted=all&r=0.

Galambos, Louis. 2001. "Global Oligopoly, Regional Authority and National Power: Crosscurrents in Pharmaceuticals Today and Tomorrow." In *Consolidation and Competition in the Pharmaceutical Industry*, Hannah Kettler, ed. London: Office of Health Economics.

Gallup. 2007. "Public Perceptions of Worldwide Malaria and TB Risks Haven't Risen," www.gallup.com/poll/27979/public-perceptions-worldwide-malaria-risks-havent-risen.aspx.

Gangte, Loon. 2012. "Interview."

GAO (Government Accountability Office). 2005. "Selection of Antiretroviral Medications Provided Under U.S. Emergency Plan is Limited," www.gao.gov/new.items/d05133.pdf.

2006. "Spending Requirement Presents Challenges for Allocating Prevention Funding Under the President's Emergency Plan for AIDS Relief," www.gao.gov/new.items/d06395.pdf.

Garrett, Laurie. 2007. "The Challenge of Global Health," www.foreignaffairs.org/20070101faessay86103/laurie-garrett/the-challenge-of-global-health.html.

2008. "The Wrong Way to Fight AIDS", *The New York Times*, July 29, www.nytimes.com/2008/07/30/opinion/30iht-edgarrett.1.14888763.html.

2012a. "Money or Die." *Foreign Affairs*, March 6, www.foreignaffairs.com/articles/137312/laurie-garrett/money-or-die.

2012b. *The End of AIDS? What Are You Smoking?*, www.lauriegarrett.com/index.php/en/blog/3214/.

Gartner, David. 2009a. "The U.S. Global AIDS Response: Norms, Interests and the Duty to Treat." Cambridge, MA: Department of Political Science, MIT.

2009b. "A Global Fund for Education: Achieving Education for All." The Brookings Institution, www.brookings.edu/research/papers/2009/08/education-gartner.

Geffen, Nathan. 2010. *Debunking Delusions: The Inside Story of the Treatment Action Campaign*. Jacana Media.

Gehring, Thomas, and Eva Ruffing. 2008. "When Arguments Prevail Over Power: The CITES Procedure for the Listing of Endangered Species." *Global Environmental Politics* 8 (2): 123–48.

Generic Pharmaceutical Association. Undated. "Bioequivalence," www.gphaonline.org/issues/bioequivalence.

Gerson, Michael. 2006. "Personal Communication," November 6.

2007. *Heroic Conservatism*. New York: HarperOne.

Gettleman, Jeffrey. 2012. "Africa's Elephants are being Slaughtered in Poaching Frenzy." *The New York Times*, September 3, sec. World/Africa, www.nytimes.com/2012/09/04/world/africa/africas-elephants-are-being-slaughtered-in-poaching-frenzy.html.

Gilead. 2012. *Gilead Sciences Announces New Collaboration with Indian Partners to Reduce Manufacturing Cost and Improve Availability of Emtricitabine-Based Antiretroviral Therapy in Developing Countries*, www.gilead.com/pr_1721615.

Gitlin, Todd. 2012. *Occupy Nation: The Roots, the Spirit, and the Promise of Occupy Wall Street*. New York: HarperCollins.

Gladwell, Malcolm. 2001. "The Mosquito Killer." *The New Yorker*, July 2, www.newyorker.com/archive/2001/07/02/010702fa_fact_gladwell.

Glickman, Lawrence B. 2009. *Buying Power: A History of Consumer Activism in America*. 1st edn. University of Chicago Press.

Global Fund. Undated. "Portfolio and Grant Performance," www.theglobalfund.org/en/performance/grantportfolio/.

2004. "Guide to the Global Fund's Policies on Procurement and Supply Management," www.who.int/hdp/publications/13h.pdf.

2006. "Guide to the Global Fund's Policies on Procurement and Supply Management," www.stoptb.org/assets/documents/gdf/drugsupply/pp_guidelines_procurement_supplymanagement_en.pdf.

2009. "Guide to the Global Fund's Policies on Procurement and Supply Management," www.theglobalfund.org/documents/psm/PSM_ProcurementSupplyManagement_Guidelines_en/.

2010a. "About the Global Fund," www.theglobalfund.org/en/about/secretariat/.

2010b. "Resource Allocation," www.theglobalfund.org/en/performance/grantportfolio/resourceallocation/.

2010c. "Global Fund Quality Assurance Policy for Pharmaceutical Products," www.theglobalfund.org/documents/psm/PSM_QAPharm_Policy_en/.

2011a. "Making a Difference – Global Fund Results Report 2011," www. theglobalfund.org/documents/publications/progress_reports/ Publication_2011Results_Report_en/.

2011b. "Procurement Support Services Progress Report: June 2009–Dec 2010," www.theglobalfund.org/documents/psm/ PSM_PSSMarch2011_Report_en/.

Gonsalves, Gregg. 2004. "Interview." ACT UP Oral History Project. MIX – The New York Lesbian & Gay Experimental Film Festival, www. actuporalhistory.org/interviews/images/gonsalves.pdf.

2011a. "Patent Pool Controversies: Part 2." *IP-Health Listserv*, http://lists. keionline.org/pipermail/ip-health_lists.keionline.org/2011-November/ 001555.html.

2011b. "No Sense of Urgency – Pressing the STOP Button on the AIDS Response." *IP-Health Listserv*, https://lists.critpath.org/pipermail/healthgap/ 2011-December/003256.html.

2012a. "ONE Pitting Global Fund Against PEPFAR?" *IP-Health Listserv*, https://lists.critpath.org/pipermail/healthgap/2012-February/003359.html.

2012b. "Interview," May 14.

Gorman, Christine. 2008. "Who Are the Health Eight (or H8)?", http:// globalhealthreport.blogspot.com/2008/04/who-are-health-eight-or-h8.html.

Gostin, Lawrence O. 2001. "Public Health, Ethics, and Human Rights: A Tribute to the Late Jonathan Mann." *Journal of Law, Medicine & Ethics* 29 (2): 121–30.

Gould, Deborah B. 2009. *Moving Politics: Emotion and Act Up's Fight Against AIDS*. University of Chicago Press.

Granich, Reuben M., Charles F. Gilks, Christopher Dye, Kevin M. De Cock, and Brian G. Williams. 2009. "Universal Voluntary HIV Testing with Immediate Antiretroviral Therapy as a Strategy for Elimination of HIV Transmission: A Mathematical Model." *The Lancet* 373 (9657): 48–57.

Granovetter, Mark. 1985. "Economic Action and Social Structure: The Problem of Embeddedness." *American Journal of Sociology* 91 (3) (November 1): 481–510.

Gray, Dylan Mohan. 2012. *Fire in the Blood*, www.fireintheblood.com/.

Grebe, Eduard. 2008. *Transnational Networks of Influence in South African AIDS Treatment Activism*. Center for Social Science Research, University of Cape Town, www.cssr.uct.ac.za/publications/working-paper/2008/transnational-networks-influence-south-african.

2011. "The Treatment Action Campaign's Struggle for AIDS Treatment in South Africa: Coalition-building Through Networks." *Journal of Southern African Studies* 37 (4): 849–68.

Greenhill, Kelly M., and Joshua W. Busby. 2008. "Ain't That a Shame? Hypocrisy, Punishment, and Weak Actor Influence in International Politics." Unpublished Paper, Harvard and Tufts Universities and the University of Texas.

Grepin, Karen. 2009. "Prevention Vs. Treament in HIV: Have We Given Prevention a Chance to Shine?" *Karen Grepin's Global Health Blog*, http:// karengrepin.com/2009/01/prevention-vs-treament-in-hiv-have-we.html.

Griffin Securities. 2005. *HIV/AIDS Industry Report*. New York, available at www. samaritanpharma.com/images/HIVINDUSTRYREPORT.pdf.

Gross, Grant. 2012. "Court Grants Stay in Google Books Case." *Computerworld*, www.computerworld.com/s/article/9231408/Court_grants_stay_in_Google_ books_case.

Gross, Robin. 2005. "Bush and Big Pharma Team Up to Discredit WHO and Generic Medicines: Drug Companies' Influence on Health Care Policy Worsens Global AIDS Crisis," www.pharmadisclose.org/pttag/ipj050503.html.

Grubb, Ian. 2010. "Personal Communication," September 14.

GSK (GlaxoSmithKline). 2011. *Corporate Responsibility Report 2011*, www.gsk. com/responsibility/downloads/GSK-CR-2011-Report.pdf.

Guardian, The. 2012. "Tanzania's Plan to Sell Ivory Stockpile Is 'Ludicrous', Say Conservationists." *The Guardian*, www.guardian.co.uk/environment/2012/ oct/09/tanzania-sell-ivory-stockpile.

Gudrais, Elizabeth. 2010. "The Social Epidemic." *Harvard Magazine* 113 (1): 22–9.

Gusterson, Hugh. 2012. "Want to Change Academic Publishing? Just Say No." *The Chronicle of Higher Education*, September 23, sec. Commentary, http:// chronicle.com/article/Want-to-Change-Academic/134546/.

Haddad, William. 2001. Speech given at the WTO/WHO Conference on Differential Pricing in Oslo, April 8–10, www.cptech.org/ip/health/who/ haddad.html.

   2004a. *"Delivery of the Generic Triple ARV to Poor Nations is Seriously Threatened by Combined Actions of the US Government, Pharma, WHO, UNICEF, UNAIDS, HHS,"* www.cptech.org/ip/health/aids/fdc/haddad03162004. html.

   2004b. "Botswana Report," http://lists.essential.org/pipermail/ip-health/2004-April/006218.html.

   2007. "Roadblocks to Generic Access," http://lists.essential.org/pipermail/ip-health/2007-November/011977.html.

   2009. "How Diverted AIDS Funds Resulted in a Million AIDS Deaths and Threaten a Million More," http://lists.essential.org/pipermail/ip-health/ 2009-April/013670.html.

   2011. "Personal Communication," June 23.

Hadden, Jennifer. 2012. "Divided Advocacy Networks: Conflict and Competition in Global Climate Change Politics." Working Paper, University of Maryland.

Hafner, Tamara, and Jeremy Shiffman. 2012. "The Emergence of Global Attention to Health Systems Strengthening." *Health Policy and Planning* (March 8), http:// heapol.oxfordjournals.org/content/early/2012/03/07/heapol.czs023.

HAI (Health Action International). 1999a. *Provisional Agenda: Compulsory Licensing of Patents and Access to Essential Medicines and Medical Technologies*. Geneva, Switzerland, www.haiweb.org/news/licensing.prog.html.

   1999b. *Increasing Access to Essential Drugs in a Globalised Economy Working Towards Solutions*. Amsterdam, Holland, www.haiweb.org/campaign/ novseminar/progr_speakers.html.

Haines, Herbert H. 1995. *Black Radicals and the Civil Rights Mainstream, 1954–1970*. University of Tennessee Press.

Hall, Peter A., and David Soskice, eds. 2001. *Varieties of Capitalism: The Institutional Foundations of Comparative Advantage*. New York: Oxford University Press.

Hamied, Yusuf. 2012. "Interview," March 12.

Harrington, Mark. 2003. "Interview." ACT UP Oral History Project. MIX – The New York Lesbian & Gay Experimental Film Festival, www.actuporalhistory.org/interviews/images/harrington.pdf.

Hawkins, Darren G. 2002. "Human Rights Norms and Networks in Authoritarian Chile." In *Restructuring World Politics: Transnational Social Movements, Networks, and Norms*, Sanjeev Khagram, James V. Riker, and Kathryn Sikkink, eds., 47–70. 1st edn. Minneapolis: University of Minnesota Press.

David A. Lake, Daniel L. Nielson, and Michael J. Tierney. 2006. *Delegation and Agency in International Organizations*. Cambridge University Press.

Health GAP Coalition. 1999. "Meeting Minutes: HIV/AIDS Forum on Africa."

2001a. "Sign-On Letter," www.healthgap.org/press_releases/01/013101_HGAP_GLAXO_signon.html.

2001b. "Regarding the Global AIDS Fund Governance and Structure," www.healthgap.org/press_releases/01/050901_LTR_GWB_AIDS_FUND.html.

2003. "Trade, Intellectual Property Rights and Patents," www.healthgap.org/camp/ftaa.html.

2004a. "NGO Letter to the Office of the Global AIDS Initiative: 385 U.S. and International Organizations Call Upon U.S. 'to Ensure That Programs Use the Most Affordable Medicines Available, and Accept the Current Drug Quality Standards of World Health Organization's Drug Prequalification Program,' in a Letter to Randall Tobias, 26 March 2004," www.healthgap.org/press_releases/04/032604_INTL_LTR_PEPFAR_Tobias.html.

2004b. "Letter to The Honorable Dr. Manmohan Singh," www.healthgap.org/press_releases/04/121604_HGAP_LTR_India_patent.pdf.

2005. "Medicine Procurement of ARVs and Other Essential Medicines in the U.S. Global AIDS Program," www.healthgap.org/press_releases/05/1105_PWATCH_HGAP_BP_PROC.pdf.

2007. "Open Letter from Clinicians and Researchers to Mile White, Abbott CEO," www.healthgap.org/camp/abbott.html.

2008. "U.S. Civil Society Letter to Members of U.S. Congress on IMF Gold Sales and Scaling up Investments in Health and Education," www.healthgap.org/camp/documents/IMFgoldsalesletter.doc.

2009. "314 Organizations Sign on to Letter to G7 Finance Ministers on Global Fund Funding Gap," www.healthgap.org/gfatm/g7letter.htm.

Hellerstein, Rebecca. 2004. "Do Pharmaceutical Firms Price Discriminate Across Rich and Poor Countries? Evidence from Antiretroviral Drug Prices," www.ny.frb.org/research/economists/hellerstein/JDE2.pdf.

Hendrix, Cullen S., and Wendy Wong. 2012. "When is the Pen Truly Mighty? Regime Type and the Efficacy of Naming and Shaming in Curbing Human Rights Abuses." *British Journal of Political Science FirstView*: 1–22.

Herek, Gregory M., John P. Capitanio, and Keith F. Widaman. 2002. "HIV-related Stigma and Knowledge in the United States: Prevalence and Trends, 1991–1999." *American Journal of Public Health* 92 (3) (March): 371–7.

Hertel, Shareen. 2006. *Unexpected Power: Conflict and Change Among Transnational Activists*. Cornell Paperbacks. Ithaca, NY: Cornell University Press, www.loc.gov/catdir/toc/ecip0613/2006014455.html.

Heywood, Mark. 2009. "South Africa's Treatment Action Campaign: Combining Law and Social Mobilization to Realize the Right to Health." *Journal of Human Rights Practice* 1 (1) (March 1): 14–36.

Hirschler, Ben. 2003. "U.S. Says Ready to Use Generic Drugs in AIDS Fight," http://lists.essential.org/pipermail/ip-health/2003-July/005007.html.

——— 2011. "Gilead Kickstarts Patent Pool for AIDS Drugs." Reuters, July 12, www.reuters.com/article/2011/07/12/us-aids-patents-idUSTRE76B0YW20110712.

Hirshman, Linda. 2012. *Victory: The Triumphant Gay Revolution*. New York: HarperCollins.

HM Treasury. 2006. "The Stern Review on the Economics of Climate Change," www.hm-treasury.gov.uk/independent_reviews/stern_review_economics_climate_change/sternreview_index.cfm.

Ho, Shirley S., Dominique Brossard, and Dietram A. Scheufele. 2007. "The Polls—Trends Public Reactions to Global Health Threats and Infectious Diseases." *Public Opinion Quarterly* 71 (4) (December 21): 671–92.

Hoag, Hannah. 2011. "The Problems with Emissions Trading." *Nature* (November 25), www.nature.com/news/the-problems-with-emissions-trading-1.9491.

Hogan, Margaret C., Kyle J. Foreman, Mohsen Naghavi, Stephanie Y. Ahn, Mengru Wang, Susanna M. Makela, Alan D. Lopez, Rafael Lozano, and Christopher J. L. Murray. 2010. "Maternal Mortality for 181 Countries, 1980–2008: A Systematic Analysis of Progress Towards Millennium Development Goal 5." *The Lancet* 375 (9726) (May 8): 1609–23.

Holmes, Charles B., William Coggin, David Jamieson, Heidi Mihm, Reuben Granich, Phillip Savio, Michael Hope et al. 2011. "Use of Generic Antiretroviral Agents and Cost Savings in PEPFAR Treatment Programs." *Journal of the American Medical Association* 304 (3): 313–20.

IFPMA (International Federation of Pharmaceutical Manufacturers Associations). 2001. "Disputed South African Law Will Not Improve Access to Medicines," www.essentialdrugs.org/edrug/archive/200104/msg00069.php.

——— 2002. "International Federation of Pharmaceutical Manufacturers Associations (IFPMA)." www.iprcommission.org/text/Views%20Articles%20Text%20Versions/IFPMA_Article_text.htm.

Indian Express. 2011. "India to Phase Out HIV Drug as per WHO Guidelines," www.indianexpress.com/news/india-to-phase-out-hiv-drug-as-per-who-guide/792362/.

Indian Generics Firm Representative. 2012. "Interview," March 14.

Individual Members of the Faculty of Harvard University. 2001. "Consensus Statement on Antiretroviral Treatment for AIDS in Poor Countries." *Topics in HIV Medicine* 9 (2) (June): 14–26.

InPharma. 2012. "Ranbaxy Taken to Task by FDA over Manufacturing Woes | InPharm," www.inpharm.com/news/171155/ranbaxy-taken-task-fda-over-manufacturing-woes.

Institute of Medicine. 2005. *Scaling Up Treatment for the Global AIDS Pandemic: Challenges and Opportunities*. Washington DC: The National Academies Press.

Interview with Pharmaceutical Executive who Works on Drug Access Issues. 2012. March 14.

IRIN News. 2010a. "KENYA: Stavudine to Be Phased Out – Gradually," www.plusnews.org/report.aspx?ReportID=87392.

2010b. "HEALTH: Control vs Elimination – the Great Malaria Debate." *IRINnews*, www.irinnews.org/report.aspx?reportid=90938.

Ismail, M. Asif. 2006. "PEPFAR Policy Hinders Treatment in Generic Terms," http://projects.publicintegrity.org/aids/report.aspx?aid=836#1.

ITPC (International Treatment Preparedness Coalition). 2011. "Concerns About the Process, Principles of Medicines Patent Pool and the Licence." *PetitionBuzz*, www.petitionbuzz.com/petitions/mppunitaid.

Jack, Andrew. 2009. "Malaria Treatment Made Cheaper." *The Financial Times*, April 17, www.ft.com/intl/cms/s/0/ce4181c6–2b74–11de-b806–00144feabdc0.html#axzz27GN9pwlM.

Jack, William, and Jean O. Lanjouw. 2005. "Financing Pharmaceutical Innovation: How Much Should Poor Countries Contribute?" *The World Bank Economic Review* 19 (1): 45–67.

James, John S. 2012. "Interview," June 18.

Joachim, Jutta M. 2007. *Agenda Setting, the UN, and NGOs: Gender Violence and Reproductive Rights*. Washington DC: Georgetown University Press.

Johnson, Krista. 2006. "Framing AIDS Mobilization and Human Rights in Post-apartheid South Africa." *Perspectives on Politics* 4 (04): 663–70.

Juneja, Sandeep. 2012. "Interview," March 12–13.

Kaiser Family Foundation. 2005. "Survey of G7 Nations on HIV Spending in Developing Countries – Chartpack – Kaiser Family Foundation," www.kff.org/hivaids/7343.cfm.

2006. "OGAC's Abstinence, Faithfulness Requirements for PEPFAR Confusing, Undercutting Other HIV-Prevention Efforts, GAO Report Says." *Daily HIV/AIDS Report*, www.kaisernetwork.org/Daily_reports/rep_index.cfm?DR_ID=36429.

2011a. "The U.S. President's Emergency Plan for AIDS Relief (PEPFAR)," www.kff.org/globalhealth/upload/8002–03.pdf.

2011b. "Disbursements for Health and All Other ODA, 2002–2009 – Kaiser Slides," http://facts.kff.org/chart.aspx?ch=2301.

2011c. "Indian Government Rejects Abbott's Patent Application For Second-Line ARV," http://globalhealth.kff.org/Daily-Reports/2011/January/04/GH-010411-India-Patent-Application.aspx.

2012a. "2012 Survey of Americans on HIV/AIDS – Kaiser Family Foundation," www.kff.org/kaiserpolls/8334.cfm.

2012b. "HIV/AIDS at 30: A Public Opinion Perspective – Kaiser Family Foundation." Accessed August 3, www.kff.org/kaiserpolls/8186.cfm.

Kaiser Health News. 2008. *PEPFAR Suspends Funding for Three Ranbaxy AIDS Drugs Banned by FDA*, www.kaiserhealthnews.org/daily-reports/2008/september/26/dr00054691.aspx.

Kantor, Mickey. 2005. *U.S. Free Trade Agreements and the Public Health*. Law Firm of Mayer Brown Row & Maw, www.who.int/entity/intellectualproperty/submissions/US%20FTAs%20and%20the%20Public%20Health.pdf.

Kaplan, Karyn. 2002. "Interview With Paisan Tan-Ud." *Gay Men's Health Crisis*, www.thebody.com/content/art13346.html.

2012. "Interview," December 14.

Kapstein, Ethan B. 2001. "The Corporate Ethics Crusade." *Foreign Affairs*, September 1, www.foreignaffairs.com/articles/57242/ethan-b-kapstein/the-corporate-ethics-crusade.

2006a. *Economic Justice in an Unfair World: Toward a Level Playing Field*. Princeton University Press.

2006b. "The New Global Slave Trade." *Foreign Affairs*, November 1.

Katzenstein, Peter J., and Nobuo Okawara. 2001. "Japan, Asian-Pacific Security, and the Case for Analytical Eclecticism." *International Security* 26 (3): 153–85.

Kaufmann, Chaim D., and Robert A. Pape. 1999. "Explaining Costly International Moral Action: Britain's Sixty-year Campaign against the Atlantic Slave Trade." *International Organization* 53 (4): 631–68.

Keck, Margaret E., and Kathryn Sikkink. 1998. *Activists Beyond Borders: Advocacy in International Politics*. Ithaca, NY: Cornell University Press.

Kelland, Kate. 2011. "Malaria Eradication No Vague Aspiration, Says Gates." Reuters, October 19, www.reuters.com/article/2011/10/19/us-malaria-gates-eradication-idUSTRE79I06620111019.

Kennedy, Ted, John McCain, Russell Feingold, Dick Durbin, Olympia Snowe, and Lincoln Chafee. 2004. "Letter to President Bush," www.healthgap.org/press_releases/04/032604_SENATE_LTR_GWB_PEPFAR.pdf.

Keohane, Robert. 1982. "The Demand for International Regimes." *International Organization* 36 (2): 325–55.

and David G. Victor. 2010. "The Regime Complex for Climate Change," http://belfercenter.ksg.harvard.edu/files/Keohane_Victor_Final_2.pdf.

Kesic, Dragan. 2011. "Strategic Development Trends in the World Pharmaceutical Industry." *Managing Global Transitions* 9 (3): 207–23.

Kidder, Tracy. 2003. *Mountains Beyond Mountains: Healing the World: The Quest of Dr. Paul Farmer*. 1st edn. New York: Random House.

Kim, Jim Yong, and Arthur Ammann. 2004. "Is the '3 by 5' Initiative the Best Approach to Tackling the HIV Pandemic?" *PLoS Med* 1 (2) (November 30): e37.

King, Brayden. 2008. "A Social Movement Perspective of Stakeholder Collective Action and Influence." *Business & Society* 47 (1) (March 1): 21–49.

King, Brayden G., and Nicholas A. Pearce. 2010. "The Contentiousness of Markets: Politics, Social Movements, and Institutional Change in Markets." *Annual Review of Sociology* 36 (1): 249–67.

King, Brayden G., and Sarah A. Soule. 2007. "Social Movements as Extra-Institutional Entrepreneurs: The Effect of Protests on Stock Price Returns." *Administrative Science Quarterly* 52 (3): 413–42.

Klotz, Audie. 1999. *Norms in International Relations: The Struggle Against Apartheid.* Ithaca, NY: Cornell University Press.

Knight, Lindsay. 2008. *UNAIDS: The First Ten Years.* UNAIDS, http://data. unaids.org/pub/Report/2008/JC1579_First_10_years_en.pdf.

Knox, Richard. 2012. "'Treatment As Prevention' Rises As Cry In HIV Fight." NPR, www.npr.org/2012/07/12/156603776/treatment-as-prevention-rises-as-cry-in-hiv-fight.

Koppell, Jonathan G. S. 2010. *World Rule: Accountability, Legitimacy, and the Design of Global Governance.* University of Chicago Press.

Koremenos, Barbara, Charles Lipson, and Duncan Snidal. 2001. "The Rational Design of International Institutions." *International Organization* 55 (4): 761–99.

Kramer, Larry. 2003. "ACT UP Oral History Project." A Program of Mix – The New York Lesbian & Gay Experimental Film Festival, www. actuporalhistory.org/interviews/images/kramer.pdf.

2012. "Happy Birthday, ACT UP, Wherever You Are." *Huffington Post,* www. huffingtonpost.com/larry-kramer/act-up_b_1382314.html.

Krauss, Kate. 2012. "Interview," May 29.

Krebs, Ronald, and Patrick Jackson. 2007. "Twisting Tongues and Twisting Arms: The Power of Political Rhetoric." *European Journal of International Relations* 13 (1): 35–66.

Kulkarni, Shefali S. 2011. "States Cut Back Efforts to Provide Drugs for HIV, AIDS." *The Washington Post,* May 23, www.washingtonpost.com/national/health/states-cut-back-efforts-to-provide-drugs-for-hiv-aids/2011/05/20/AFYGRK9G_story.html.

La Guardia, Anton, and Toby Hamden. 2001. "Bush Defies Europe over Pollution: US Rejects Kyoto as 'It Makes No Sense'." *The Daily Telegraph,* March 30.

Lancet, The. 2004. "The Important World of Drug Prequalification." 364 (9448): 1830.

Lanjouw, Jean O. 2003. "Intellectual Property and the Availability of Pharmaceuticals in Poor Countries." *Innovation Policy and the Economy* 3 (January 1): 91–129, doi:10.2307/25056154.

Laurent, Christian, Charles Kouanfack, Sinata Koulla-Shiro, Nathalie Nkoué, Anke Bourgeois, Alexandra Calmy, Bernadette Lactuock *et al.* 2004. "Effectiveness and Safety of a Generic Fixed-dose Combination of Nevirapine, Stavudine, and Lamivudine in HIV-1-infected Adults in Cameroon: Open-label Multicentre Trial." *The Lancet* 364 (9428): 29–34.

Laxminarayan, Ramanan, Elli Klein, and David Smith. 2008. *Impact of Malaria Controls on ACTS Demand.* World Bank, http://siteresources.worldbank.org/HEALTHNUTRITIONANDPOPULATION/Resources/281627–1095698140167/LaxminarayanMalariaControlACTs.pdf.

Lefkowitz, Jay. 2009. "AIDS and the President – An Inside Account." Commentary, www.commentarymagazine.com/viewarticle.cfm/aids-and-the-president–an-inside-account-14057.

Legro, Jeffrey W. 2005. *Rethinking The World: Great Power Strategies and International Order.* Ithaca, NY: Cornell University Press.

Levey, Bob. 2003. "Q&A with Bob Levey: Interview with Paul Zeitz." *The Washington Post*, April 15, www.washingtonpost.com/wp-srv/liveonline/03/regular/metro/levey/r_metro_levey041603.htm.

Lewin, Tamar. 2012. "Harvard and M.I.T. Offer Free Online Courses." *The New York Times*, May 2, sec. Education, www.nytimes.com/2012/05/03/education/harvard-and-mit-team-up-to-offer-free-online-courses.html.

Lieberman, Evan S. 2009. *Boundaries of Contagion: How Ethnic Politics Have Shaped Government Responses to AIDS.* 1st edn. Princeton University Press.

Lilongwe Times. 2010. "W.H.O. Launches New ART Guidelines," www.lilongwetimes.com/life-style/health/391-who-launches-new-art-guidelines.

Lindsey, Daryl. 2001. "The AIDS-drug Warrior." *Salon,* www.salon.com/2001/06/18/love_9/.

Lite, Jordan. 2008. "What Is Artemisinin?: Scientific American." *Scientific American,* www.scientificamerican.com/article.cfm?id=artemisinin-coartem-malaria-novartis.

Litsios, Socrates. 2002. "Malaria Control and the Future of International Public Health." In *Contextual Determinants of Malaria*, Elizabeth A. Casman and Hadi Dowlatabadi, eds., 292–330. Washington DC: Resources for the Future.

Liu, Deborah, and Soon Jim Lim. 2003. *GlaxoSmithKline and AIDS Drug Policy.* Stanford Graduate School of Business.

Love, James. 1999a. "AIDS Activists Circulate Sign-on Letter on African Trade Bills," http://lists.essential.org/pharm-policy/msg00027.html.

  1999b. "BMS Press Briefing on HIV/Africa Initiative," http://lists.essential.org/pharm-policy/msg00074.html.

  2001a. "Comment on Attaran/Gillespie-White and PhRMA Patent Surveys," http://lists.essential.org/pipermail/ip-health/2001-October/002097.html.

  2001b. "Affidavit of James Packard Love." CPTech.

  2003. "Interview (Extended Interview from the Film, *Pills Profits Protest*, directed by Anne-christine d'Adesky and Ann T. Rossetti)."

  2007. "Recent Examples of the Use of Compulsory Licenses on Patents." Knowledge Ecology International, www.keionline.org/misc-docs/recent_cls_8mar07.pdf.

  2009. "Personal Communication," December 4.

  2011. "KEI Comments on the ITPC Letter to the Medicines Patent Pool Foundation and UNITAID," http://keionline.org/node/1294.

Lozano, Rafael, Haidong Wang, Kyle J. Foreman, Julie Knoll Rajaratnam, Mohsen Naghavi, Jake R. Marcus, Laura Dwyer-Lindgren, *et al.* 2011. "Progress Towards Millennium Development Goals 4 and 5 on Maternal and Child Mortality: An Updated Systematic Analysis." *The Lancet* 378 (9797) (September 24): 1139–65.

Lucchini, Stéphane, Boubou Cisse, Ségolène Duran, Marie de Cenival, Caroline Comiti, Marion Gaudry, and Jean-Paul Moatti. 2003. "Decrease in Prices of Antiretroviral Drugs for Developing Countries: From Political 'Philanthropy' to Regulated Markets?" In *Economics of AIDS and Access to HIV/AIDS Care in Developing Countries: Issues and Challenges*, Jean-Paul Moatti, Benjamin Coriat, Yves Souteyrand, Tony Barnett, Jérôme

Dumoulin, and Yves-Antoine Flori, eds., 169–212. Paris: Collection Sciences Sociales et Sida.

Luders, Joseph. 2006. "The Economics of Movement Success: Business Responses to Civil Rights Mobilization." *American Journal of Sociology* 111 (4) (January 1): 963–98.

Lueck, Sarah. 2004a. "White House Gets Pressure on AIDS Plan: Activists, Drug Firms Duel Over Use of Funds For Generic Combination Drugs in Africa." *The Wall Street Journal*, www.aegis.org/news/wsj/2004/WJ040306.htm.

2004b. "White House Aims To Answer Critics Of Its AIDS Fight," http://lists. essential.org/pipermail/ip-health/2004-April/006332.html.

Maenza, J., and C. Flexner. 1998. "Combination Antiretroviral Therapy for HIV Infection." *American Family Physician* 57 (11) (June): 2789–98.

Magaziner, Ira. 2004. "Conference: Provoking Hope: A Brown University HIV/AIDS Symposium: Keynote April 24, 2004," www.kaisernetwork.org/health_cast/ uploaded_files/042404_brown_keynote.pdf.

2012. "Interview," February 24.

Majumdar, Bappa. 2009. "India Patent Rejections Welcomed by HIV/AIDS Groups," www.reuters.com/article/2009/09/09/us-india-hiv-drugs-idUSTRE5881G420090909.

Malaria No More. Undated. *Who We Are*, www.malarianomore.org/who-we-are.

Malkin, Elisabeth. 2006. "At World Forum, Support Erodes for Private Management of Water." *The New York Times*, March 20, sec. International/Americas, www. nytimes.com/2006/03/20/international/americas/20water.html.

Mann, Jonathan M. 1996. "Health and Human Rights." *BMJ: British Medical Journal* 312 (7036) (April 13): 924–5.

1999. *Health and Human Rights: A Reader*. New York: Taylor & Francis.

Lawrence Gostin, Sofia Gruskin, Troyen Brennan, and Zita Lazzarini. 1994. "Health and Human Rights." *Health and Human Rights* 1 (1): 6–23.

Marks, S. P. 2001. "Jonathan Mann's Legacy to the 21st Century: The Human Rights Imperative for Public Health." *The Journal of Law, Medicine & Ethics: a Journal of the American Society of Law, Medicine & Ethics* 29 (2): 131–8.

Martin, Jerome. 2011. "First Thoughts on the Petition to the Medicines Patent Pool Foundation," http://lists.keionline.org/pipermail/ip-health_lists. keionline.org/2011-October/001393.html.

Martin, Stephen. 2000. "The Theory of Contestable Markets." Lafayette, IN: Dept. of Economics, Purdue University.

Marx, Karl. 1978. *Das Kapital*. London: Penguin Press Edition.

Matthews, Duncan. 2011. *Intellectual Property, Human Rights and Development: The Role of NGOs and Social Movements*. Cheltenham: Edward Elgar Publishing.

Maxmen, Amy. 2012. "Malaria Subsidy Pilot Soars, but Some See Turbulence Ahead." *Nature Medicine* 18 (5): 634–5.

McAdam, Doug, John D. McCarthy, and Mayer N. Zald. 1996. *Comparative Perspectives on Social Movements: Political Opportunities, Mobilizing Structures, and Cultural Framings*. Cambridge University Press.

McCright, Aaron M., and Riley E. Dunlap. 2011. "Cool Dudes: The Denial of Climate Change Among Conservative White Males in the United States." *Global Environmental Change* 21: 1163–7.

McDonnell, Margaret Reilly. 2007. *Case Study of the Campaigns Leading to The President's Emergency Plan for AIDS Relief*. U.S. Coalition for Child Survival, www.child-survival.org/downloads/toolkit/Case-PEPFAR.pdf.

McLean, Bethany. 2006. "The Power of Philanthropy," http://money.cnn.com/magazines/fortune/fortune_archive/2006/09/18/8386185/index.htm.

McNeil Jr., Donald G. 2001. "Indian Company Offers to Supply AIDS Drugs at Low Cost in Africa – New York Times." *The New York Times*, February 6, www.nytimes.com/2001/02/07/world/indian-company-offers-to-supply-aids-drugs-at-low-cost-in-africa.html?pagewanted=all&src=pm.

2002. "New List of Safe AIDS Drugs, Despite Industry Lobby," *The New York Times*, March 20, http://www.nytimes.com/2002/03/21/world/new-list-of-safe-aids-drugs-despite-industry-lobby.html.

2005. "A Path to Cheaper AIDS Drugs for Poor Nations," *The New York Times*, January 26, www.nytimes.com/2005/01/26/health/26aids.html.

2010. "Global Fight Against AIDS Reports Failure at Fund-Raising." *The New York Times*, October 5, www.nytimes.com/2010/10/06/world/africa/06aids.html.

2011. "Gilead to Share 4 AIDS and Hepatitis Drugs With Patent Pool." *The New York Times*, July 12, www.nytimes.com/2011/07/12/health/12global.html.

2012a. "Global Fund's Executive Director Steps Down." *The New York Times*, January 24, www.nytimes.com/2012/01/25/health/global-funds-executive-director-steps-down.html.

2012b. "Change Rattles Leading Health-Funding Agency." *The New York Times*, November 15, sec. Health, www.nytimes.com/2012/11/16/health/change-rattles-leading-health-funding-agency.html.

Mearsheimer, John J. 1994. "The False Promise of International Institutions." *International Security* 19 (3): 5–49.

Medicines for Malaria Venture. 2012. *MMV at a Glance*, www.mmv.org/newsroom/publications/mmv-glance.

Messac, Luke. 2008. *Lazarus at America's Doorstep: Elites and Framing in Federal Appropriations for Global AIDS Relief*. Cambridge, MA: Harvard University Press.

Milano, Mark. 2007. "Interview." ACT UP Oral History Project. MIX – The New York Lesbian & Gay Experimental Film Festival, www.actuporalhistory.org/interviews/images/milano.pdf.

2012. "Interview," July 14.

Miller, Candace M., Mpefe Ketlhapile, Heather Rybasack-Smith, and Sydney Rosen. 2010. "Why Are Antiretroviral Treatment Patients Lost to Follow-up? A Qualitative Study from South Africa." *Tropical Medicine & International Health* 15: 48–54.

Ministry of Foreign Affairs of Japan. 2000. *Japan's Initiative in the Fight Against Infectious and Parasitic Diseases on the Occasion of the Kyushu-Okinawa G8 Summit ("Okinawa ID (Infectious Diseases) Initiative")*, www.mofa.go.jp/policy/oda/summit/infection.html.

Morin, Jean-Frederic. 2006. "Tripping up TRIPS Debates IP and Health in Bilateral Agreements." *International Journal of Intellectual Property Management* 1 (1–2): 37–53.

MSF (Médecin Sans Frontières). 1999. "People With Aids Are Dying Because of Lack of Access To Life-Saving Drugs," www.msfaccess.org/resources/press-releases/445.

2000a. "MSF Calls On Davos Leaders To Stop People Dying of Market Failure – Business CEOs & Politicians Must Take Action To Restart R&D," www.msfaccess.org/resources/press-releases/454.

2000b. *MSF Statement on New UNAIDS Proposal and Clinton's Executive Order on Access to HIV/AIDS Medicines*, www.doctorswithoutborders.org/press/release_print.cfm?id=598.

2000c. "MSF Calls for Replication and Expansion of Successful Efforts to Reduce AIDS Drug Prices," www.msfaccess.org/resources/press-releases/437.

2011. "TRIPS, TRIPS Plus and Doha." *MSF Access Campaign*, http://msfaccess.org/our-work/overcoming-barriers-access/article/1363.

Mukherjee, Rupali. 2011. "AIDS Drug Patents by Abbot, BMS Rejected." *The Times Of India*, January 13, http://articles.timesofindia.indiatimes.com/2011–01–13/india-business/28379392_1_leena-menghaney-ritonavir-patent-applications.

Mukherjee, Siddhartha. 2010. *The Emperor of All Maladies: A Biography of Cancer.* Reprint. New York: Simon & Schuster.

Nadelmann, Ethan A. 1990. "Global Prohibition Regimes: The Evolution of Norms in International Society." *International Organization* 44 (04): 479–526.

NASTAD. 2011. *ADAPs with Waiting Lists (9,066 Individuals in 11 States*, as of September 8, 2011)*, www.nastad.org/Docs/094006_ADAP%20Watch%20update%20-%209.9.11.pdf.

2012. *ADAPs with Waiting Lists (2,030 Individuals in 9 States*, as of July 12, 2012)*, www.nastad.org/Docs/095939_ADAP%20Watch%20update%20-%207.16.12.pdf.

Nesmith, Jeff. 2004. "Anti-AIDS Coalition Scolds U.S. White House's Refusal to Back Cheap Drugs Irks Group," http://lists.essential.org/pipermail/ip-health/2004-April/006211.html.

Netherlands Environmental Assessment Agency. 2012. *Total GHG Emissions (CO_2, CH_4, N_2O, HFCs, PFCs, SF_6) in 1990, 2000, 2005 and 2008*, http://edgar.jrc.ec.europa.eu/overview.php.

New, William. 2012. *Johnson & Johnson Denies Patent Pool Licences For HIV Medicines For The Poor. IP-Watch*, www.ip-watch.org/2012/01/12/johnson-johnson-denies-patent-pool-licences-for-hiv-medicines-for-the-poor/.

New York Times, The. 1989. "AZT's Inhuman Cost – New York Times." *New York Times*, August 27, www.nytimes.com/1989/08/28/opinion/azt-s-inhuman-cost.html.

2005. "How Not to Roll Back Malaria," October 16, www.nytimes.com/2005/10/16/opinion/16sun1.html.

Nexon, Dan. 2012. "The Duck of Minerva: Open Access and IR Journals." *The Duck of Minerva*, http://duckofminerva.blogspot.com/2012/06/open-access.html.

Nguyen-Krug, Helena, and Hans V. Hogerzeil. 2006. "Human Rights: A Potentially Powerful Force for Essential Medicines." *Bulletin of the World Health Organization* 84 (5): 410–1.

Nicolaou, Stavros. 2012. "Interview," April 3.

Nordhaus, William. 2006. "The Stern Review on the Economics of Climate Change," www.econ.yale.edu/~nordhaus/homepage/SternReviewD2.pdf.

North, Douglass Cecil. 1990. *Institutions, Institutional Change, and Economic Performance: The Political Economy of Institutions and Decisions*. Cambridge, New York: Cambridge University Press.

Nunn, Amy. 2008. *The Politics and History of AIDS Treatment in Brazil*. New York: Springer.

O'Rourke, Dara. 2005. "Market Movements: Nongovernmental Organization Strategies to Influence Global Production and Consumption." *Journal of Industrial Ecology* 9 (1–2): 115–28.

Obelisk Seven Blog. 2010. "Global Warming: The Frameworks Institute on Why the Deniers Are Winning the Argument," http://obeliskseven.blogspot.com/2010/11/global-warming-frameworks-institute-on.html.

Odell, John S., and Susan Sell. 2006. "Reframing the Issue: The WTO Coalition on Intellectual Property and Public Health, 2001." In *Negotiating Trade: Developing Countries in the WTO and NAFTA*, ed. John S. Odell. Cambridge University Press.

OECD (Organization for Economic Cooperation and Development). 2008. "Pharmaceutical Pricing Policies in a Global Market," www.oecd.org/health/pharmaceuticalpricingpoliciesinaglobalmarket.htm.

Office of the U.S. Global AIDS Coordinator. 2007. "The Power of Partnerships: The President's Emergency Plan for AIDS Relief Third Annual Report to Congress," www.pepfar.gov/press/c21604.htm.

    2008. "The Power of Partnerships: The U.S. President's Emergency Plan for AIDS Relief," www.pepfar.gov/documents/organization/100029.pdf.

    2010. "Saving Lives Through Smart Investments: Latest PEPFAR Results," www.pepfar.gov/documents/organization/153723.pdf.

    2012. *Report on Costs of Treatment in the President's Emergency Plan for AIDS Relief (PEPFAR)*, www.pepfar.gov/documents/organization/188493.pdf.

Oliver, J. Eric, and Taeku Lee. 2005. "Public Opinion and the Politics of Obesity in America." *Journal of Health Politics, Policy and Law* 30 (5) (October 1): 923–54.

ONE. 2007. "ONE Campaign and DATA to Merge, Creating World Class Advocacy Organization to Fight Extreme Poverty," www.one.org/c/us/pressrelease/123/.

Orbinski, James. 1999. "Nobel Lecture" December 10, Oslo, Norway, www.nobelprize.org/nobel_prizes/peace/laureates/1999/msf-lecture.html.

Over, Mead. 2008. "Prevention Failure: The Ballooning Entitlement Burden of U.S. Global AIDS Treatment Spending and What to Do About It – Working Paper 144," www.cgdev.org/content/publications/detail/15973/.

    2011. *Achieving an AIDS Transition: Preventing Infections to Sustain Treatment*. 1st edn. Washington DC: Center for Global Development.

Oxfam. 2001. *Cut the Cost: How World Trade Rules Threaten the Health of Poor People*. Oxfam.

    2011. *Oxfam Reaction to Global Partnership for Education Donor Commitments Pledged Today*, www.oxfam.org/en/pressroom/reactions/global-partnership-education-donor-commitments.

Payne, Keith. 2010. "Why Is the Death of One Million a Statistic?" www. psychologytoday.com/blog/life-autopilot/201003/why-is-the-death-one-million-statistic.

Payne, Rodger A. 2001. "Persuasion, Frames and Norm Construction." *European Journal of International Relations* 7 (1): 37–61.

PBS Frontline. 2010. "The Spill." *FRONTLINE,* www.pbs.org/wgbh/pages/frontline/the-spill/.

2012a. "People Living with AIDS," www.facebook.com/photo.php?fbid=10150925611491641&set=a.491930816640.259623.45168721640&type=1&theater.

2012b. "Race and America's HIV Epidemic – ENDGAME: AIDS in Black America – FRONTLINE," *FRONTLINE,* www.pbs.org/wgbh/pages/frontline/endgame-aids-in-black-america/.

Pearl, Daniel, and Alix Freedman. 2001. "Altruism, Politics and Bottom Line Intersect at Indian Generics Firm." *Wall Street Journal,* March 12, www.aegis.com/news/wsj/2001/WJ010308.html.

Pécoul, Bernard. 2012. "Interview," May 10.

Perez-Casas, Carmen. 2011. "Personal Communication."

Perriëns, Joseph. 2010. "Personal Communication."

Pew Research Center. 2012. "The American-Western European Values Gap." *Pew Global Attitudes Project,* www.pewglobal.org/2011/11/17/the-american-western-european-values-gap/.

Pfeifer, Lauren. 2011. "New Name, New Start: The Global Partnership for Education." *ONE Campaign,* www.one.org/blog/2011/09/21/new-name-new-start-the-global-partnership-for-education/.

Philipson, Tomas J., and Anupam B. Jena. 2005. *Who Benefits from New Medical Technologies? Estimates of Consumer and Producer Surpluses for HIV/AIDS Drugs.* NBER Working Paper. National Bureau of Economic Research, Inc, http://ideas.repec.org/p/nbr/nberwo/11810.html.

Physicians for Human Rights. 2005. *Statement for Group of 8 Meeting in July 2005: Health Workforces Must Be Supported to Achieve the Millennium Development Goals,* www.healthgap.org/press_releases/05/0705_PHR_INTL_LTR_G8_HCW.pdf.

Pianin, Eric. 2001. "EPA Chief Lobbied on Warming Before Bush's Emissions Switch: Memo Details Whitman's Plea for Presidential Commitment." *Washington Post,* March 27.

Piot, Peter. 2009. "Interview," January 28.

2012. *No Time to Lose: A Life in Pursuit of Deadly Viruses.* 1st edn. New York, London: W. W. Norton & Company.

Pitt, Catherine, Giulia Greco, Timothy Powell-Jackson, and Anne Mills. 2010. "Countdown to 2015: Assessment of Official Development Assistance to Maternal, Newborn, and Child Health, 2003–08." *The Lancet* 376 (9751) (October 30): 1485–96.

PLoS Medicine Editors, The. 2009. "Time for a 'Third Wave' of Malaria Activism to Tackle the Drug Stock-out Crisis." *PLoS Med* 6 (11) (November 24): e1000188.

Plumley, Ben. 2010. "Personal Communication," July 9.

Pogge, Thomas W. 2005. "Human Rights and Global Health: A Research Program." *Metaphilosophy* 36 (1–2): 182–209.

Polanyi, Karl. 1944. *The Great Transformation: The Political and Economic Origins of Our Time*. 2nd edn. Boston: Beacon Press.

Pollack, Andrew. 2012. "F.D.A. Approves Once-a-Day Pill for H.I.V." *The New York Times*, August 27, sec. Business Day, www.nytimes.com/2012/08/28/business/fda-approves-once-a-day-pill-for-hiv.html.

Population Action International. 2008. "U.S. HIV/AIDS and Family Planning/Reproductive Health Assistance: A Growing Disparity within PEPFAR Focus Countries," http://209.68.15.158/Issues/U.S._Policies_and_Funding/FPRH/fprh.pdf./

Porter, Michael E. 1980. *Competitive Strategy: Techniques for Analyzing Industries and Competitors*. 1st edn. New York: Free Press.
   2008. "The Five Competitive Forces That Shape Strategy." *Harvard Business Review*, January.

Provost, Claire. 2012. "World Water Forum Declaration Falls Short on Human Rights, Claim Experts." *The Guardian*, www.guardian.co.uk/global-development/2012/mar/14/world-water-forum-declaration-human-rights.

Quick, Jonathan D., and Eric Olawolu Moore. 2010. "Global Access to Essential Medicines." In *Routledge Handbook of Global Public Health*, Richard Parker and Marni Sommer, eds., 421–32. Abingdon, NY: Routledge.

Ragavan, Srividhya. 2004. "The Jekyll and Hyde Story of International Trade: The Supreme Court in PhRMA v. Walsh and the TRIPs Agreement." *University of Richmond Law Review* 38 (4): 777–838.

Rao, Hayagreeva. 2008. *Market Rebels: How Activists Make or Break Radical Innovations*. Princeton University Press.

Rauch, Jonathan. 2007. "This Is Not Charity," www.theatlantic.com/magazine/archive/2007/10/-ldquo-this-is-not-charity-rdquo/6197/.

Rawls, John. 1999. *A Theory of Justice*. Rev. edn. Cambridge, MA: Belknap Press of Harvard University Press.

Reich, Michael R. 1987. "Essential Drugs: Economics and Politics in International Health." *Health Policy* 8 (1) (August): 39–57.
   and R. Govindaraj. 1998. "Dilemmas in Drug Development for Tropical Diseases. Experiences with Praziquantel." *Health Policy (Amsterdam, Netherlands)* 44 (1) (April): 1–18.

ReliefWeb. 2012. *Global Fund-led Initiative Slashes Cost of anti-Malaria Medicines in Many African Countries*, http://reliefweb.int/report/world/global-fund-led-initiative-slashes-cost-anti-malaria-medicines-many-african-countries.

RESULTS. 2012. "Asking Another Advocate to Write About the World Bank's Broken Promise on Global Education." *RESULTS*, www.results.org/take_action/global_laser_talk_september_2012/.

Reuters. 2012a. "Lawsuit Between Google, Authors in U.S. Suspended Pending Appeal." *Yahoo! News*, http://news.yahoo.com/lawsuit-between-google-authors-u-suspended-pending-appeal-170438010–sector.html.
   2012b. "GlaxoSmithKline to Reveal More Drug Secrets." *The New York Times*, October 11, www.nytimes.com/reuters/2012/10/11/business/11reuters-glaxosmithkline-data.html.

Revkin, Andrew. 2012. "A Story Exposes How the Chinese Government Is Fueling Elephant Slaughter." *Dot Earth Blog*, http://dotearth.blogs.nytimes.com/2012/09/14/a-report-exposes-how-the-chinese-government-is-fueling-elephant-slaughter/.

Rice, Condoleezza. 2011. *No Higher Honor: A Memoir of My Years in Washington.* Random House Digital, Inc.

Rick Warren News. 2008. "President George W. Bush Receives 'International Medla of Peace' That Coincides with PEPFAR Milestone on World AIDS Day". www.rickwarrennews.com/081201_forum.htm.

Ripin, David. 2012. "Interview," January 24.

Risse, Thomas, Stephen C. Ropp, and Kathryn Sikkink. 1999. *The Power of Human Rights: International Norms and Domestic Change.* Cambridge University Press.

Rodrik, Dani. 2002. *Feasible Globalizations.* Working Paper. National Bureau of Economic Research, www.nber.org/papers/w9129.

Roemer-Mahler, Anne. 2010a. "Business Strategy and Access to Medicines in Developing Countries." *Global Health Governance* 4 (1): 1–14.

2010b. "Business Conflict and Global Politics: The Pharmaceutical Industry and the Global Governance of Intellectual Property." *Review of International Political Economy* 20 (1): 121–52.

Rosenberg, Tina. 2001. "Look at Brazil." *The New York Times,* www.nytimes.com/2001/01/28/magazine/look-at-brazil.html?pagewanted=all&src=pm.

Ruger, Jennifer Prah, and Derek Yach. 2008. "The Global Role of the World Health Organization." *Global Health Governance* 2 (2): 1–11.

Russell, Asia. 2012. "Interview," June 26.

Rustin, Bayard. 1964. "From Protest to Politics: The Future of the Civil Rights Movement Commentary Magazine," www.commentarymagazine.com/article/from-protest-to-politics-the-future-of-the-civil-rights-movement/.

Saad, Lydia. 2009. "Increased Number Think Global Warming is 'Exaggerated'," www.gallup.com/poll/116590/Increased-Number-Think-Global-Warming-Exaggerated.aspx.

Saba, Joseph. 1998. *Drug Access Initiative.* UNAIDS.

Sabot, Oliver, Justin M. Cohen, Michelle S. Hsiang, James G. Kahn, Suprotik Basu, Linhua Tang, Bin Zheng *et al.* 2010. "Costs and Financial Feasibility of Malaria Elimination." *The Lancet* 376 (9752) (November): 1604–15.

Sack, Kevin. 2010. "Economy Wreaks Havoc on Federal AIDS Drug Program." *The New York Times,* June 30, www.nytimes.com/2010/07/01/us/01aidsdrugs.html.

Samb, Badara. 2010. "Interview," September 13.

Saunders, Dudley. 2003. "Interview." ACT UP Oral History Project. MIX – The New York Lesbian & Gay Experimental Film Festival, www.actuporalhistory.org/interviews/images/saunders.pdf.

Sawyer, Eric. 1996. "Remarks at Opening Ceremony," AIDS Conference Vancouver, Canada, http://www.actupny.org/Vancouver/sawyerspeech.html.

2002. "An ACT UP founder 'acts up' for Africa's access to AIDS." In *From ACT UP to the WTO: Urban Protest and Community Building in the Era of Globalization,* ed. Benjamin Heim Shepard, 88–102. London, New York: Verso.

2004. "Interview." ACT UP Oral History Project. MIX – The New York Lesbian & Gay Experimental Film Festival. http://www.actuporalhistory.org/interviews/images/sawyer.pdf.

2012. "Interview," July 10.

Schelling, Thomas. 1960. *The Strategy of Conflict.* Cambridge, MA: Harvard University Press.

Scherer, F. M. 1993. "Pricing, Profits, and Technological Progress in the Pharmaceutical Industry." *Journal of Economic Perspectives* 7 (3): 97–115.

and Jayashree Watal. 2002. "Post-TRIPS Options for Access to Patented Medicines in Developing Nations." *Journal of International Economic Law* 5 (4) (December 1): 913–39.

Schocken, Celina. Undated. "Overview of the Global Fund to Fight AIDS, Tuberculosis and Malaria," www.cgdev.org/section/initiatives/_active/hivmonitor/funding/gf_overview.

Schoofs, Mark. 2003. "Clinton Program Would Help Poor Nations Get AIDS Drugs," www.aegis.com/news/wsj/2003/WJ031008.html.

2011. "Researchers Manipulate Drug's Chemistry in Bid to Lower Treatment Cost." *The Wall Street Journal*, May 13, http://online.wsj.com/article/SB10001424052748703730804576319480990825422.html.

Schurman, Rachel. 2004. "Fighting 'Frankenfoods': Industry Opportunity Structures and the Efficacy of the Anti-Biotech Movement in Western Europe." *Social Problems* 51 (2) (May 1): 243–68.

Schwartländer, Bernhard, Ian Grubb, and Jos Perriëns. 2006. "The 10-year Struggle to Provide Antiretroviral Treatment to People with HIV in the Developing World." *The Lancet* 368 (9534): 541–6.

Schweitzer, Stuart O. 2006. *Pharmaceutical Economics and Policy.* 2nd edn. Oxford University Press.

SCMS (Supply Chain Management System). Undated. "FAQ" http://scms.pfscm.org/scms/about/faq.

Scouflaire, Sophie-Marie, Cécile Macé, and Daniel Berman. 2003. *Surmounting Challenges: Procurement of Antiretroviral Medicines in Low- and Middle-income Countries: The Experience of Médecins Sans Frontières.* Geneva: WHO.

Sealy, Geraldine. 2005. "An Epidemic Failure." *Rolling Stone*, June 2, http://web.archive.org/web/20060511000548/http://www.rollingstone.com/politics/story/7371950/an_epidemic_failure.

Sell, Susan K. 2001. "TRIPS and the Access to Medicines Campaign." *Wisconsin International Law Journal* 20: 481–522.

and Aseem Prakash. 2004. "Using Ideas Strategically: The Contest Between Business and NGO Networks in Intellectual Property Rights." *International Studies Quarterly* 48 (1): 143–75.

Seuba, Xavier. 2006. "A Human Rights Approach to the WHO Model List of Essential Medicines." *Bulletin of the World Health Organization* 84 (5): 405–6.

Shadlen, Kenneth C. 2007. "The Political Economy of AIDS Treatment: Intellectual Property and the Transformation of Generic Supply." *International Studies Quarterly* 51 (3): 559–81.

2009. "The Politics of Patents and Drugs in Brazil and Mexico: The Industrial Bases of Health Policies." *Comparative Politics* 42 (1): 41–58. doi:10.5129/001041509X12911362972791.

Samira Guennif, Alenka Guzman, and N. Lalitha. 2012. *Intellectual Property, Pharmaceuticals, and Public Health: Access to Drugs in Developing Countries.* Kenneth C. Shadlen, Samira Guennif, Alenka Guzman, and N. Lalitha, eds. Cheltenham: Edward Elgar Publishing.

Shiffman, Jeremy. 2006. "HIV/AIDS and the Rest of the Global Health Agenda." *The Lancet* 84 (12): 923.

2008. "Has Donor Prioritization of HIV/AIDS Displaced Aid for Other Health Issues?" *Health Policy and Planning* 23 (2) (March 1): 95–100.

2009. "A Social Explanation for the Rise and Fall of Global Health Issues." *Bulletin of the World Health Organization* 87 (8) (August 1): 608–13.

2010. "Issue Attention in Global Health: The Case of Newborn Survival." *The Lancet* 375 (9730) (June): 2045–9.

Shiffman, Jeremy, and Kathryn Quissell. 2012. "Family Planning: a Political Issue." *The Lancet* 380 (9837) (July 14): 181–5.

Shiffman, Jeremy, and Stephanie Smith. 2007. "Generation of Political Priority for Global Health Initiatives: A Framework and Case Study of Maternal Mortality." *The Lancet* 370 (9595): 1370–9.

Sikkink, Kathryn. 1986. "Codes of Conduct for Transnational Corporations: The Case of the WHO/UNICEF Code." *International Organization* 40 (4) (October 1): 815–40.

Singhal, Arvind, and Everett M. Rogers. 2003. *Combating AIDS: Communication Strategies in Action*. New Delhi: Sage.

Slaughter, Anne-Marie. 2004. *A New World Order*. Princeton University Press.

Smith, N. Craig. 1990. *Morality and the Market: Consumer Pressure from Corporate Accountability*. 1st edn. London: Routledge.

and Anne Duncan. 2005. "GlaxoSmithKline and Developing Country Access to Essential Medicines (A)." *Journal of Business Ethics Education* 2 (1): 97–122.

Smith, N. Craig, and John A. Quelch. 1996. *Ethics in Marketing*. Homewood, IL: Richard D Irwin.

Smith, Raymond A., and Patricia A. Siplon. 2006. *Drugs into Bodies: Global AIDS Treatment Activism*. Westport, CT: Praeger.

Somberg, John C. 2006. "The Pharmaceutical Revolution: Drug Discovery and Development." In *The Process of New Drug Discovery and Development*, Charles Smith and James O'Donnell, eds., 547–64. New York: Informa Healthcare.

Sorkin, Andrew Ross. 2012. "Occupy Wall Street: A Frenzy That Fizzled." *The New York Times*, September 18, http://query.nytimes.com/gst/fullpage.html.

Soule, Sarah Anne. 2009. *Contention and Corporate Social Responsibility*. Cambridge Studies in Contentious Politics. New York: Cambridge University Press.

Spar, Debora L., and Lane T. La Mure. 2003. "The Power of Activism: Assessing the Impact of NGOs on Global Business." *California Management Review* 45 (3) (April 1): 78–101.

Sridhar, Devi, Sanjeev Khagram, and Tikki Pang. 2010. "Are Existing Governance Structures Equipped to Deal with Today's Global Health Challenges? – Towards Systematic Coherence in Scaling Up." *Global Health Governance* 2 (2): 1–25.

Staley, Peter. 2008. "Are Millions Becoming HIV Positive Because Of ACT UP Paris?" *POZ*, http://blogs.poz.com/peter/archives/2008/07/are_millions_be.html.

Steinbrook, R., and J. M. Drazen. 2001. "AIDS – Will the Next 20 Years Be Different?" *The New England Journal of Medicine* 344 (23) (June 7): 1781–2.

Stone, Brad. 2012. "Worldreader: Taking the E-Book Revolution to Africa."
    BusinessWeek: Technology, September 6, www.businessweek.com/articles/
    2012–09–06/worldreader-taking-the-e-book-revolution-to-africa.
Stonebraker, Jeffrey S. 2002. "How Bayer Makes Decisions to Develop New
    Drugs." *Interfaces* 32 (6) (November 1): 77–90.
Strom, Stephanie. 2011. "Mission Accomplished, Nonprofits Close." *The New
    York Times*, April 1, sec. Business Day, www.nytimes.com/2011/04/02/
    business/02charity.html.
Sturchio, Jeff. 2003. *"Partnership for Action: An Update on the Expansion of Access to
    HIV Care and Treatment in Africa by the Companies Involved in the Accelerating
    Access Initiative Since May 2000."* The Accelerating Access Initiative: Lessons
    Learned from a Public/Private Collaboration BCIU Round Table United
    Nations General Assembly High-Level Meeting on HIV/AIDS.
    2004. "Partnership for Action: The Experience of the Accelerating Access
    Initiatve, 2000–04, and Lessons Learned." In *Delivering Essential Medicines*,
    Amir Attaran and Brigitte Granville, eds., 116–51. London: Royal Institute
    of International Affairs.
    2009. "Interview," December 3.
    2013. "Personal Communication," January 8.
Suleman, Fatima. 2001. "Further Slashes of AIDS Drugs Prices," www.hst.org.
    za/news/further-slashes-aids-drugs-prices.
Sun, Lena H. 2012. "Shift in Strategy to Treatment as Prevention for HIV/
    AIDS." *The Washington Post*, July 23, www.washingtonpost.com/national/
    health-science/shift-in-strategy-to-treatment-as-prevention-for-hivaids/
    2012/07/20/gJQAfjZbyW_story.html.
Sundstrom, Lisa McIntosh. 2005. "Foreign Assistance, International Norms,
    and NGO Development: Lessons from the Russian Campaign."
    International Organization 59: 419–49.
Szymanski, Katie. 2000. *The Boys in the Band*. Scoop News, www.scoop.co.nz/
    stories/WO0009/S00146.htm.
't Hoen, Ellen. 2002. "TRIPS, Pharmaceutical Patents, and Access to Essential
    Medicines: a Long Way from Seattle to Doha." *Chicago Journal of
    International Law* 3 (1): 27–46.
    2009. *The Global Politics of Pharmaceutical Monopoly Power*. Diemen,
    Netherlands: AMB.
    2010. "Interview," September 13.
    Jonathan Berger, Alexandra Calmy, and Suerie Moon. 2011. "Driving a
    Decade of Change: HIV/AIDS, Patents and Access to Medicines for All."
    Journal of the International AIDS Society 14 (15): 1–12.
Tanner, Marcel, and Don de Savigny. 2008. "Malaria Eradication Back on the
    Table." *Bulletin of the World Health Organization* 86 (2) (February): 82.
Tarrow, Sidney G. 2005. *The New Transnational Activism. Cambridge Studies in
    Contentious Politics*. New York: Cambridge University Press, www.loc.gov/
    catdir/toc/ecip056/2005000307.html.
Thomas, John R. 2001. *HIV/AIDS Drugs, Patents and the TRIPS Agreement: Issues
    and Options*. Congressional Research Service, Library of Congress.
Thrupkaew, Noy. 2012. "Ending Demand Won't Stop Prostitution." *The New
    York Times*, September 22, www.nytimes.com/2012/09/23/opinion/sunday/
    ending-demand-wont-stop-prostitution.html.

Timberg, Craig, and Daniel Halperin. 2012. *Tinderbox: How the West Sparked the AIDS Epidemic and How the World Can Finally Overcome It.* 1st edn. Penguin Group US.

Tobias, Randall. 2004a. "Remarks on The Five-Year Strategy for the President's Emergency Plan for AIDS Relief," http://2001-2009.state.gov/s/gac/rl/rm/2004/29771.htm.

2004b. "Hearings Before a Subcommittee of the Committee on Appropriations United States Senate One Hundred Eighth Congress Second Session on H.R. 4818/S. 2812," http://ftp.resource.org/gpo.gov/hearings/108s/92146.txt.

2004c. "Interview on the Jim Lehrer NewsHour," http://2001-2009.state.gov/s/gac/rl/rm/2004/32606.htm.

Torres, Mary Ann. 2002. "Human Right to Health, National Courts, and Access to HIV/AIDS Treatment: A Case Study from Venezuela," *Chicago Journal of International Law* 3: 105–14.

Tren, Richard, and Roger Bate. 2006. *Brazil's AIDS Program: A Costly Success.* Health Policy Outlook. American Enterprise Institute.

Trouiller, Patrice, Piero Olliaro, Els Torreele, James Orbinski, Richard Laing, and Nathan Ford. 2002. "Drug Development for Neglected Diseases: A Deficient Market and a Public-health Policy Failure." *The Lancet* 359 (9324) (June 22): 2188–94.

Tsebelis, George. 2002. *Veto Players: How Political Institutions Work.* New York: Russell Sage Foundation.

Tufts Center for the Study of Drug Development. 2010. *Outlook 2010,* http://csdd.tufts.edu/_documents/www/Outlook2010.pdf.

Tuller, David. 2010. "Following Trail of Lost AIDS Patients in Africa." *The New York Times,* October 25, www.nytimes.com/2010/10/26/health/26cases.html.

US Federal Trade Commission. 1999. *The Pharmaceutical Industry.* Washington DC.

UNAIDS (Joint United Nations Programme on HIV/AIDS). 2004. "'Three Ones' Key Principles," http://data.unaids.org/UNA-docs/three-ones_keyprinciples_en.pdf.

2008. "2008 Report on the Global AIDS Epidemic," www.unaids.org/en/KnowledgeCentre/HIVData/GlobalReport/2008/default.asp.

2010. "Key Facts: Progress in Low- and Middle-Income Countries by Region," www.who.int/entity/hiv/pub/2010progressreport/key_facts_en.pdf.

2011a. "AIDS at 30: Nations at the Crossroads," www.unaids.org/unaids_resources/aidsat30/aids-at-30.pdf.

2011b. *UNAIDS 2011 World AIDS Day Report.* Geneva: UNAIDS, www.unaids.org/en/resources/publications/2011/name,63525,en.asp.

2012a. *Together We Will End AIDS,* www.unaids.org/en/media/unaids/contentassets/documents/epidemiology/2012/20120718_togetherwewillendaids_en.pdf.

2012b. *More Than 80 Countries Increase Their Domestic Investments for AIDS by over 50% Between 2006 and 2011,* www.unaids.org/en/resources/presscentre/pressreleaseandstatementarchive/2012/july/20120718prunaidsreport/.

and WHO (World Health Organization). 2011. "Using TRIPS Flexibilities to Improve Access to HIV Treatment." http://www.unaids.org/en/media/

unaids/contentassets/documents/unaidspublication/2011/JC2049_Policy Brief_TRIPS_en.pdf.

UNICEF (United Nations (International) Children's (Emergency) Fund). 2007. "UNICEF Procurement of HIV/AIDS-Related Supplies." http://www.unicef.org/supply/files/Procurement_of_HA_supplies.pdf.

UNITAID. 2011. "HIV/AIDS Fact Sheet." http://www.unitaid.eu/images/Factsheets/EN_HIV_Factsheet_May2011.pdf.

UN (United Nations). 2001. *Declaration of Commitment on HIV/AIDS*. United Nations General Assembly Special Assembly on HIV/AIDS, http://data.unaids.org/publications/irc-pub03/aidsdeclaration_en.pdf.

2012a. "Every Woman Every Child," www.everywomaneverychild.org/about.

2012b. *Millennium Development Goals: 2012 Progress Chart*, www.un.org/millenniumgoals/pdf/2012_Progress_E.pdf.

2012c. "Unprecedented Global Health Movement Yields Gains for Women's and Children's Health." *MarketWatch*, www.marketwatch.com/story/unprecedented-global-health-movement-yields-gains-for-womens-and-childrens-health-2012-09-26.

2012d. "UN Commission Sets Out Plan to Make Life-saving Health Supplies More Accessible," www.everywomaneverychild.org/component/content/article/1-about/409-un-commission-sets-out-plan-to-make-life-saving-health-supplies-more-accessible.

2012e. "United Nations Millennium Development Goals." Accessed September 23, www.un.org/millenniumgoals/maternal.shtml.

University of California San Francisco. 2011. "AIDS Treatment," www.ucsfhealth.org/conditions/aids/treatment.html.

Van Evera, Stephen. 1997. *Guide to Methods for Students of Political Science*. Ithaca, NY: Cornell University Press.

Van Noorden, Richard. 2011. "European Carbon Market Plummets." *European Carbon Market Plummets*, http://blogs.nature.com/news/2011/11/european_carbon_market_plummet.html.

Van Zyl, Andre. 2011a. "Ensuring Quality Medicines: A Decade of Prequalification." *WHO Drug Information* 25 (3): 231–9.

2011b. "Personal Communication," July 30.

Victor, David G., Charles F. Kennel, and Veerabhadran Ramanathan. 2012. "The Climate Threat We Can Beat." *Foreign Affairs*, May 1.

Waltz, Kenneth Neal. 1979. *Theory of International Politics*. Reading, MA: Addison-Wesley Pub. Co.

Waning, Brenda, Ellen Diedrichsen, and Suerie Moon. 2010. "A Lifeline to Treatment: The Role of Indian Generic Manufacturers in Supplying Antiretroviral Medicines to Developing Countries." *Journal of the International AIDS Society* 13 (35).

Waning, Brenda, Warren Kaplan, Matthew P. Fox, Mariah Boyd-Boffa, Alexis C. King, Danielle A. Lawrence, Lyne Soucy, Sapna Mahajan, Hubert G. Leufkens, and Manjusha Gokhale. 2010. "Temporal Trends in Generic and Brand Prices of Antiretroviral Medicines Procured with Donor Funds in Developing Countries." *Journal of Generic Medicines: The Business Journal for the Generic Medicines Sector* 7 (2): 159–75.

Waning, Brenda, Warren Kaplan, Alexis King, Danielle Lawrence, Hubert Leufkens, and Matthew Fox. 2009. "Global Strategies to Reduce the Price of Antiretroviral Medicines: Evidence from Transactional Databases." *Bulletin of the World Health Organization* 87 (7): 520–8.

Waning, Brenda, Margaret Kyle, Ellen Diedrichsen, Lyne Soucy, Jenny Hochstadt, Till Bärnighausen, and Suerie Moon. 2010. "Intervening in Global Markets to Improve Access to HIV/AIDS Treatment: An Analysis of International Policies and the Dynamics of Global Antiretroviral Medicines Markets." *Globalization and Health* 6 (9): 1–19.

Washington Post–Kaiser Family Foundation. 2012. "2012 HIV/AIDS Poll – Washington Post–Kaiser Family Foundation." *The Washington Post*, www.washingtonpost.com/politics/polling/2012-hivaids-poll-washington-postkaiser-family/2012/07/24/gJQA3TGt0W_page.html.

Waxman, Henry. 2004. "Letter to President Bush," www.healthgap.org/press_releases/04/032604_Waxman_GWB_LTR.pdf.

2007. "Letter to Mark Dybul, U.S. Global AIDS Coordinator," http://oversight-archive.waxman.house.gov/documents/20070419155613.pdf.

Welink, Jan. 2010. "WHO Prequalification Programme," www.who.int/entity/medicines/areas/quality_safety/regulation_legislation/icdra/WF-2-Dec.pdf.

WHO (World Health Organization). Undated. "Inspections," http://apps.who.int/prequal/assessment_inspect/info_inspection.htm.

2002. "Scaling up Antiretroviral Therapy in Resource-limited Settings," www.who.int/hiv/pub/guidelines/pub18/en/index.html.

2003. "Scaling up Antiretroviral Therapy in Resource-limited Settings: Treatment Guidelines for a Public Health Approach," www.who.int/3by5/publications/documents/arv_guidelines/en/index.html.

2004a. "Removal of Antiretroviral Products from the WHO List of Prequalified Medicines," http://apps.who.int/prequal/info_press/pq_news_01Sep2004.htm.

2004b. "Two CIPLA AIDS Medicines Back on WHO's List of Prequalified Medicines," http://apps.who.int/prequal/info_press/pq_news_30Nov2004.htm.

2004c. "Hetero Drugs Ltd. Withdraws Antiretrovirals," http://apps.who.int/prequal/info_press/pq_news_19Nov2004.htm.

2004d. "Ranbaxy Withdraws All Its Antiretroviral Medicines from WHO's List of Prequalified Products," http://apps.who.int/prequal/info_press/pq_news_09Nov2004.htm.

2006. "Antiretroviral Therapy for HIV Infection in Adults and Adolescents: Recommendations for a Public Health Approach (2006 Revision)," www.who.int/hiv/pub/arv/adult/en/index.html.

2008. "Fact Sheet: Top Ten Causes of Death," www.who.int/mediacentre/factsheets/fs310_2008.pdf.

2009a. "WHO | Towards Universal Access: Scaling up Priority HIV/AIDS Interventions in the Health Sector," www.who.int/hiv/pub/2009progressreport/en/.

2009b. "Rapid Advice: Antiretroviral Therapy for HIV Infection in Adults and Adolescents," www.who.int/hiv/pub/arv/advice/en/index.html.

2009c. "Diarrhoeal Disease," www.who.int/mediacentre/factsheets/fs330/en/index.html.

2010a. "More Than Five Million People Receiving HIV Treatment," www.who.int/mediacentre/news/releases/2010/hiv_treament_20100719/en/index.html.

2010b. "Antiretroviral Therapy for HIV Infection in Adults and Adolescents: Recommendations for a Public Health Approach – 2010 Rev," www.who.int/hiv/pub/arv/adult2010/en/index.html.

2010c. "The WHO Prequalification Programme and the Medicines Patent Pool: A Primer," http://apps.who.int/prequal/info_general/documents/FAQ/PQ_PatentPool.pdf.

2010d. *Every Woman and Every Child: Global Strategy for Women's and Children's Health,* www.who.int/pmnch/events/2010/commitments_summary092910.pdf.

2010e. "WHO | World Malaria Report 2010," www.who.int/malaria/world_malaria_report_2010/en/index.html.

2011a. "Prequalification Programme," http://apps.who.int/prequal/.

2011b. "Guideline on Submission of Documentation for Prequalification of Multisource (generic) Finished Pharmaceutical Products (FPPs) Approved by Stringent Regulatory Authorities (SRAs)," http://apps.who.int/prequal/info_applicants/Guidelines/PQProcGenericSRA_July2011.pdf.

2011c. "WHO Prequalification of Medicines Programme (PQP) Facts and Figures for 2010," http://apps.who.int/medicinedocs/documents/s18635en/s18635en.pdf.

2011d. "WHO | The Top 10 Causes of Death," www.who.int/mediacentre/factsheets/fs310/en/index.html.

2012a. "Essential Medicines Selection: WHO Expert Committees," www.who.int/selection_medicines/committees/en/index.html.

2012b. "WHO List of Prequalified Medicinal Products," http://apps.who.int/prequal/query/ProductRegistry.aspx?list=ha.

2012c. "WHO | Maternal Mortality," www.who.int/mediacentre/factsheets/fs348/en/index.html.

2012d. "WHO | 'Strategic Use' of HIV Medicines Could Help End Transmission of Virus," www.who.int/mediacentre/news/releases/2012/hiv_medication_20120718/en/index.html.

and UNAIDS. 2002. "Accelerating Access Initiative: Widening Access to Care and Support for People Living with HIV/AIDS. Progress Report," www.who.int/hiv/pub/prev_care/aai/en/.

Will, Kurt Dieter. 1991. *"The Global Politics of AIDS: The World Health Organization and the International Regime for AIDS."* Charleston: Department of Government and International Studies, University of South Carolina.

Williamson, Oliver E. 1983. *Markets and Hierarchies: Analysis and Antitrust Implications.* Macmillan US.

Wolfe, Maxine. 2004. "Interview." ACT UP Oral History Project. MIX – The New York Lesbian & Gay Experimental Film Festival, www.actuporalhistory.org/interviews/images/wolfe.pdf.

Wong, Wendy. 2012a. "The Role of Formal and Informal Rules in the Internal Lives of International NGOs." Paper presented at International Studies Association. San Diego, CA.

2012b. *Internal Affairs: How the Structure of NGOs Transforms Human Rights.* Ithaca, NY: Cornell University Press.

World Bank. 2003. "Instructions for the Procurement of Specialized Medicines for HIV/AIDS Programs," http://web.worldbank.org/WBSITE/ EXTERNAL/PROJECTS/PROCUREMENT/0,contentMDK: 20109126~pagePK:84269~piPK:60001558~ theSitePK:84266~isCURL: Y~isCURL:Y,00.html.

2007. "Forest Carbon Partnership Facility."

WorldPublicOpinion.org. Undated. "Aid for HIV/AIDS Crisis in Africa," www. americans-world.org/digest/regional_issues/africa/africa3a.cfm.

WTO (World Trade Organization). Undated. "TRIPS: Agreement on Trade-Related Aspects of Intellectual Property Rights," www.wto.org/english/ tratop_e/trips_e/t_agm3_e.htm.

2001. "Declaration on the TRIPS Agreement and Public Health," www.wto. org/english/thewto_e/minist_e/min01_e/mindecl_trips_e.htm.

Yale AIDS Network. 2003. "University IP Policies and Access to Medicines," www.yale.edu/aidsnetwork/Spring%202003%20Univ%20Policies.ppt.

Yekutiel, Perez. 1981. "Lessons from the Big Eradication Campaigns." *World Health Forum* 2 (4): 465–90.

York, Dan. 1999. *A Discussion and Critique of Market Transformation: Challenges and Perspectives.* Madison: Energy Center of Wisconsin.

Youde, Jeremy. 2008. "Is Universal Access to Antiretroviral Drugs an Emerging International Norm?" *Journal of International Relations and Development* 11 (4): 415–40.

Yurday, Erin. 2004. *Strategic Activism: The Rainforest Action Network.* Stanford Graduate School of Business.

Zald, Mayer. 1996. "Culture, Ideology and Strategic Framing." In *Comparative Perspectives on Social Movements*, Doug McAdam, John D. McCarthy, and Mayer Zald, eds., 261–74. Cambridge University Press.

Zaller, John. 1992. *The Nature and Origins of Mass Opinion.* Cambridge, New York: Cambridge University Press.

Zimbabwe Broadcasting Corporation. 2011. "Stavudine to Be Phased Out," www.zbc.co.zw/news-categories/health/9945-stavudine-to-be-phased-out. html.

Zimmerman, Rachel. 2002. "World Health Organization Prepares List of 'Quality' AIDS Medications," www.aegis.com/news/wsj/2002/WJ020306. html.

Index

Note: Page numbers with the suffix 'n' indicate a note, with appropriate number, and 't' a table.